Clinical Advances in Head and Neck Imaging including Dentistry

Editor

Erich Sorantin

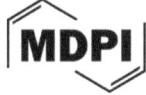

Basel • Beijing • Wuhan • Barcelona • Belgrade • Novi Sad • Cluj • Manchester

Editor
Erich Sorantin
Department of Radiology
Medical University of Graz
Graz
Austria

Editorial Office
MDPI AG
Grosspeteranlage 5
4052 Basel, Switzerland

This is a reprint of articles from the Special Issue published online in the open access journal *Journal of Clinical Medicine* (ISSN 2077-0383) (available at: https://www.mdpi.com/journal/jcm/special_issues/G8LV42N253).

For citation purposes, cite each article independently as indicated on the article page online and as indicated below:

Lastname, A.A.; Lastname, B.B. Article Title. *Journal Name* **Year**, *Volume Number*, Page Range.

ISBN 978-3-7258-2545-5 (Hbk)
ISBN 978-3-7258-2546-2 (PDF)
doi.org/10.3390/books978-3-7258-2546-2

Cover image courtesy of Erich Sorantin

© 2024 by the authors. Articles in this book are Open Access and distributed under the Creative Commons Attribution (CC BY) license. The book as a whole is distributed by MDPI under the terms and conditions of the Creative Commons Attribution-NonCommercial-NoDerivs (CC BY-NC-ND) license.

Contents

About the Editor vii

Rieke Lisa Meister, Michael Groth, Shuo Zhang, Jan-Hendrik Buhk and Jochen Herrmann
Evaluation of Artifact Appearance and Burden in Pediatric Brain Tumor MR Imaging with Compressed Sensing in Comparison to Conventional Parallel Imaging Acceleration
Reprinted from: *J. Clin. Med.* **2023**, *12*, 5732, doi:10.3390/jcm12175732 1

Petra Rugani, Iva Brcic, Marton Magyar, Uwe Yacine Schwarze, Norbert Jakse and Kurt Ebeleseder
Pulp Revascularization in an Autotransplanted Mature Tooth: Visualization with Magnetic Resonance Imaging and Histopathologic Correlation
Reprinted from: *J. Clin. Med.* **2023**, *12*, 6008, doi:10.3390/jcm12186008 13

Sotirios Petsaros, Emmanouil Chatzipetros, Catherine Donta, Pantelis Karaiskos, Argiro Boziari, Evangelos Papadakis and Christos Angelopoulos
Scattered Radiation Distribution Utilizing Three Different Cone-Beam Computed Tomography Devices for Maxillofacial Diagnostics: A Research Study
Reprinted from: *J. Clin. Med.* **2023**, *12*, 6199, doi:10.3390/jcm12196199 25

Natalia Kazimierczak, Wojciech Kazimierczak, Zbigniew Serafin, Paweł Nowicki, Adam Lemanowicz, Katarzyna Nadolska and Joanna Janiszewska-Olszowska
Correlation Analysis of Nasal Septum Deviation and Results of AI-Driven Automated 3D Cephalometric Analysis
Reprinted from: *J. Clin. Med.* **2023**, *12*, 6621, doi:10.3390/jcm12206621 37

Lea Stursa, Brigitte Wendl, Norbert Jakse, Margit Pichelmayer, Frank Weiland, Veronica Antipova and Barbara Kirnbauer
Accuracy of Palatal Orthodontic Mini-Implants Placed Using Fully Digital Planned Insertion Guides: A Cadaver Study
Reprinted from: *J. Clin. Med.* **2023**, *12*, 6782, doi:10.3390/jcm12216782 51

Marcus Rieder, Bernhard Remschmidt, Vera Schrempf, Matthäus Schwaiger, Norbert Jakse and Barbara Kirnbauer
Neurosensory Deficits of the Mandibular Nerve Following Extraction of Impacted Lower Third Molars—A Retrospective Study
Reprinted from: *J. Clin. Med.* **2023**, *12*, 7661, doi:10.3390/jcm12247661 62

Daniel Poszytek and Bartłomiej Górski
Relationship between the Status of Third Molars and the Occurrence of Dental and Periodontal Lesions in Adjacent Second Molars in the Polish Population: A Radiological Retrospective Observational Study
Reprinted from: *J. Clin. Med.* **2024**, *13*, 20, doi:10.3390/jcm13010020 74

Jana Di Rosso, Andreas Krasser, Sebastian Tschauner, Helmuth Guss and Erich Sorantin
Bismuth Shielding in Head Computed Tomography—Still Necessary?
Reprinted from: *J. Clin. Med.* **2024**, *13*, 25, doi:10.3390/jcm13010025 88

Arnela Hadzic, Martin Urschler, Jan-Niclas Aaron Press, Regina Riedl, Petra Rugani, Darko Štern and Barbara Kirnbauer
Evaluating a Periapical Lesion Detection CNN on a Clinically Representative CBCT Dataset—A Validation Study
Reprinted from: *J. Clin. Med.* **2024**, *13*, 197, doi:10.3390/jcm13010197 99

Natalia Kazimierczak, Wojciech Kazimierczak, Zbigniew Serafin, Paweł Nowicki, Jakub Nożewski and Joanna Janiszewska-Olszowska
AI in Orthodontics: Revolutionizing Diagnostics and Treatment Planning—A Comprehensive Review
Reprinted from: *J. Clin. Med.* **2024**, *13*, 344, doi:10.3390/jcm13020344 . . . . **112**

Petra Rugani, Katharina Weingartner and Norbert Jakse
Influence of the Tube Angle on the Measurement Accuracy of Peri-Implant Bone Defects in Rectangular Intraoral X-ray Imaging
Reprinted from: *J. Clin. Med.* **2024**, *13*, 391, doi:10.3390/jcm13020391 . . . . **131**

Milda Pucėtaitė, Davide Farina, Silvija Ryškienė, Dalia Mitraitė, Rytis Tarasevičius, Saulius Lukoševičius, et al.
The Diagnostic Value of CEUS in Assessing Non-Ossified Thyroid Cartilage Invasion in Patients with Laryngeal Squamous Cell Carcinoma
Reprinted from: *J. Clin. Med.* **2024**, *13*, 891, doi:10.3390/jcm13030891 . . . . **145**

Zachary Abramson, Chris Oh, Martha Wells, Asim F. Choudhri and Matthew T. Whitehead
CT and MR Appearance of Teeth: Analysis of Anatomy and Embryology and Implications for Disease
Reprinted from: *J. Clin. Med.* **2024**, *13*, 1187, doi:10.3390/jcm13051187 . . . . **156**

About the Editor

Erich Sorantin

Erich Sorantin, MD was born in 1957 and, after finishing high school, he studied Medicine at the University of Vienna, graduating in 1982. Afterwards, he worked in several hospitals, completed his training as a general practitioner and became fully qualified as a pediatrician and radiologist. In 1988, he joined the team at the Department of Radiology, Medical University Graz, where he became a faculty member in 1994 and earned his professorship in 2002. From 2013 to 2022, he served as the acting Head of the Division of Pediatric Radiology, the Department of Radiology, Medical University Graz. Moreover, he coordinates a multi-institutional, multidisciplinary academic network in Central Europe, which focuses on the biomedical imaging and technology transfer of advanced pediatric care as well as radiation protection. Additionally, Dr. Sorantin served as a Consultant for computer graphics for the medical vendor Siemens, concentrating on virtual endoscopic techniques, for approximately eight years. During this period, two products were brought to the market: the Virtuoso3D and the Leonardo Workstation. Dr. Sorantin has received several awards, and in 2018, he obtained a PhD honoris causa in Informatics from the Faculty of Science, Univ.of Szeged/HU. Dr. Sorantin retired at the end of 2022 and is now working as a Consultant for pediatric radiology as well as freelancer for medical informatics. In addition, he remains an active researcher and publisher. He has been married since 1984 and has three sons and three grandchildren.

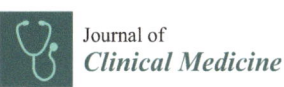

Article

Evaluation of Artifact Appearance and Burden in Pediatric Brain Tumor MR Imaging with Compressed Sensing in Comparison to Conventional Parallel Imaging Acceleration

Rieke Lisa Meister [1,2,*], Michael Groth [3], Shuo Zhang [4], Jan-Hendrik Buhk [5] and Jochen Herrmann [1]

1. Department of Diagnostic and Interventional Radiology and Nuclear Medicine, Section of Pediatric Radiology, University Medical Center Hamburg-Eppendorf, 20251 Hamburg, Germany
2. Department of Medical Imaging, Southland Hospital, Invercargill 9812, New Zealand
3. Department of Radiology, St. Marienhospital Vechta, 49377 Vechta, Germany
4. Philips Healthcare, 22335 Hamburg, Germany; zhang.shuo@philips.com
5. Department of Neuroradiology, Asklepios Kliniken St. Georg und Wandsbek, 22043 Hamburg, Germany
* Correspondence: rieke.meister@southerndhb.govt.nz

Abstract: Clinical magnetic resonance imaging (MRI) aims for the highest possible image quality, while balancing the need for acceptable examination time, reasonable signal-to-noise ratio (SNR), and lowest artifact burden. With a recently introduced imaging acceleration technique, compressed sensing, the acquisition speed and image quality of pediatric brain tumor exams can be improved. However, little attention has been paid to its impact on method-related artifacts in pediatric brain MRI. This study assessed the overall artifact burden and artifact appearances in a standardized pediatric brain tumor MRI by comparing conventional parallel imaging acceleration with compressed sensing. This showed that compressed sensing resulted in fewer physiological artifacts in the FLAIR sequence, and a reduction in technical artifacts in the 3D T1 TFE sequences. Only a slight difference was noted in the T2 TSE sequence. A relatively new range of artifacts, which are likely technique-related, was noted in the 3D T1 TFE sequences. In conclusion, by equipping a basic pediatric brain tumor protocol for 3T MRI with compressed sensing, the overall burden of common artifacts can be reduced. However, attention should be paid to novel compressed-sensing-specific artifacts.

Keywords: compressed SENSE; acceleration technique; image quality; brain neoplasms; children

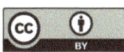

1. Introduction

Magnetic resonance imaging (MRI) is considered the gold standard for neuro-oncologic brain imaging [1,2]. Recent technical advances in imaging acceleration have shown clear clinical benefits in a reduction of scan times and improvement of image quality [3–5]. In children, shorter examination times are particularly desired to keep sedation duration at a minimum, to minimize the exposure time to radiofrequency-induced energy deposition, and to ensure maximum patient compliance [6–9].

In this context, different imaging strategies have been integrated into various pediatric imaging schemes over the last several years, demonstrating promising results in children [10–13]. A common approach is the use of compressed sensing (CS) as an imaging acceleration technique based on variable density sampling, sparsifying transformation, and iterative reconstruction [14]. Since CS was made available for clinical use, little attention has been paid to its effects on common image artifacts so far [15], which are known to have a high impact on image quality and diagnostic confidence.

In the process of equipping our brain tumor protocol with compressed sensing, and assessing image quality during and after implementation, we found that there was a noticeable change in the artifact burden and appearance. Recognition of artifacts related to compressed sensing seemed important in order to avoid misinterpretation.

This study aimed to assess the overall artifact burden and artifact appearances in a standardized pediatric brain tumor MRI by comparing conventional parallel imaging acceleration with CS.

2. Materials and Methods

Study population: All children with brain tumors who underwent a brain MRI examination with compressed sensing at our institution between October and December 2019 and who had undergone at least one previous examination using the standard protocol without compressed sensing were retrospectively identified. Of 60 patients, 38 were excluded as one of their two protocols had been modified regarding the number of acquired sequences and overall length of the protocol beyond purely introducing CS. The study cohort included 22 patients, aged 2.3–18.8 years at the time of their CS MRI examination [13]. All children had been diagnosed with varying brain tumor entities (mainly astrocytoma, medulloblastoma, and ependymoma) and had undergone different therapeutic pathways at the time of imaging (surgery, radiation therapy, chemotherapy, or multimodality therapy). Five patients below the age of five years were examined under general anesthesia. For details regarding patient data see Supplementary Materials [13].

MRI Protocol: MRI examinations were performed on a 3.0 Tesla whole-body clinical MRI system (Ingenia, software release R5.6, Philips, Best, The Netherlands). A standard 32-channel receiver head coil (Philips) was used. Ear plugs and noise canceling headphones were given to all patients. Foam pads were used to minimize head motion. Some children preferred to listen to music or watch a movie during their examination. All unsedated patients were instructed to keep still during examinations to avoid movement artifacts.

The pediatric brain tumor MR protocol included both unenhanced and contrast enhanced 3D T1-weighted turbo-field-echo (TFE) sequences with similar technical parameters acquired in the sagittal plane with reconstructions in the axial and coronal planes; an axial fluid-attenuated inversion recovery (FLAIR) sequence; and an axial T2-weighted turbo-spin-echo (TSE) sequence [13,16]. Gadolinium was used as an intravenous contrast agent with a dosage of 0.2 mL Gadoteric Acid (Dotagraf^R, Jenapharm, Germany)/kg body weight, and enhanced 3D T1 TFE sequences were obtained 3 min after contrast injection.

Sensitivity encoding (SENSE) was applied for conventional parallel imaging acceleration and was combined with the CS principle for 'Compressed SENSE' acceleration, the latter employing L1 regularization after wavelet sparsifying transformation and iterative reconstruction. Both acceleration techniques (SENSE and CS) were implemented in the vendor software. Imaging parameters for adaptation of the basic MRI brain tumor protocol to compressed sensing were optimized according to visual observation to ensure best diagnostic image quality, the comparative results of which were published elsewhere [13]. Key imaging parameters are given in Table 1 [13].

Table 1. Comparison of sequence data for the SENSE and compressed sensing (CS) pediatric brain tumor protocols.

	3D T1 TFE		T2 TSE		FLAIR	
	SENSE	CS	SENSE	CS	SENSE	CS
Scan time (min:sec)	03:38	03:00	03:36	02:07	03:51	02:38
Acceleration	SENSE 1.2 × 2.2	3.3	-	1.3	SENSE 1.8 × 1.3	4.5
TR/TE (ms)	8.3/3.8	8.6/4.0	3000/80	3954/80	11,000/125	4800/396
TI delay (ms)	956.8	989.9	-	-	2800	1650
SNR^a (arbitrary)	167.0	145.7	155.3	189.3	205.3	222.3
FOV (mm^3)	240 × 240 × 175	240 × 240 × 175	230 × 182 × 152	230 × 182 × 152	230 × 183 × 138	230 × 179 × 152
Voxel size [ACQ] (mm^3)	1.0 × 1.0 × 1.0	0.85 × 0.85 × 0.85	0.55 × 0.65 × 3.0	0.55 × 0.65 × 3.0	0.65 × 0.87 × 3.0	0.75 × 0.75 × 3.3
Voxel size [REC] (mm^3)	0.9 × 0.9 × 1.0	0.43 × 0.43 × 0.43	0.4 × 0.4 × 3.0	0.4 × 0.4 × 3.0	0.34 × 0.34 × 3.0	0.34 × 0.34 × 3.3

SENSE sensitivity encoding, CS compressed sensing sensitivity encoding, 3D three-dimensional, TFE turbo field echo, TSE turbo spin echo, FLAIR fluid-attenuated inversion recovery, TR repetition time, TE echo time, TI inversion time, SNR signal-to-noise ratio, FOV field of view, ACQ voxel acquisition voxel size, REC voxel reconstruction voxel size. SNR^a (in arbitrary units) measurements were conducted in a standard phantom with separate noise maps (for details, see text).

Image analysis: Two pediatric radiologists, with 16 years (JH) and 13 years (MG) of experience, evaluated artifact burden and strength of artifacts during a consensus reading. Readers were blinded for clinical information and technical parameters. In total, 176 sequences were viewed in random order via Centricity PACS Universal Viewer (GE Web Client Version 6.0, Chicago, IL, USA).

Image artifacts were categorized as either physiology-related (motion, ringing, CSF flow, pulsation/ghosting), physics-related (chemical shift, susceptibility effects), or technique-related [17–19]. The latter included acceleration technique (e.g., compressed sensing)-specific artifacts that have been described in the literature [15].

Detailed description of artifact types is given in Supplementary Table S2 [15,17,18,20]. Using a 3-point scale, artifacts were rated according to their strength. The scale incorporated information regarding the amount of regional extension and diagnostic disturbance (0 points, no artifacts; 1 point, light artifacts with most underlying or adjacent structures visible, small or focal appearance, only slight diagnostic impairment; 2 points, strong artifacts, underlying or adjacent structures not clearly visible, extensive or multifocal appearance, substantial impairment of diagnostic assessment). For each of the four sequences and for both acceleration protocols (SENSE vs. CS), artifact frequency and artifact strength were determined. For each artifact type, the artifact frequency and the mean artifact strength were calculated. To assure comparable quantitative image quality between both protocols, separate phantom data-based noise maps were acquired for each of the sequences [21], with comparable measured signal-to-noise-ratio (SNR) values.

Statistical Analysis: Statistical analyses were computed with Excel (Version 16.44, 2020, Microsoft Corporation, Redmond, WA, USA), using a paired Wilcoxon test for numeric variables of artifact strength and summarized artifact strength scores to compare corresponding data sets of each of the sequences for both protocols under the assumption that there was no statistical difference (H0) [11–13,22]. A p-value < 0.05 was considered statistically significant. Data of scores are given as categorical values with n = absolute number of affected scans of all 22 patients including percentage, artifact strength scores given as sum of absolute values with mean $\pm$ 1 standard deviation, and summarized artifact strength scores given as mean value $\pm$ 1 standard deviation.

3. Results

In total, an overall reduction in artifact burden was noted for the compressed sensing (CS) protocol, with the four sequences benefiting to different extents with respect to the various artifacts. Results are summarized in Tables 2–5.

A significant decrease in disruptive artifacts was noted for CS 3D T1 TFE pre-contrast (overall $p < 0.001$) and post-contrast (overall $p < 0.001$) images, which is mainly attributable to a reduction in physiological and technical artifacts over the basal ganglia and the cortex. Ghosting and pulsation artifacts of vascular structures were eliminated ($p = 0.002$ for pre-contrast, $p < 0.001$ for post-contrast 3D T1 TFE; see Figure 1), followed by a reduction in grid-like reconstruction artifacts ($p = 0.008$ and $p = 0.029$, respectively; see Figure 2).

In addition, CS-specific artifacts were noted in both unenhanced and enhanced CS 3D T1 TFE sequences. A "Wavy-lines" artifact occurred in two examinations in CS 3D T1 TFE post-contrast with a broad, wavy pattern of distortion in the horizontal direction over the rostral frontal lobes (Figure 3). Similar but considerably smaller artifacts were seen next to typical susceptibility artifacts caused by a shunt device.

The "Starry-sky" artifact occurred in all of the unenhanced CS 3D T1 TFE sequences, but only occasionally in the enhanced equivalents. It presented as dotted salt-and-pepper-like noise, mainly at the center of the k-space, but with no preference for specific tissue types or anatomical structures (Figure 4).

Table 2. Evaluation of artifact occurrence and strength in 3D T1 TFE.

Artifact Category	Type of Artifact	SENSE Scans Affected n (%)	SENSE Artifact Strength Sum Score (Mean ± SD)	Compressed Sensing (CS) Scans Affected n (%)	Compressed Sensing (CS) Artifact Strength Sum Score (Mean ± SD)	p
Physiology-related	Motion	2 (9%)	2 (0.09 ± 0.29)	0	0	0.180
	Ringing	11 (50%)	14 (0.64 ± 0.73)	10 (45%)	10 (0.45 ± 0.61)	0.010
	CSF flow	0	0	0	0	0
Physics-related	Pulsation/ghosting	12 (55%)	15 (0.68 ± 0.72)	0	0	0.002
	Chemical shift	22 (100%)	30 (1.36 ± 0.49)	22 (100%)	36 (1.64 ± 0.49)	0.030
	Susceptibility effects	21 (95%)	35 (1.59 ± 0.59)	21 (95%)	34 (1.55 ± 0.60)	0.285
	Straight bands	10 (45%)	10 (0.45 ± 0.51)	1 (5%)	1 (0.05 ± 0.21)	0.008
Technique-related	Starry sky	0	0	22 (100%)	33 (1.50 ± 0.51)	
	Wax layer	0	0	1 (5%)	1 (0.05 ± 0.21)	
	Wavy lines	0	0	1 (5%)	1 (0.05 ± 0.21)	
Overall			4.82 ± 1.50		3.68 ± 1.04 *	<0.001

SENSE sensitivity encoding, CS compressed sensing sensitivity encoding, 3D three-dimensional, TFE turbo field echo, CSF cerebro-spinal fluid. Scans affected are given as absolute number of scans (n) and percentage of scans. Artifact strength given as numeric score summarizing all 22 scans with mean ± SD (artifact strength 0–2 points per scan; maximum artifact strength sum score per sequence and artifact 44 points; see Table S2). The mean overall score summarizes the artifact burden from all artifact types' strength scores with values given as mean ± SD. * The CS-specific artifacts are not included in the mean overall score as they did not occur in the SENSE protocol.

Table 3. Evaluation of artifact occurrence and strength in 3D T1 TFE post-contrast.

Artifact Category	Type of Artifact	SENSE Scans Affected n (%)	SENSE Artifact Strength Sum Score (Mean ± SD)	Compressed Sensing (CS) Scans Affected n (%)	Compressed Sensing (CS) Artifact Strength Sum Score (Mean ± SD)	p
Physiology-related	Motion	4 (18%)	6 (0.27 ± 0.63)	1 (5%)	1 (0.05 ± 0.21)	0.066
	Ringing	14 (64%)	19 (0.64 ± 0.73)	11 (55%)	14 (0.45 ± 0.51)	0.060
	CSF flow	0	0	1 (5%)	2 (0.09 ± 0.43)	0.317
Physics-related	Pulsation/ghosting	17 (77%)	23 (1.05 ± 0.72)	0	0	<0.001
	Chemical shift	22 (100%)	31 (1.41 ± 0.50)	22 (100%)	31 (1.41 ± 0.50)	0.354
	Susceptibility effects	21 (95%)	37 (1.68 ± 0.57)	21 (95%)	35 (1.59 ± 0.59)	0.180
	Straight bands	9 (41%)	10 (0.45 ± 0.60)	2 (9%)	2 (0.09 ± 0.29)	0.029
Technique-related	Starry sky	0	0	12 (55%)	14 (0.45 ± 0.51)	
	Wax layer	0	0	11 (50%)	11 (0.50 ± 0.51)	
	Wavy lines	0	0	2 (9%)	2 (0.09 ± 0.43)	
Overall			5.73 ± 1.72		3.86 ± 1.21 *	<0.001

SENSE sensitivity encoding, CS compressed sensing sensitivity encoding, 3D three-dimensional, TFE turbo field echo, CSF cerebro-spinal fluid. Scans affected are given as absolute number of scans (n) and percentage of scans. Artifact strength given as numeric score summarizing all 22 scans with mean ± SD (artifact strength 0–2 points per scan; maximum artifact strength sum score per sequence and artifact 44 points; see Table S2). The mean overall score summarizes the artifact burden from all artifact types' strength scores with values given as mean ± SD. * The CS-specific artifacts are not included in the mean overall score as they did not occur in the SENSE protocol.

Table 4. Evaluation of artifact occurrence and strength in T2 TSE.

Artifact Category	Type of Artifact	SENSE Scans Affected n (%)	SENSE Artifact Strength Sum Score (Mean ± SD)	Compressed Sensing (CS) Scans Affected n (%)	Compressed Sensing (CS) Artifact Strength Sum Score (Mean ± SD)	p
Physiology-related	Motion	3 (14%)	4 (0.18 ± 0.50)	3 (14%)	3 (0.14 ± 0.35)	0.423
	Ringing	9 (41%)	12 (0.55 ± 0.74)	10 (45%)	12 (0.55 ± 0.67)	0.192
	CSF flow	22 (100%)	38 (1.73 ± 0.46)	22 (100%)	41 (1.86 ± 0.35)	0.080
	Pulsation/ghosting	17 (77%)	22 (1.00 ± 0.69)	20 (91%)	26 (1.18 ± 0.59)	0.041

Table 4. Cont.

Artifact Category	Type of Artifact	SENSE		Compressed Sensing (CS)		p
		Scans Affected n (%)	Artifact Strength Sum Score (Mean ± SD)	Scans Affected n (%)	Artifact Strength Sum Score (Mean ± SD)	
Physics-related	Chemical shift	1 (5%)	1 (0.05 ± 0.21)	1 (5%)	1 (0.05 ± 0.21)	0
	Susceptibility effects	19 (86%)	23 (1.05 ± 0.58)	19 (86%)	23 (1.05 ± 0.58)	0
Technique-related	Straight bands	0	0	0	0	
	Starry sky	0	0	0	0	
	Wax layer	0	0	0	0	
	Wavy lines	0	0	0	0	
Overall			4.55 ± 1.53		4.82 ± 1.10 *	0.018

SENSE sensitivity encoding, CS compressed sensing sensitivity encoding, 3D three-dimensional, TFE turbo field echo, CSF cerebro-spinal fluid. Scans affected are given as absolute number of scans (n) and percentage of scans. Artifact strength given as numeric score summarizing all 22 scans with mean ± SD (artifact strength 0–2 points per scan; maximum artifact strength sum score per sequence and artifact 44 points; see Table S2). The mean overall score summarizes the artifact burden from all artifact types' strength scores with values given as mean ± SD. * The CS-specific artifacts are not included in the mean overall score as they did not occur in the SENSE protocol.

Table 5. Evaluation of artifact occurrence and strength in FLAIR.

Artifact Category	Type of Artifact	SENSE		Compressed Sensing (CS)		p
		Scans Affected n (%)	Artifact Strength Sum Score (Mean ± SD)	Scans Affected n (%)	Artifact Strength Sum Score (Mean ± SD)	
Physiology-related	Motion	10 (45%)	11 (0.50 ± 0.60)	0	0	0.005
	Ringing	21 (95%)	24 (1.09 ± 0.43)	6 (27%)	6 (0.27 ± 0.46)	<0.001
	CSF flow	22 (100%)	43 (1.95 ± 0.21)	8 (36%)	8 (0.36 ± 0.49)	<0.001
	Pulsation/ghosting	18 (82%)	30 (1.36 ± 0.79)	0	0	<0.001
Physics-related	Chemical shift	6 (27%)	(0.27 ± 0.46)	0	0	0.028
	Susceptibility effects	19 (86%)	20 (0.91 ± 0.43)	19 (86%)	23 (1.05 ± 0.58)	0.109
Technique-related	Straight bands	0	0	0	0	
	Starry sky	0	0	0	0	
	Wax layer	0	0	0	0	
	Wavy lines	0	0	0	0	
Overall			6.09 ± 1.72		1.68 ± 0.72 *	<0.001

SENSE sensitivity encoding, CS compressed sensing sensitivity encoding, 3D three-dimensional, TFE turbo field echo, CSF cerebro-spinal fluid. Scans affected are given as absolute number of scans (n) and percentage of scans. Artifact strength given as numeric score summarizing all 22 scans with mean ± SD (artifact strength 0–2 points per scan; maximum artifact strength sum score per sequence and artifact 44 points; see Table S2). The mean overall score summarizes the artifact burden from all artifact types' strength scores with values given as mean ± SD. * The CS-specific artifacts are not included in the mean overall score as they did not occur in the SENSE protocol.

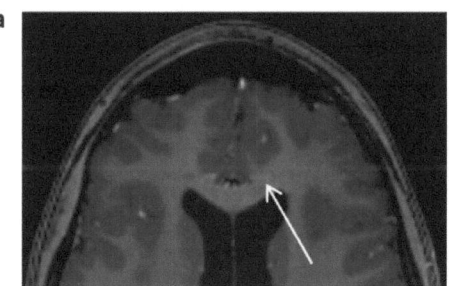

Figure 1. Cont.

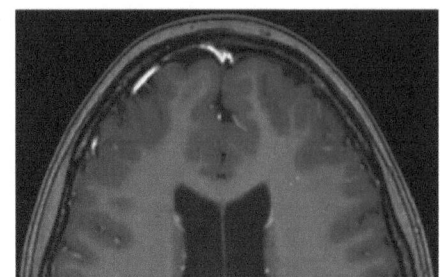

Figure 1. Enhanced 3D T1 TFE images of a 12-year-old male patient with non-germinomatous germ cell tumor (not shown). Pulsation artifact of anterior cerebral artery in phase-encoding direction noted in SENSE 3D T1 TFE ((**a**), arrow); not seen in follow-up imaging with CS 3D T1 TFE (**b**).

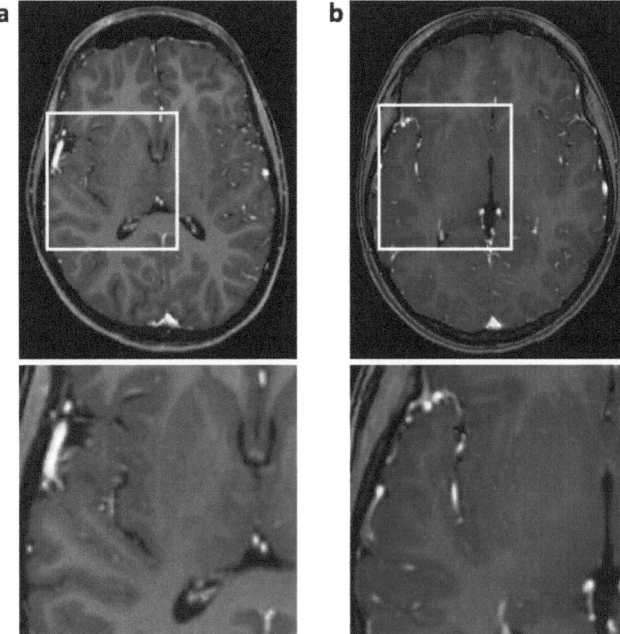

Figure 2. Enhanced 3D T1 TFE images of an 18-year-old male patient with ganglioglioma (not shown). Reconstruction artifact with thin oblique geometrical streaks is seen in SENSE 3D T1 TFE ((**a**), post-surgery); not present in CS 3D T1 TFE (**b**). White box indicates magnification.

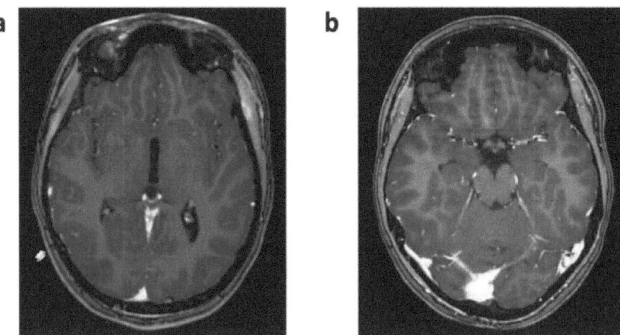

Figure 3. *Cont.*

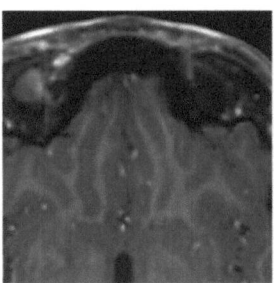
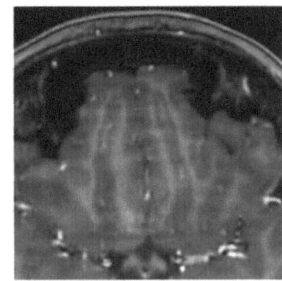

Figure 3. Enhanced 3D T1 TFE images of a 13-year-old female patient with astrocytoma (not shown). "Wavy-lines" artifact with prominent wavy signal distortion over frontal lobes in CS 3D T1 TFE (**b**) was not seen in SENSE 3D T1 TFE (**a**) study prior.

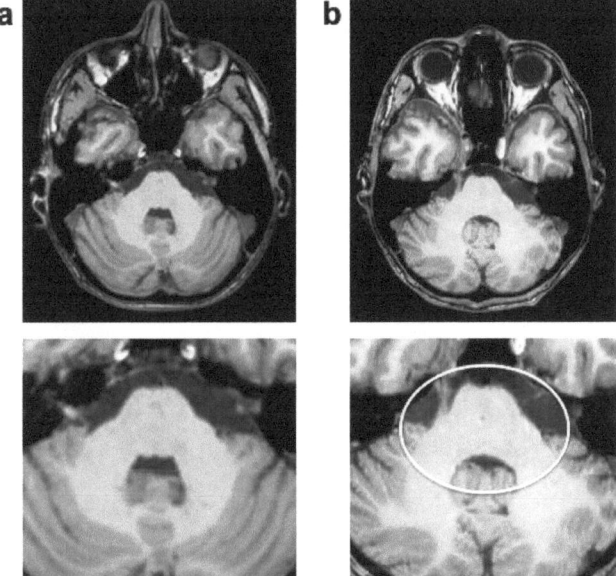

Figure 4. Unenhanced 3D T1 TFE images of a 6-year-old male patient with astrocytoma (not shown). "Starry-sky" artifact presenting as subtle salt-and-pepper-like noisiness in central structures of the acquired volume in CS (**b**); not present in previous SENSE imaging (**a**). White circle indicates artifact.

The "Wax-layer" artifact presented as patchy inhomogeneous blurring of brain structure mainly in post-contrast CS 3D T1 TFE (Figure 5).

The CS FLAIR benefited mostly from a reduction in physiological artifacts (overall $p < 0.001$), namely, an improved suppression of cerebro-spinal fluid flow artifacts ($p < 0.001$) and elimination of the dependent ghosting artifacts ($p < 0.001$; see Figure 6). CS FLAIR was the only sequence to demonstrate a significant decrease in motion artifacts ($p = 0.005$) caused by head or eye movement. However, CS FLAIR images were deemed slightly noisier than standard images on visual inspection.

The CS T2 TSE, on the other hand, showed less subjective noising, but the remainder of the artifacts, including CSF-related phenomena, were deemed comparable.

Ringing or truncation artifacts occurred in SENSE and CS 3D T1 TFE and T2 TSE. In CS 3D T1 TFE, ringing became less intense ($p = 0.010$), while it remained comparable in T2 TSE.

No significant differences were noticed for susceptibility effects and chemical shift artifacts between the two groups.

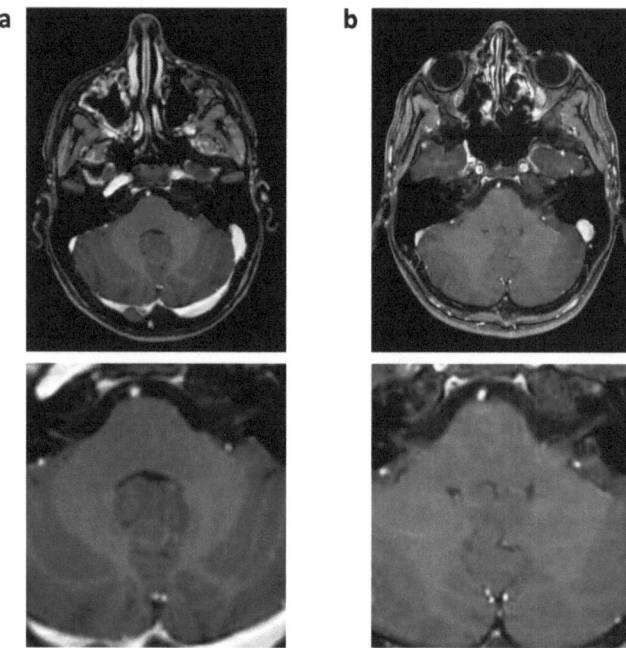

Figure 5. Enhanced 3D T1 TFE images of a 12-year-old male patient with non-germinomatous germ cell tumor (not shown). Wax-layer artifact presenting as patchy to blurred signal inhomogeneity in the pons and cerebellum in CS (**b**); not present in previous SENSE study (**a**).

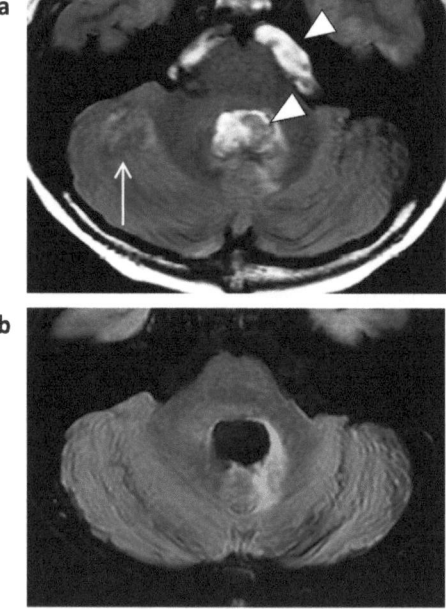

Figure 6. FLAIR images of a 5-year-old male patient with astrocytoma (post-resection). Bright CSF-flow-related enhancement (FRE, arrowheads) in fourth ventricle and prepontine cisterns is seen in SENSE FLAIR (**a**), not present in CS FLAIR (**b**). As a consequence, the CSF-dependent ghosting artifacts (arrow) did not occur.

4. Discussion

Our study on pediatric brain tumor MR imaging showed that overall artifact burden can be reduced using CS acceleration in comparison to standard parallel imaging acceleration. To the best of our knowledge, the effects of compressed sensing on artifact types and artifact load have not been systematically studied in pediatric brain tumor MR imaging before.

While a number of other studies have described challenges and potential artifacts arising from neuroimaging with 3 Tesla MRI and implementation of compressed sensing and/or SENSE [11,15,23,24], the potential effect of acceleration techniques on artifact appearance in pediatric MR imaging protocols has only been investigated to a limited extent and mainly with regards to abdominal imaging [9,25].

MR brain tumor imaging relies on the best possible image quality in order to maximize diagnostic confidence, but pediatric neuroimaging is often challenging in patients with small body volumes. Acceleration techniques that maintain or even improve image quality are therefore highly desired [14]. Also, pathologic findings often are of millimeter size and can be found in areas which are frequently altered by artifacts, e.g., in periventricular localization, adjacent to surgical sites, or next to surgical material and shunt devices [26,27]. Thus, the appearance of artifacts in these particular areas has the potential to affect diagnostic confidence.

Some neuro-oncologic patients might show limited compliance due to their altered state of consciousness, or physical impairment caused by the primary disease or treatment, resulting in motion artifacts, as patients are not able to keep their head still for a long period of time. The same problem is seen in young children, who often are anxious or bored during an MR examination, and in sedated children who present with uncontrolled movement of head or limbs. This challenge in oncologic and pediatric MR imaging can be addressed by the choice of movement-robust sequences and a reduction of scan time; however, these effects might be observed best in examination protocols with longer duration. In our study, a significant reduction in motion artifacts was seen in the CS FLAIR sequence, which was shortened most significantly by compressed sensing implementation [13].

Especially younger pediatric patients often demonstrate pronounced CSF flow artifacts. Their CSF circulation can differ from that of adult patients as it is affected by physiological parameters such as respiratory rate, arterial pulsation, and blood pressure [28,29]. Ghosting of these artifacts, as frequently seen in the posterior fossa, heavily disguises the detectability of local pathologic findings. In children, pathologic findings in the posterior fossa also occur often due to the statistically high likelihood of pediatric primary CNS tumors originating around the fourth ventricle.

With adequate suppression of the CSF signal by reduced TR and TI, such ghosting artifacts and signal loss [17] that occurred at basal cisterns, the third ventricle, and the foramen of Monro were dramatically reduced in the CS FLAIR sequence, whereas there was no apparent difference in T2 sequences under comparable parameter settings.

Interestingly, in 3D T1 gradient echo sequences, ghosting artifacts not related to CSF flow but to pulsation of the arteries of the circle of Willis were also eliminated in the CS protocol. This can be explained by the incoherent sampling pattern used in compressed sensing instead of the regular periodic undersampling in conventional SENSE [4,30,31]. The decrease in reconstruction artifacts in CS 3D T1 TFE sequences might be caused by the CS-specific L1 reconstruction algorithm in combination with the incoherent sampling pattern, which is designed to minimize disruptive signals.

A higher spatial resolution in CS 3D T1 TFE also contributed to a reduction in ringing artifacts that occurred at anatomical borders where signal intensity changed abruptly. The significant decrease in ringing artifacts in CS FLAIR may be due to better fat suppression.

The technical foundation of the CS 3D T1 TFE sequence serves as a potential explanation for CS-specific artifacts as well. Again, the mathematical random varying density undersampling scheme in CS could explain the frequently occurring "Starry-sky" artifact, as the center of the k-space might be too sparsely represented, resulting in too few coefficients during the mathematical iterative image reconstruction process [30,32]. Its strength of occurrence showed no correlation with the field of view or head volume, as it was observed in examinations of all patients with different body sizes. Although the "Starry-sky" artifact was found to be only slightly disruptive and therefore not deemed diagnostically impactful, further careful adjustment of the CS factor in accordance with the SNR might help to reduce the strength of this artifact. A potential cause of the wax-layer artifact could be a strong denoising level, where large sparsity in general is assumed in the algorithm. Still, as the CS denoising settings remained unchanged for all patients over the period of the study, and the artifact appeared only sporadically within our population, subtle patient motion could also have caused this particular artifact, as it typically creates blurring or smearing in compressed sensing imaging. The "Wavy-lines" artifact's close anatomical relation to the air-filled paranasal sinuses and shunt devices indicates a correlation with larger gradients between different types of tissue, contributing to field inhomogeneity. Although Sartoretti et al. described a strong correlation between a similar streaky linear artifact and having a smaller reconstruction voxel size than acquisition voxel size [15], the "Wavy-lines" artifact does not appear to be caused by this, as voxel sizes remained comparable during our study.

The balance between image quality and noise depends on coil sensitivity and the acceleration factor [32–34]. With regards to subjective noisiness, it aims for the most beneficial compromise during the compressed sensing implementation process, with the aim of optimizing general image quality and examination time for overall protocol improvement [13]. As quantitative noise evaluation did not show significant differences between the two protocols but the subjective noisiness of T2 TSE and FLAIR sequences differed, there is still space for further adjustment of the denoising factor, acceleration factor, and TR.

There were limitations to our study that need to be outlined. The small study cohort with $n = 22$ patients might not cover the full extent of potential artifacts in brain MRI. Total blinding of protocols was not possible due to the distinct image impression of conventional parallel imaging and CS usage, which could easily be identified by an experienced reader. Additional adjustments of the CS FLAIR sequence parameters regarding CSF suppression might disguise the effects of CS on CSF artifact appearance; however, these amendments were deemed necessary in the context of compressed sensing implementation in order to achieve superior image quality [13]. Prior to the study, an optimization of sequences was conducted during a pilot phase based on the previous experience of other centers and the recent literature [3,5,9,12,22,35–39].

5. Conclusions

In conclusion, CS contributes to a reduction in overall artifact burden and even the elimination of certain physiology-related artifacts in dedicated pediatric brain tumor MRI. However, to a lesser extent, the introduction of CS can also add new artifacts. Readers not familiar with CS therefore need to become accustomed to CS-specific artifacts to avoid pitfalls in interpretation. The artifact burden observed while utilizing iterative reconstruction algorithms should be monitored and regularly addressed during the optimization process. Future studies are needed to further investigate the artifact impact on diagnostic performance.

Supplementary Materials: The following supporting information can be downloaded at: https://www.mdpi.com/article/10.3390/jcm12175732/s1, Table S1: Patient demographics; Table S2: Description of artifacts assessed in this study.

Author Contributions: Conceptualization, R.L.M., J.H., M.G. and S.Z.; methodology, R.L.M.; software, S.Z.; validation, J.H. and J.-H.B.; formal analysis, J.H. and M.G.; data curation, R.L.M.; writing—original draft preparation, R.L.M.; writing—review and editing, J.H., M.G., S.Z. and J.-H.B.; supervision, J.H. All authors have read and agreed to the published version of the manuscript.

Funding: This research received no external funding.

Institutional Review Board Statement: This retrospective study was approved by the institutional review board with a waiver for informed consent (Ethikkommission Ärztekammer Hamburg; ref: WF-840/20) and was conducted in accordance with the Declaration of Helsinki.

Informed Consent Statement: Not applicable.

Data Availability Statement: Data are available on request.

Acknowledgments: The authors would like to thank Malcolm Gill for assistance in proofreading the manuscript.

Conflicts of Interest: The authors declare no conflict of interest. S.Z. is a Philips employee.

References

1. Fink, J.R.; Muzi, M.; Peck, M.; Krohn, K.A. Multimodality Brain Tumor Imaging: MR Imaging, PET, and PET/MR Imaging. *J. Nucl. Med.* **2015**, *56*, 1554–1561. [CrossRef]
2. Villanueva-Meyer, J.E.; Mabray, M.C.; Cha, S. Current Clinical Brain Tumor Imaging. *Neurosurgery* **2017**, *81*, 397–415. [CrossRef]
3. Sartoretti, E.; Sartoretti, T.; Binkert, C.; Najafi, A.; Schwenk, Á.; Hinnen, M.; van Smoorenburg, L.; Eichenberger, B.; Sartoretti-Schefer, S. Reduction of procedure times in routine clinical practice with Compressed SENSE magnetic resonance imaging technique. *PLoS ONE* **2019**, *14*, e0214887. [CrossRef] [PubMed]
4. Hollingsworth, K.G. Reducing acquisition time in clinical MRI by data undersampling and compressed sensing reconstruction. *Phys. Med. Biol.* **2015**, *60*, R297. [CrossRef] [PubMed]
5. Vranic, J.E.; Cross, N.M.; Wang, Y.; Hippe, D.S.; de Weerdt, E.; Mossa-Basha, M. Compressed Sensing-Sensitivity Encoding (CS-SENSE) Accelerated Brain Imaging: Reduced Scan Time without Reduced Image Quality. *AJNR Am. J. Neuroradiol.* **2019**, *40*, 92–98. [CrossRef] [PubMed]
6. Barkovich, M.J.; Li, Y.; Desikan, R.S.; Barkovich, A.J.; Xu, D. Challenges in pediatric neuroimaging. *Neuroimage* **2019**, *185*, 793–801. [CrossRef] [PubMed]
7. Machata, A.M.; Willschke, H.; Kabon, B.; Prayer, D.; Marhofer, P. Effect of brain magnetic resonance imaging on body core temperature in sedated infants and children. *Br. J. Anaesth.* **2009**, *102*, 385–389. [CrossRef]
8. Salerno, S.; Granata, C.; Trapenese, M.; Cannata, V.; Curione, D.; Espagnet, M.C.R.; Magistrelli, A.; Tomà, P. Is MRI imaging in pediatric age totally safe? A critical reprisal. *Radiol. Med.* **2018**, *123*, 695–702. [CrossRef]
9. Serai, S.D.; Hu, H.H.; Ahmad, R.; White, S.; Pednekar, A.; Anupindi, S.A.; Lee, E.Y. Newly Developed Methods for Reducing Motion Artifacts in Pediatric Abdominal MRI: Tips and Pearls. *AJR Am. J. Roentgenol.* **2020**, *214*, 1042–1053. [CrossRef]
10. Ahmad, R.; Hu, H.H.; Krishnamurthy, R.; Krishnamurthy, R. Reducing sedation for pediatric body MRI using accelerated and abbreviated imaging protocols. *Pediatr. Radiol.* **2018**, *48*, 37–49. [CrossRef]
11. Vasanawala, S.S.; Alley, M.T.; Hargreaves, B.A.; Barth, R.A.; Pauly, J.M.; Lustig, M. Improved pediatric MR imaging with compressed sensing. *Radiology* **2010**, *256*, 607–616. [CrossRef]
12. Zhang, T.; Cheng, J.Y.; Potnick, A.G.; Barth, R.A.; Alley, M.T.; Uecker, M.; Lustig, M.; Pauly, J.M.; Vasanawala, S.S. Fast pediatric 3D free-breathing abdominal dynamic contrast enhanced MRI with high spatiotemporal resolution. *J. Magn. Reson. Imaging* **2015**, *41*, 460–473. [CrossRef] [PubMed]
13. Meister, R.L.; Groth, M.; Jurgens, J.H.W.; Zhang, S.; Buhk, J.H.; Herrmann, J. Compressed SENSE in Pediatric Brain Tumor MR Imaging: Assessment of Image Quality, Examination Time and Energy Release. *Clin. Neuroradiol.* **2022**, *32*, 725–733. [CrossRef] [PubMed]
14. Kozak, B.M.; Jaimes, C.; Kirsch, J.; Gee, M.S. MRI Techniques to Decrease Imaging Times in Children. *Radiographics* **2020**, *40*, 485–502. [CrossRef] [PubMed]
15. Sartoretti, T.; Reischauer, C.; Sartoretti, E.; Binkert, C.; Najafi, A.; Sartoretti-Schefer, S. Common artefacts encountered on images acquired with combined compressed sensing and SENSE. *Insights Imaging* **2018**, *9*, 1107–1115. [CrossRef]
16. Thust, S.C.; Heiland, S.; Falini, A.; Jäger, H.R.; Waldman, A.D.; Sundgren, P.C.; Godi, C.; Katsaros, V.K.; Ramos, A.; Bargallo, N.; et al. Glioma imaging in Europe: A survey of 220 centres and recommendations for best clinical practice. *Eur. Radiol.* **2018**, *28*, 3306–3317. [CrossRef]
17. Heiland, S. From A as in Aliasing to Z as in Zipper: Artifacts in MRI. *Clin. Neuroradiol.* **2008**, *18*, 25–36. [CrossRef]
18. Lisanti, C.; Carlin, C.; Banks, K.P.; Wang, D. Normal MRI appearance and motion-related phenomena of CSF. *AJR Am. J. Roentgenol.* **2007**, *188*, 716–725. [CrossRef]
19. Dietrich, O.; Reiser, M.F.; Schoenberg, S.O. Artifacts in 3-T MRI: Physical background and reduction strategies. *Eur. J. Radiol.* **2008**, *65*, 29–35. [CrossRef]
20. Zhuo, J.; Gullapalli, R.P. AAPM/RSNA physics tutorial for residents: MR artifacts, safety, and quality control. In *Radiographics*; 2006; Volume 26, pp. 275–297. [CrossRef] [PubMed]
21. Foley, J.R.; Broadbent, D.A.; Fent, G.J.; Garg, P.; Brown, L.A.; Chew, P.G.; Dobson, L.E.; Swoboda, P.P.; Plein, S.; Higgins, D.M.; et al. Clinical evaluation of two dark blood methods of late gadolinium quantification of ischemic scar. *J. Magn. Reson. Imaging* **2019**, *50*, 146–152. [CrossRef]

22. Zhang, T.; Chowdhury, S.; Lustig, M.; Barth, R.A.; Alley, M.T.; Grafendorfer, T.; Calderon, P.D.; Robb, F.J.; Pauly, J.M.; Vasanawala, S.S. Clinical performance of contrast enhanced abdominal pediatric MRI with fast combined parallel imaging compressed sensing reconstruction. *J. Magn. Reson. Imaging* **2014**, *40*, 13–25. [CrossRef] [PubMed]
23. Vargas, M.I.; Delavelle, J.; Kohler, R.; Becker, C.D.; Lovblad, K. Brain and spine MRI artifacts at 3Tesla. *J. Neuroradiol.* **2009**, *36*, 74–81. [CrossRef] [PubMed]
24. Sharma, S.D.; Fong, C.L.; Tzung, B.S.; Law, M.; Nayak, K.S. Clinical image quality assessment of accelerated magnetic resonance neuroimaging using compressed sensing. *Investig. Radiol.* **2013**, *48*, 638–645. [CrossRef] [PubMed]
25. Jaimes, C.; Kirsch, J.E.; Gee, M.S. Fast, free-breathing and motion-minimized techniques for pediatric body magnetic resonance imaging. *Pediatr. Radiol.* **2018**, *48*, 1197–1208. [CrossRef]
26. Chaskis, C.; Neyns, B.; Michotte, A.; De Ridder, M.; Everaert, H. Pseudoprogression after radiotherapy with concurrent temozolomide for high-grade glioma: Clinical observations and working recommendations. *Surg. Neurol.* **2009**, *72*, 423–428. [CrossRef]
27. Pasqualetti, F.; Malfatti, G.; Cantarella, M.; Gonnelli, A.; Montrone, S.; Montemurro, N.; Gadducci, G.; Giannini, N.; Pesaresi, I.; Perrini, P.; et al. Role of magnetic resonance imaging following postoperative radiotherapy in clinical decision-making of patients with high-grade glioma. *Radiol. Med.* **2022**, *127*, 803–808. [CrossRef]
28. Dreha-Kulaczewski, S.; Konopka, M.; Joseph, A.A.; Kollmeier, J.; Merboldt, K.-D.; Ludwig, H.-C.; Gärtner, J.; Frahm, J. Respiration and the watershed of spinal CSF flow in humans. *Sci. Rep.* **2018**, *8*, 5594. [CrossRef]
29. Mestre, H.; Tithof, J.; Du, T.; Song, W.; Peng, W.; Sweeney, A.M.; Olveda, G.; Thomas, J.H.; Nedergaard, M.; Kelley, D.H. Flow of cerebrospinal fluid is driven by arterial pulsations and is reduced in hypertension. *Nat. Commun.* **2018**, *9*, 4878. [CrossRef]
30. Lustig, M.; Donoho, D.; Pauly, J.M. Sparse MRI: The application of compressed sensing for rapid MR imaging. *Magn. Reson. Med.* **2007**, *58*, 1182–1195. [CrossRef]
31. Lustig, M.; Donoho, D.L.; Santos, J.M.; Pauly, J.M. Compressed Sensing MRI. *IEEE Signal Process. Mag.* **2008**, *25*, 72–82. [CrossRef]
32. Liang, D.; Liu, B.; Wang, J.; Ying, L. Accelerating SENSE using compressed sensing. *Magn. Reson. Med.* **2009**, *62*, 1574–1584. [CrossRef] [PubMed]
33. Pruessmann, K.P.; Weiger, M.; Scheidegger, M.B. SENSE: Sensitivity encoding for fast MRI. *Magn. Reson. Med.* **1999**, *42*, 952–962. [CrossRef]
34. Geethanath, S.; Reddy, R.; Konar, A.S.; Imam, S.; Sundaresan, R.; DR, R.B.; Venkatesan, R. Compressed sensing MRI: A review. *Crit. Rev. Biomed. Eng.* **2013**, *41*, 183–204. [CrossRef] [PubMed]
35. Jaspan, O.N.; Fleysher, R.; Lipton, M.L. Compressed sensing MRI: A review of the clinical literature. *Br. J. Radiol.* **2015**, *88*, 20150487. [CrossRef] [PubMed]
36. Yoon, J.K.; Kim, M.J.; Lee, S. Compressed Sensing and Parallel Imaging for Double Hepatic Arterial Phase Acquisition in Gadoxetate-Enhanced Dynamic Liver Magnetic Resonance Imaging. *Investig. Radiol.* **2019**, *54*, 374–382. [CrossRef]
37. Toledano-Massiah, S.; Sayadi, A.; de Boer, R.; Gelderblom, J.; Mahdjoub, R.; Gerber, S.; Zuber, M.; Zins, M.; Hodel, J. Accuracy of the Compressed Sensing Accelerated 3D-FLAIR Sequence for the Detection of MS Plaques at 3T. *AJNR Am. J. Neuroradiol.* **2018**, *39*, 454–458. [CrossRef]
38. He, M.; Xu, J.; Sun, Z.; Wang, S.; Zhu, L.; Wang, X.; Wang, J.; Feng, F.; Xue, H.; Jin, Z. Comparison and evaluation of the efficacy of compressed SENSE (CS) and gradient- and spin-echo (GRASE) in breath-hold (BH) magnetic resonance cholangiopancreatography (MRCP). *J. Magn. Reson. Imaging* **2020**, *51*, 824–832. [CrossRef]
39. Woodfield, J.; Kealey, S. Magnetic resonance imaging acquisition techniques intended to decrease movement artefact in paediatric brain imaging: A systematic review. *Pediatr. Radiol.* **2015**, *45*, 1271–1281. [CrossRef]

Disclaimer/Publisher's Note: The statements, opinions and data contained in all publications are solely those of the individual author(s) and contributor(s) and not of MDPI and/or the editor(s). MDPI and/or the editor(s) disclaim responsibility for any injury to people or property resulting from any ideas, methods, instructions or products referred to in the content.

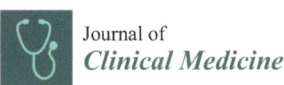

Case Report

Pulp Revascularization in an Autotransplanted Mature Tooth: Visualization with Magnetic Resonance Imaging and Histopathologic Correlation

Petra Rugani [1,*], Iva Brcic [2], Marton Magyar [3], Uwe Yacine Schwarze [4,5], Norbert Jakse [1] and Kurt Ebeleseder [6]

1. Department of Dental Medicine and Oral Health, Division of Oral Surgery and Orthodontics, Medical University of Graz, Billrothgasse 4, 8010 Graz, Austria
2. Diagnostic and Research Institute of Pathology, Comprehensive Cancer Centre Graz, Medical University of Graz, 8010 Graz, Austria; iva.brcic@medunigraz.at
3. Department of Radiology, Division of Neuroradiology, Vascular and Interventional Radiology, Medical University of Graz, 8010 Graz, Austria; marton.magyar@medunigraz.at
4. Department of Dentistry and Oral Health, Division of Oral Surgery and Orthodontics, Medical University of Graz, 8010 Graz, Austria; uwe.schwarze@medunigraz.at
5. Department of Orthopedics and Traumatology, Musculo-Skeletal Research Unit for Biomaterials, Medical University of Graz, 8036 Graz, Austria
6. Department of Dental Medicine and Oral Health, Division of Prosthodontics, Restorative Dentistry and Periodontology, Medical University of Graz, 8010 Graz, Austria; kurt.ebeleseder@medunigraz.at
* Correspondence: petra.rugani@medunigraz.at; Tel.: +43-316-385-13486

Abstract: Autotransplantation of a mature tooth usually leads to pulpal necrosis. Root canal treatment is recommended to prevent related inflammatory complications a few weeks after surgery. Extraoral root-end resection may facilitate reperfusion and obviate root canal treatment, but cannot be pictured with conventional dental radiography at this point in time. In the case of a lower mature transplanted molar, contrast-enhanced magnetic resonance imaging proved to be a feasible method for visualizing pulp revascularization just 4 weeks after autotransplantation. Consequently, root canal treatment was obviated. Nevertheless, the tooth had to be extracted 18 months postoperatively due to external cervical root resorption, probably caused by the extraction trauma. This allowed the histological processing and examination of the newly generated intracanal tissue. Uninflamed fibrovascular connective tissue was found, while odontoblasts or cementoblast-like cells were absent. These findings indicated that it was most likely stem cells from the bone marrow and the periodontal ligament that drove the regeneration.

Keywords: autotransplantation; magnetic resonance imaging; cone-beam computed tomography; histopathology

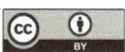

1. Introduction

Tooth autotransplantation (AT) is defined as repositioning of a tooth or tooth germ in the same patient's mouth. It has been an accepted method since the 1980s. Success is defined by two main aspects: Periodontal and endodontic healing of the transplant at the recipient site.

A prerequisite for periodontal healing is a gentle surgical technique. Especially, damage of the root cementum has to be avoided. Thorough preoperative planning and the application of surgical templates have proven to be beneficial [1]. Endodontic healing after AT is defined as an ingrowth of new tissue through the apical foramen into the pulp canal and pulp chamber of the transplant (pulp revascularization, PRV). PRV in immature transplanted teeth with a developing root is common and is probably facilitated by the large diameter of the apical foramen and the high number of apical stem cells [2,3]. A small diameter of 0.2–0.4 mm however, as found in the apical constrictions of mature premolars, reduces the chances of PRV to almost zero [4]. As a failed PRV is mostly combined with endodontic infection, rapid external infection-related root resorption can follow. Consequently, in mature teeth root canal treatment is recommended within 7–14 days after AT [5,6].

Assessment and evidence of successful PRV is therefore a critical issue for further treatment of autotransplanted teeth. Two aspects have to be considered: First, successful PRV should not be disturbed by an unnecessary endodontic intervention and second, root resorption has to be avoided in cases of failed PRV. Traditionally, PRV is assessed indirectly. First by ruling out necrosis (i.e., lack of signs indicating infection related root resorption) and later by pulp canal obliteration (PCO) on intraoral radiographs and/or clinically by the regained sensitivity of the tooth.

A more recent approach aims to show PRV directly via magnetic resonance imaging (MRI) with or without the use of a contrast agent [7–10]. In mature teeth, with a high risk of pulp necrosis, this verification may obviate the need for prophylactic root canal treatment several weeks after surgery.

Several case reports [11,12] and recent studies [13,14] indicated that extra-oral root end resection (EORER) might promote PRV in autotransplanted teeth and thus prevent endodontic complications. We hereby report for the first time on histological findings that might help to understand the biological process underlying the PRV of autotransplanted apically resected mature teeth (ATMT-EORER). Contrast-enhanced MRI was applied for non-invasive success control.

2. Report

The PRICE reporting guidelines were followed in the preparation of this report [15].

A 28-year-old male white patient was referred by his orthodontist with pericoronitis at the partially impacted lower right third molar. Removal of tooth 48 (FDI (World Dental Federation)) and orthodontic therapy to resolve crowding was intended. In his past medical history, he had lost the left lower first molar three years prior to admission due to apical periodontitis. Due to aplasia of tooth 45, the deciduous tooth 85 was still present but its roots were severely resorbed (Figure 1). In the course of the treatment planning, the decision was made to transplant the partially impacted tooth 48 in the position of the missing second premolar as an alternative to implant placement.

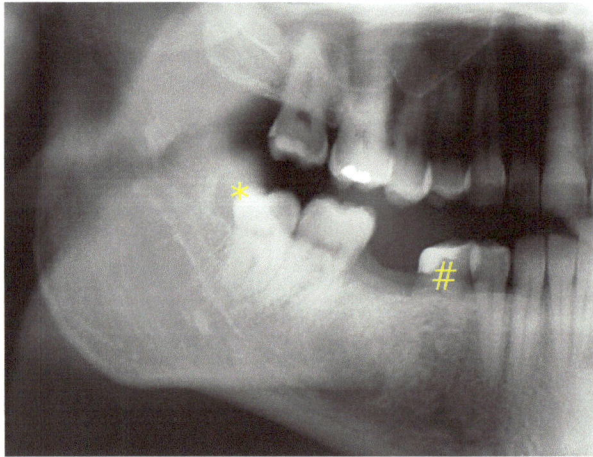

Figure 1. Initial panoramic radiograph; * Signs for pericoronitis tooth 48 as indication for tooth removal; # Deciduous tooth 85 with heavy restoration and severely resorbed roots and a poor long-term prognosis.

The patient was in good general health but was a smoker. He gave informed consent to autotransplantation, knowing that prognosis was reduced due to the mature multi-rooted donor tooth.

In the preoperative analysis, a CBCT (Cone beam computed tomography) scan was obtained using Planmeca ProMax 3D Max (Planmeca OY, Helsinki, Finland), with a voxel size of 0.2 mm and standard settings to confirm the integrity of the donor tooth and adequate dimensions of the recipient site. CBCT data were then segmented using the coDiagnostiX^{TM} software (Version 9.0, Dental Wings GmbH, Chemnitz, Germany) to create a virtual 3D replica of the tooth transplant. This model was 3D printed to serve as a reference for recipient-site preparation (Figure 2).

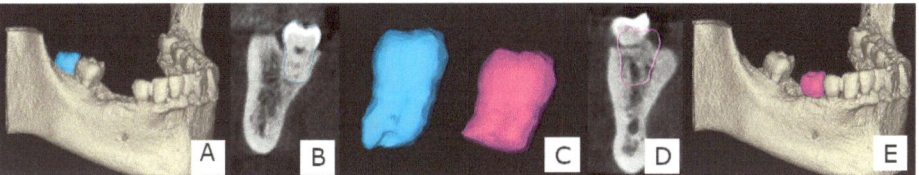

Figure 2. (**A**,**B**) Segmentation of the tooth transplant (blue) (**C**) segmented donor (blue) and planned transplant after EORER (pink) (**D**,**E**) Planned transplant at the recipient site (pink).

The surgery was performed under local anesthesia (Ultracain Dental Forte 1:100,000; Sanofi-Aventis GmbH, Vienna, Austria). Tooth 85 was removed and a local mucoperiosteal flap was raised at the recipient site. The recipient socket was prepared using an implant drill kit (Frialit II, Dentsply Sirona Austria GmbH, Vienna, Austria). Sufficient enlargement was verified using the printed graft replica. (Figure 3A) Thereafter, pericoronal osteotomy was performed (Figure 3C) and tooth 48 was extracted as gently as possible. Care was taken not to damage the root cement, but because of the impaction elevators had to be used as well. The root tip was resected (EORER, Figure 3C) with 40,000 rpm under water cooling with a diamond disc. As a result, the apical opening increased to >1 mm. (Figure 3D) There was no additional extracorporeal treatment of either pulp or cementum. Subsequently, the graft was gently inserted into its new socket. (Figures 3E and 4) After insertion, the flap was closed and the transplant was fixed in the socket using sutures (Figure 3F).

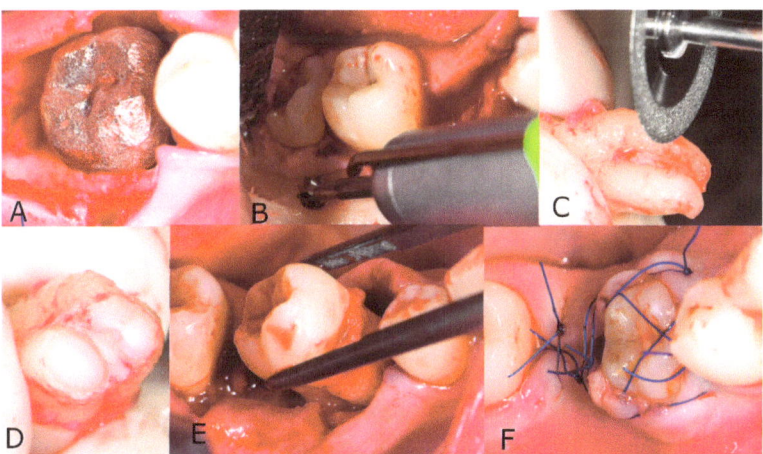

Figure 3. Autotransplantation (**A**) Tooth replica fitted in the prepared new socket (**B**) Osteotomy to remove the graft tooth 48 (**C**) Root-end resection of the transplant (**D**) Enlarged apical opening (**E**) Re-insertion of the graft into the new socket (**F**) Wound closure.

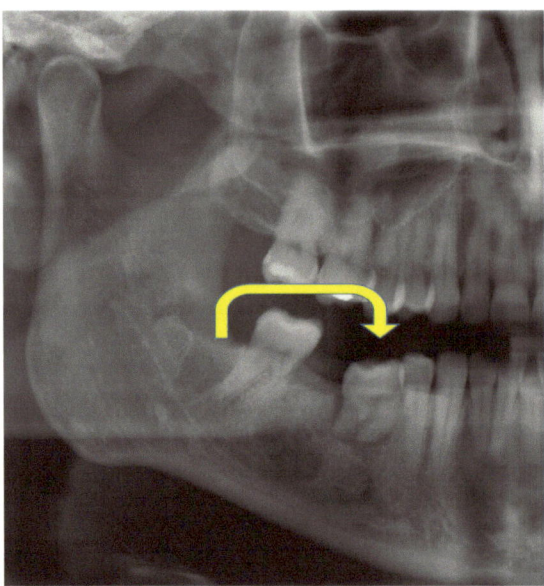

Figure 4. Postoperative panoramic radiograph. After removal of the deciduous tooth 85 the wisdom tooth and surgical preparation of the recipient socket tooth 48 had been transplanted (Yellow arrow). Note the shorter roots of the transplant after EORER.

A flexible wire-composite splint was bonded to the vestibular enamel of the transplant and the neighboring teeth. The metallic component of the splint was a twistflex wire (GAC Wildcat Wire 0.0175-inch, Ortho-Care, Shipley, UK).

The patient received perioperative antibiotic prophylaxis for 4 days (cephalexin administered thrice daily for 4 days; Ospexin® 1000 mg, Sandoz GmbH, Kundl, Austria) and antiphlogistic therapy was prescribed for 2–5 days (dexibuprofen administered thrice daily for 2–3 days; Seractil® forte 400 mg, Gebro Pharma GmbH, Fieberbrunn, Austria). Sutures were removed after 1 week, the wire splint after 4 weeks.

The patient was recalled every three months during the first year. The endodontic status of the transplant was assessed during each follow-up. The following clinical endodontic data were obtained:

- Presence/absence of local swelling or sinus tract
- Sensitivity to percussion
- Pulpal sensitivity to an electric pulp tester (Digitest®, Parkell, NY, USA).

Intraoral radiographs were obtained using the rectangular technique with appropriate film holders. The presence of pulp obliteration (a sign of revascularization), external infection-related root resorption, or apical radiolucency (signs of infected pulp necrosis) were investigated (Figure 5).

Contrast-enhanced magnetic resonance imaging (MRI) was performed immediately after splint removal to assess revascularization using a contrast medium (Gadobutrol, Gadovist®, Bayer, Leverkusen, Germany; Figure 6 right). 3D T1 and T2 sequences were obtained with and without contrast agent to detect the accumulation of the contrast agent (Siemens Magnetom Prismafit, T1 Starvibe 0.7 mm 3D with contrast agent). The good local resolution allowed a significant magnification of the transplanted teeth and thus, an assessment of the small volume pulp in all three dimensions. A head and neck radiologist with more than 10 years of experience was responsible for the interpretation of the images.

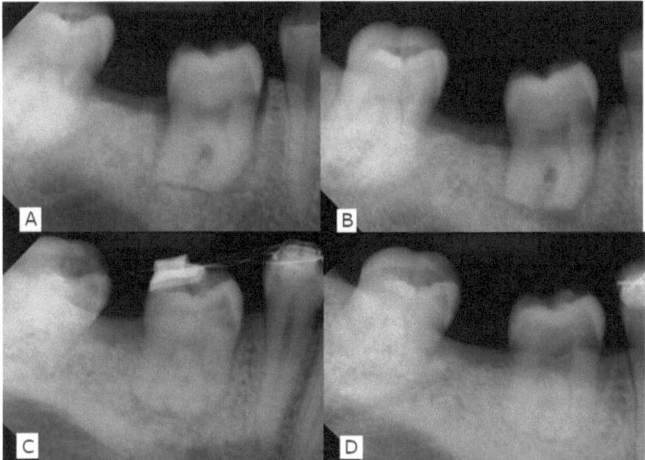

Figure 5. Radiographic follow-up with intraoral radiographs. (**A**) postop (**B**) 3 months postop beginning formation of the periodontal ligament space, no signs for external root resorption (**C**) 12 months postop, visible obliteration of the pulp chamber (**D**) 18 months postop radiolucent lesion in the pulp chamber.

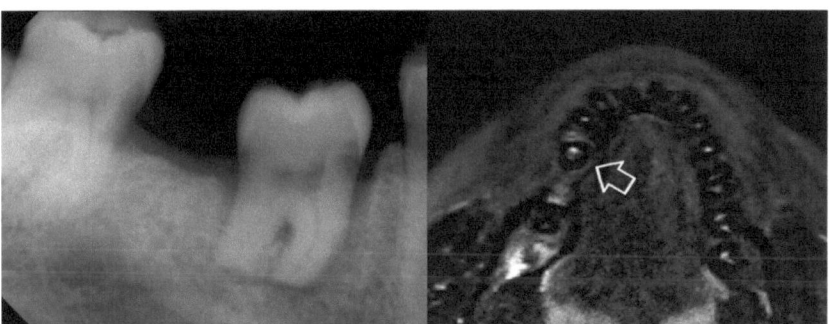

Figure 6. Radiographic control 4 weeks postoperatively. (**Left**), intraoral radiograph with still-missing signs of PDL regeneration or reperfusion. (**Right**), contrast-enhanced MRI with uptake of the contrast medium in the pulp chamber (arrow) already confirming reperfusion.

Electromechanical tapping (Periotest®, Medizintechnik Gulden, Modautal, Germany) was performed to assess tooth mobility and values were compared to neighboring corresponding teeth, respectively. Periotest values were similar and were slightly positive after 12 months (+3).

The postoperative course was uneventful. The MRI showed enhancement of the contrast agent in the pulp chamber four weeks postoperatively (Figure 2B) and sensitivity was restored three months after surgery. Orthodontic therapy was initiated after the 9-month-recall with the transplanted tooth engaged in tooth movement.

After 18 months, the patient presented with a buccal swelling with purulent drainage (Figure 7A) over the cervical aspect of the transplant. The CBCT scan revealed external resorption in the subgingival part of the crown, especially the dental neck (Figure 7C). As a consequence of its reduced prognosis, the tooth was extracted with the patient's consent.

The extracted tooth was fixed in 4% phosphate-buffered formaldehyde pH 7 immediately after extraction. After this, the tooth was rinsed in tap water then dehydrated in ascending grades of ethanol (40%, 70%, 80% 96% 3 times absolute for analysis). Infiltration with a light curing resin (Technovit 7200, Kulzer, Hanaus, Germany) was performed in ascending grades mixed with ethanol absolute for analysis (30:70, 50:50, 70:30, 3 times pure Technovit 7200). Finally, the tooth was embedded in the same resin and processed into undecalcified thin ground sections with a thickness of about 100 µm, according to the Karl Donath method [16], using machines from EXAKT (EXAKT Apparatebau, Norderstedt, Germany) and Walter Messner (Walter Messner GmbH, Oststeinbek, Germany). A section was stained with basic fuchsin methylene blue and Azur II [17].

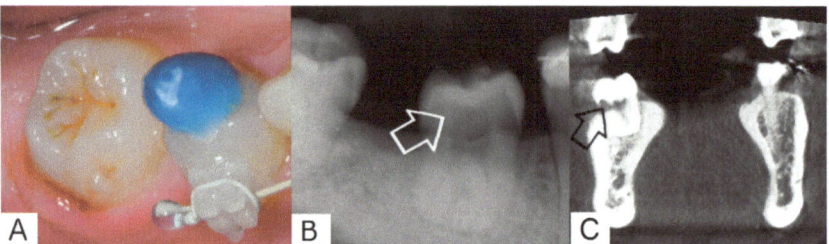

Figure 7. 18-month follow-up. (**A**). Clinical picture with signs of inflammation (bleeding and suppuration from the gingival margin) (**B**). Intraoral radiograph with suspect radiolucency in the crown of the transplant (white arrow) (**C**). Native CBCT (resolution 0.2 mm) The arrow shows the buccal resorption in the subgingival part of the crown of the transplanted tooth, but otherwise a regular periodontal ligament space and no further signs of external root resorption.

A specialist in pathology assessed the stained section. Histology confirmed the presence of fibrovascular connective tissue in the root canal (Figures 8 and 9). Resorptive lacunae and cementum damage were observed on the root surface (Figure 9A,B). At the apical section of the root, a layer of bone-like tissue was directly deposited on the canal dentin walls (Figure 9C,D) with focal dentin resorption (also known as replacement resorption, Figure 9D,E). In addition, osteocytes with slender cytoplasmic processes extending in all directions were present in the bone-like tissue (Figure 9E). In contrast, odontoblasts (Figure 9E) and cementoblast-like cells were absent.

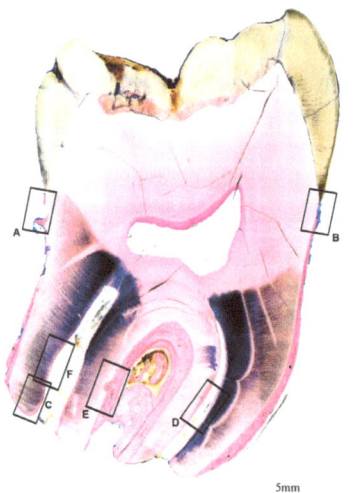

Figure 8. Low power image of an explanted/extracted tooth 18 months after transplantation. The enamel is ulcerated. Resorptive lacunae and cementum damage are visible at the root surface. The canal lumen is composed of vascularized fibro-connective tissue. Bony islands are also present. Details marked with rectangles A–F are shown in Figure 9.

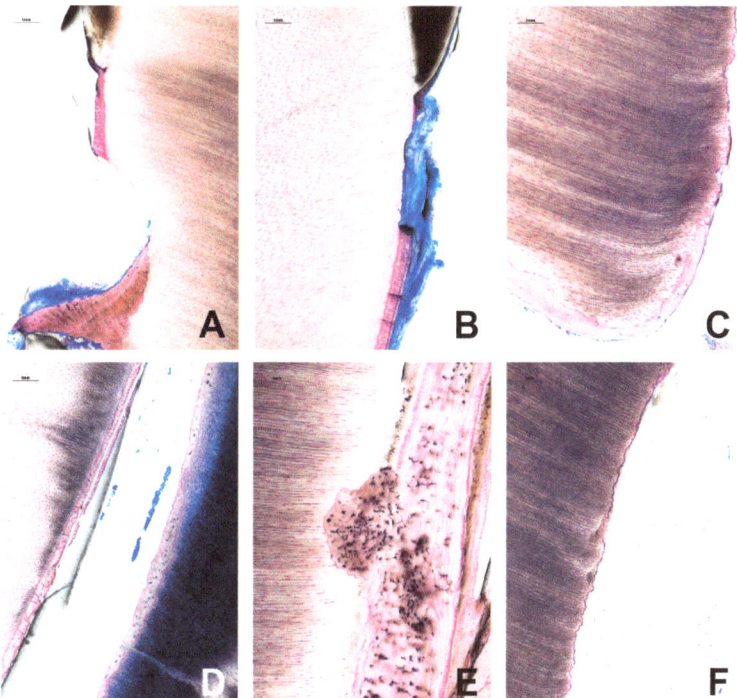

Figure 9. Higher power image of an explanted/extracted tooth 18 months after transplantation. (**A,B**) Resorptive lacunae and cementum damage on the root surface. (**C,D**) A layer of bone-like tissue is directly deposited on the canal dentin walls at the apical section of the root. (**E**) Dentin resorption. Osteocytes with slender, cytoplasmic processes radiating in all direction are present in the bone-like tissue. (**F**) Odontoblast-like cells are not found in the canal dentin walls.

3. Discussion

Revascularization occurred in a transplanted mature third molar after ATMT-EORER, proven by contrast-enhanced MRI 4 weeks after surgery. MRI brought immediate clarity on the PRV process in the tooth and could eliminate the risk of missing the early radiological signs of root resorption.

The application of the modern possibilities of cross-sectional imaging data is essential for a high success rate of the autotransplantation of teeth. CBCT- or MSCT-derived dicom data is used to create replicas of the transplant. The use of these replicas for recipient site preparation ensures two key factors for successful periodontal healing: minimal extraoral time and optimal fitting of the transplant, hence minimal damage of the active cells of the root surface. MRI on the other hand, has proven capable of showing revascularization and endodontic healing at an early stage, which is decisive for the further therapeutic procedure.

Display of pulpal perfusion with MRI has already been described in 2001 by Ploder et al. [7] using a 1.0 Tesla unit. Shortly after, Kress et al. [18] demonstrated that it was possible to produce MR images showing the perfusion of dental pulp in vivo, but that the analysis solely composed of non-contrast-enhanced sequences was not conclusive. They reported that the comparison of signal intensities before and after contrast agent administration showed the most significant difference between vital and avital teeth.

Assaf et al. [10] concluded that by application of 3T, PRV can be adequately visualized using fsT1w and fsT2w sequences, even without the use of contrast media, with scanning times of up to 20 min. They applied this protocol after replantation of avulsed teeth in children. There is a considerable risk that the pulp of the transplanted teeth may necrotize without adequate blood supply, therefore the MRI without contrast was able to detect avital teeth well. In our daily clinical setting, patients are examined in 30-min slots, limiting the maximum duration of the examination. For this reason, it was not feasible to perform native, high-resolution sequences lasting up to 20 min. Another consideration is that the longer the image acquisition time, the greater the chance that there will be motion artefacts.

Furthermore, MRI does not provide interpretable results if artefact causing elements are present. Especially orthodontic devices and dental implants cause major distortions. [19] Allergy to the contrast agent and claustrophobia are further contraindications. The application of contrast agents in children especially might raise concerns. In our facility, only macrocyclic gadolinium-based MRI contrast agents in single doses are used. Usually, patients are only examined once. In the MRI machines for pediatric examinations, Gadobutrol (Gadovist®; Bayer Healthcare, Leverkusen, Germany) is applied. So far, patients have experienced solely mild (mild itching) but no severe side effects.

All children are informed about the examination and possible side effects of MRI and MRI contrast media effects in the presence of their parents or guardians. In addition, known allergies and kidney disease are considered as contraindications. Several recent studies are consistent with our findings regarding the high safety of gadolinium-based macrocyclic MRI contrast agents [20–22].

In future studies, it would be interesting to evaluate the extent to which the vascular supply of the pulp can be determined using arterial spin labelling (ASL). This method would theoretically allow the measurement of local blood perfusion/supply without the need for intravenous contrast administration. A major limitation in imaging transplanted teeth is the small volume of the area examined at submillimeter resolution and, consequently, the length of the sequences applied. This is compounded by the small amount of signaling tissue in the oral area, especially in the pulp.

In our case, each motion reduced 3D T1 sequence took about 6:52 min, despite a 64-channel head coil and a 3T MRI machine. In patients with avital pulp, there was no measurable signal enhancement in the T1 sequence after gadolinium administration (Figure 10). In comparison, vital re-implanted teeth showed significant contrast uptake, similar to the other healthy teeth (Figure 11). It is to be expected that older and 1.5T machines with non-optimized coils will take significantly longer to produce reasonably good images with a good signal-to-noise ratio. Nevertheless, it is a good method for examining the vitality of the transplanted teeth and is well tolerated by our patients.

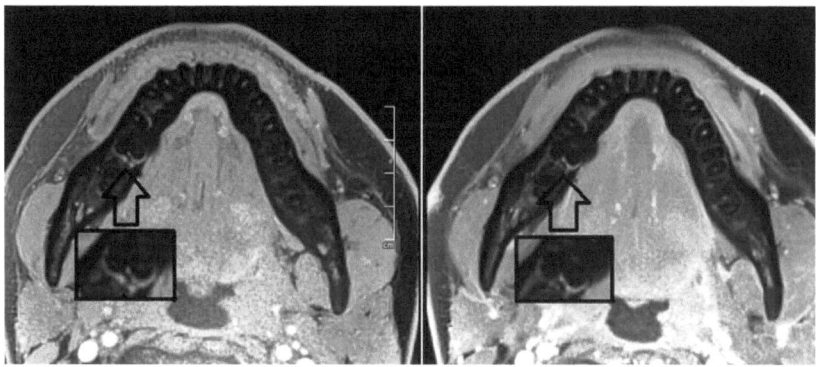

Figure 10. T1-weighted MRI on our 3T scanner, left without contrast and right with contrast. There is no significant T1 signal enhancement in the pulp in both native and post-contrast imaging. Note: Healthy teeth show clear and measurable contrast enhancement after magnification. The black arrow shows the region of interest with the image below magnified.

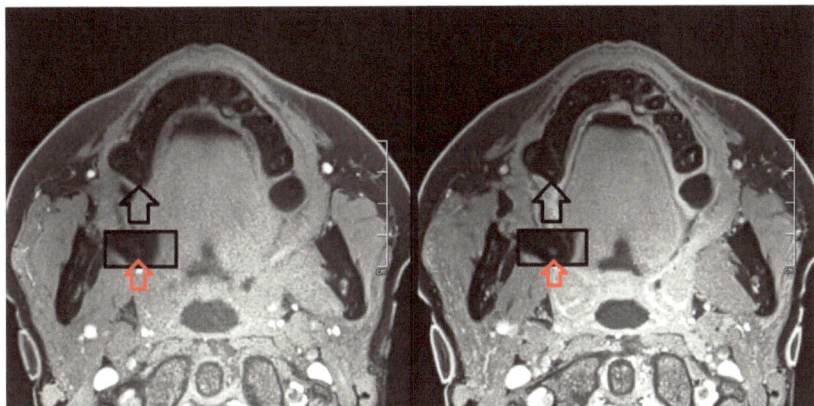

Figure 11. T1-weighted 3T MRI left, without, right, with contrast enhancement in the same patient at our hospital. The enhancement is clearly visible as a white spot in the pulp area after magnification on the right image. The black arrow shows the region of interest, the red arrow on the magnified image shows the pulp without and with contrast enhancement.

The transplanted tooth developed a resorptive lesion beneath the buccal cervical margin. Given the configuration of this lesion, it was obviously caused by trauma to the root cementum through the use of luxators during extraction and it worsened the prognosis for this case. In consultation with the patient, it was decided to remove the tooth. Consequently, the opportunity arose to have the transplant examined histologically.

ATMT-EORER has been described in animal studies [23,24] and was first implemented in humans by Jakse et al. [11]. To date, there have been only few reports regarding similar procedures and the mechanisms underlying pulpal healing have not been clarified yet. The histological assessment of an autotransplanted mature human tooth demonstrating these mechanisms is unique. Revascularization is mostly studied in animal trials, predominantly in studies addressing regenerative endodontics (RET). A review by Fang et al. [1] identified only two studies with histological examinations of intracanal tissues after RET [25,26]. Nevertheless, revascularization is a critical issue after transplantation, as its failure usually leads to endodontic infection and rapid external root resorption and possibly loss of the transplant.

Tooth germs with open apices have a greater ability to revascularize. This is clearly demonstrated by the consistently high success rates of pulpal healing in the autotransplantation of immature teeth with 2/3–3/4 developed roots [24,27–29].

Three mechanisms have to be considered to explain the highly predictable endodontic healing in immature transplants:

(a) A larger diameter of the apical foramen facilitates cell migration and ingrowth of new vessels into the ischemic pulp space.
(b) Immature teeth display a shorter root; therefore, the migration distance for the ingrown tissue is short.
(c) Immature teeth are endowed with more and a larger spectrum of stem cells.

The influence of stem/progenitor cells has been widely discussed in regenerative endodontic treatment (RET), where the term revascularization refers to the ingrowth of new tissue into a formerly infected root canal. Therefore, bleeding is provoked from the periapical tissue by introducing instruments below the apical constriction. The technique delivers undifferentiated mesenchymal stem cells into the root canal systems of adult patients with mature teeth [30].

In RET, these stem/progenitor cells might be derived from the periodontal ligament (PDL), apical papilla, Hertwig epithelial root sheath, or may be bone marrow mesenchymal stem cells or even surviving dental pulp stem cells [31].

After autotransplantation with root-end resection and hence the removal of the apical papilla, bone marrow stem cells, possibly triggered by the preparation of the recipient site, and stem cells from the PDL most likely drove the intracanal repair process in the present study. The use of tooth replicas for recipient site preparation significantly reduces the extraoral time of the transplant; as a consequence, it may be a key factor in the preservation of vital PDL cells for revascularization. Axin2 expressing cells have been identified in PDL [32]. Axin2+ mesenchymal PDL cells were described as key progenitor cell sources and might play a vital role in postnatal cementogenesis [33].

The mechanism of cell homing [3,34,35] addresses the availability of feasible stem cells beyond local availability. This aspect needs to be investigated in future studies.

The extracted molar subjected to histologic evaluation showed no cementum-like tissue in the revascularized root canals, but bone-like tissue with osteocytes in lacunae. This finding is consistent with the literature [36]. In our case, intracanal cementum was not observed. However, studies on the histologic features of revascularized teeth are rare, with animal trials predominantly animal trials addressing RET [2].

An early study by Skoglund and Tronstad [37] showed that the odontoblastic layer rarely survived in transplanted dog teeth, which was corroborated by Yamauchi et al. [38] after investigating RET in dog teeth. The mineralized tissue inside the canal was characterized by intracanal cement (IC) and bony islands. Wang et al. [39] identified IC, bony islands, and fibrous connective tissue (intracanal periodontal ligament) and hypothesized that different tissue types co-exist in the canal lumen. Furthermore, they reported the presence of lymphocyte infiltration next to IC and concluded that inflammation might stimulate the differentiation of stem/progenitor cells into cementoblasts.

The presented histology indicates that in cases of ATMT- EORER, pulp canal obliteration is presumably caused by the ingrowth of IC and not by reparative dentin. Still, the result is a functional tooth entailing no need for root canal treatment. Pulp canal obliteration is a sure sign of revascularization. Still, it takes several months until it can be proofed on radiographs. By then an endodontic infection may already have destroyed the transplant through rapid external infection-related root resorption. As contrast-enhanced-MRI can bring immediate clarity as soon as four weeks after surgery, it represents a preferable method that does not involve any additional harm to the patient. With an examination time of about 7 min for the T1 sequence, it can be easily integrated into clinical routine and evidence of reperfusion can reduce the number of check-ups required. Nevertheless, the application of MRI for dental purposes is confined by the limited availability of modern machines and highly skilled staff. For this reason, the routine application of the method can currently only be carried out at specialized facilities. Picturing the vascular supply of the pulp with other methods like arterial spin labelling (ASL) to avoid the need for intravenous contrast administration may be a matter of future research and developments.

A further shortcoming of the presented study is its limited perspective of the histological investigation, as only one case is assessed. In addition, relevant details may have been lost during cutting.

4. Conclusions

If applicable, contrast-enhanced MRI is a feasible method to demonstrate PRV of transplanted teeth and thus to ensure a good prognosis, even of mature transplanted teeth. Histologically, the intracanal tissue of the presented tooth showed no odontoblasts, but fibrovascular connective tissue. These results indicate that PRV in transplanted root-end resected teeth is driven by bone marrow stem cells and stem cells from the periodontal ligament. Likewise, pulp canal obliteration is presumably caused by the ingrowth of intracanal cementum or bone and not by reparative dentin.

Author Contributions: Conceptualization, P.R., methodology, P.R., I.B., M.M. and U.Y.S.; validation, N.J. and K.E.; formal analysis, N.J. and K.E.; investigation, P.R.; resources, N.J.; data curation, P.R., I.B., M.M. and U.Y.S.; writing—original draft preparation, P.R., I.B., M.M. and U.Y.S.; writing—review and editing, N.J. and K.E.; visualization, P.R., I.B., M.M. and U.Y.S.; supervision, N.J. and K.E.; project administration, P.R. All authors have read and agreed to the published version of the manuscript.

Funding: This research received no external funding.

Institutional Review Board Statement: The current study was conducted according to the guidelines of the Declaration of Helsinki. Ethical approval was obtained from the ethics committee of the Medical University of Graz (reference number: IRB00002556; review board number 30-519 ex 17/18 date: 29 January 2019).

Informed Consent Statement: Informed consent was obtained from the subject involved in the study.

Data Availability Statement: The data that support the findings of this study are available from the corresponding author upon reasonable request. The data are not publicly available due to privacy or ethical restrictions.

Acknowledgments: CBCT planning and data segmentation performed by Barbara Kirnbauer, Medical University of Graz, Austria.

Conflicts of Interest: The authors declare no conflict of interest.

References

1. Verweij, J.P.; van Westerveld, K.J.H.; Anssari Moin, D.; Mensink, G.; van Merkesteyn, J.P.R. Autotransplantation With a 3-Dimensionally Printed Replica of the Donor Tooth Minimizes Extra-Alveolar Time and Intraoperative Fitting Attempts: A Multicenter Prospective Study of 100 Transplanted Teeth. *J. Oral. Maxillofac. Surg.* **2020**, *78*, 35–43. [CrossRef]
2. Fang, Y.; Wang, X.; Zhu, J.; Su, C.; Yang, Y.; Meng, L. Influence of apical diameter on the outcome of regenerative endodontic treatment in teeth with pulp necrosis: A review. *J. Endod.* **2018**, *44*, 414–431. [CrossRef]
3. Kim, J.Y.; Xin, X.; Moioli, E.K.; Chung, J.; Lee, C.H.; Chen, M.; Fu, S.Y. Regeneration of dental-pulp-like tissue by chemotaxis—Induced cell homing. *Tissue Eng. A* **2010**, *16*, 3023–3031. [CrossRef]
4. Wolf, T.G.; Kim, P.; Campus, G.; Stiebritz, M.; Siegrist, M.; Briseño-Marroquín, B. 3-Dimensional analysis and systematic review of root canal morphology and physiological foramen geometry of 109 mandibular first premolars by micro-computed tomography in a mixed Swiss-German population. *J. Endod.* **2020**, *46*, 801–809. [CrossRef]
5. Kokai, S.; Kanno, Z.; Koike, S.; Uesugi, S.; Takahashi, Y.; Ono, T.; Soma, K. Retrospective study of 100 autotransplanted teeth with complete root formation and subsequent orthodontic treatment. *Am. J. Orthod. Dentofac. Orthop.* **2015**, *148*, 982–989. [CrossRef] [PubMed]
6. Tsukiboshi, M. Autotransplantation of teeth: Requirements for predictable success. *Dent. Traumatol.* **2002**, *18*, 157–180. [CrossRef] [PubMed]
7. Ploder, O.; Partik, B.; Rand, T.; Fock, N.; Voracek, M.; Undt, G.; Baumann, A. Reperfusion of autotransplanted teeth—Comparison of clinical measurements by means of dental magnetic resonance imaging. *Oral. Surg. Oral. Med. Oral. Pathol. Oral. Radiol. Endodontology* **2001**, *92*, 335–340. [CrossRef] [PubMed]
8. Nakashima, M.; Akamine, A. The Application of Tissue Engineering to Regeneration of Pulp and Dentin in Endodontics. *J. Endod.* **2005**, *31*, 711–718. [CrossRef] [PubMed]
9. Annibali, S.; Bellavia, D.; Ottolenghi, L.; Cicconetti, A.; Cristalli, M.P.; Quaranta, R.; Pilloni, A. Micro-CT and PET analysis of bone regeneration induced by biodegradable scaffolds as carriers for dental pulp stem cells in a rat model of calvarial "critical size" defect: Preliminary data. *J. Biomed. Mater. Res. Part. B Appl. Biomater.* **2013**, *102*, 815–825. [CrossRef]
10. Assaf, A.T.; Zrnc, T.A.; Remus, C.C.; Khokale, A.; Habermann, C.R.; Schulze, D.; Fiehler, J.; Heiland, M.; Sedlacik, J.; Friedrich, R.E. Early detection of pulp necrosis and dental vitality after traumatic dental injuries in children and adolescents by 3-Tesla magnetic resonance imaging. *J. Cranio Maxillofac. Surg.* **2015**, *43*, 1088–1093. [CrossRef]
11. Jakse, N.; Ruckenstuhl, M.; Rugani, P.; Kirnbauer, B.; Sokolowski, A.; Ebeleseder, K. Influence of extraoral apicoectomy on revascularization of an autotransplanted tooth: A case report. *J. Endod.* **2018**, *44*, 1298–1302. [CrossRef]
12. Gaviño Orduña, J.F.; García García, M.; Dominguez, P.; Caviedes Bucheli, J.; Martin Biedma, B.; Abella Sans, F.; Manzanares Céspedes, M.C. Successful pulp revascularization of an autotransplantated mature premolar with fragile fracture apicoectomy and plasma rich in growth factors: A 3-year follow-up. *Int. Endod. J.* **2020**, *53*, 421–433. [CrossRef]
13. Raabe, C.; Bornstein, M.M.; Ducommun, J.; Sendi, P.; Von Arx, T.; Janner, S.F.M. A retrospective analysis of autotransplanted teeth including an evaluation of a novel surgical technique. *Clin. Oral. Investig.* **2021**, *25*, 3513–3525. [CrossRef]
14. Rugani, P.; Kirnbauer, B.; Mischak, I.; Ebeleseder, K.; Jakse, N. Extraoral Root-End Resection May Promote Pulpal Revascularization in Autotransplanted Mature Teeth—A Retrospective Study. *J. Clin. Med.* **2022**, *11*, 7199. [CrossRef]
15. Nagendrababu, V.; Chong, B.S.; McCabe, P.; Shah, P.K.; Priya, E.; Jayaraman, J.; Pulikkotil, S.J.; Dummer, P.M.H. PRICE 2020 guidelines for reporting case reports in Endodontics: Explanation and elaboration. *Int. Endod. J.* **2020**, *53*, 922–947. [CrossRef]

16. Donath, K. [The separating thin section technique for the production of histological preparations from tissues and materials that cannot be sectioned: Description of apparatus and methods] German. Die Trenn-Dünnschliff-Technik zur Herstellung histologischer Präparate von nicht schneidbaren Geweben und Materialien. *Präparator* **1998**, *34*, 197–206.
17. Laczko, J.; Levai, G. A simple differential staining method for semi-thin sections of ossyfying cartilage and bone tissue embedded in epoxy resin. *Mikroskopie* **1975**, *31*, 1–4.
18. Kress, B.; Buhl, Y.; Anders, L.; Stippich, C.; Palm, F.; Bähren, W.; Sartor, K. Quantitative analysis of MRI signal intensity as a tool for evaluating tooth pulp vitality. *Dentomaxillofac. Radiol.* **2004**, *33*, 241–244. [CrossRef] [PubMed]
19. Reda, R.; Zanza, A.; Mazzoni, A.; Cicconetti, A.; Testarelli, L.; Di Nardo, D. An Update of the Possible Applications of Magnetic Resonance Imaging (MRI) in Dentistry: A Literature Review. *J. Imaging* **2021**, *7*, 75. [CrossRef]
20. Shah, R.; D'Arco, F.; Soares, B.; Cooper, J.; Brierley, J. Use of gadolinium contrast agents in paediatric population: Donald Rumsfeld meets Hippocrates! *Br. J. Radiol.* **2019**, *92*, 20180746. [CrossRef] [PubMed]
21. Prince, M.R.; Lee, H.G.; Lee, C.H.; Youn, S.W.; Lee, I.H.; Yoon, W.; Yang, W.; Wang, H.; Wang, J.; Shih, T.T.; et al. Safety of gadobutrol in over 23,000 patients: The GARDIAN study, a global multicentre, prospective, non-interventional study. *Eur. Radiol.* **2017**, *27*, 286–295. [CrossRef]
22. Heshmatzadeh Behzadi, A.; McDonald, J. Gadolinium-based contrast agents for imaging of the central nervous system: A multicenter European prospective study. *Medicine* **2022**, *101*, e30163. [CrossRef]
23. Skoglund, A. Pulpal changes in replanted and autotransplanted apicoectomized mature teeth of dogs. *Int. J. Oral. Surg.* **1981**, *10*, 111–121.
24. Skoglund, A. Vascular changes in replanted and autotransplanted apicoectomized mature teeth of dogs. *Int. J. Oral. Surg.* **1981**, *10*, 100–110. [CrossRef]
25. Nosrat, A.; Kolahdouzan, A.; Hosseini, F.; Mehrizi, E.A.; Verma, P.; Torabinejad, M. Histologic outcomes of uninfected human immature teeth treated with regenerative endodontics: 2 case reports. *J. Endod.* **2015**, *41*, 1725–1729. [CrossRef]
26. Martin, G.; Ricucci, D.; Gibbs, J.L.; Lin, L.M. Histological findings of revascularized/revitalized immature permanent molar with apical periodontitis using platelet-rich plasma. *J. Endod.* **2013**, *39*, 138–144. [CrossRef] [PubMed]
27. Andreasen, J.O.; Paulsen, H.U.; Yu, Z.; Schwartz, O. A long-term study of 370 autotransplanted premolars. Part III. Periodontal healing subsequent to transplantation. *Eur. J. Orthod.* **1990**, *12*, 25–37. [CrossRef]
28. Filippi, A. [Tooth transplantation] German. *Quintessenz* **2008**, *59*, 497–504.
29. Paulsen, H.U.; Andreasen, J.O.; Schwartz, O. Pulp and periodontal healing, root development and root resorption subsequent to transplantation and orthodontic rotation: A long-term study of autotransplanted premolars. *Am. J. Orthod. Dentofac. Orthop.* **1995**, *108*, 630–640. [CrossRef]
30. Chrepa, V.; Henry, M.A.; Daniel, B.J.; Diogenes, A. Delivery of Apical Mesenchymal Stem Cells into Root Canals of Mature Teeth. *J. Dent. Res.* **2015**, *12*, 1653–1659. [CrossRef] [PubMed]
31. Lei, L.; Chen, Y.; Zhou, R.; Huang, X.; Cai, Z. Histologic and Immunohistochemical Findings of a Human Immature Permanent Tooth with Apical Periodontitis after Regenerative Endodontic Treatment. *J. Endod.* **2015**, *41*, 1172–1179. [CrossRef] [PubMed]
32. Yuan, X.; Pei, X.; Zhao, Y.; Tulu, U.S.; Liu, B.; Helms, J.A. A Wnt-Responsive PDL Population Effectuates Extraction Socket Healing. *J. Dent. Res.* **2018**, *7*, 803–809. [CrossRef] [PubMed]
33. Xie, X.; Wang, J.; Wang, K.; Li, C.; Zhang, S.; Jing, D.; Xu, C.; Wang, X.; Zhao, H.; Feng, J.Q. Axin2+-Mesenchymal PDL Cells, Instead of K14+ Epithelial Cells, Play a Key Role in Rapid Cementum Growth. *J. Dent. Res.* **2019**, *11*, 1262–1270. [CrossRef]
34. Eramo, S.; Natali, A.; Pinna, R.; Milia, E. Dental pulp regeneration via cell homing. *Int. Endod. J.* **2018**, *51*, 405–419. [CrossRef]
35. Ahmed, G.M.; Abouauf, E.A.; AbuBakr, N.; Fouad, A.M.; Dörfer, C.E.; Fawzy El-Sayed, K.M. Cell-Based Transplantation versus Cell Homing Approaches for Pulp-Dentin Complex Regeneration. *Stem Cells Int.* **2021**, *8483668*. [CrossRef] [PubMed]
36. Yanpiset, K.; Trope, M. Pulp revascularization of replanted immature dog teeth after different treatment methods. *Endod. Dent. Traumatol.* **2000**, *16*, 211–217. [CrossRef]
37. Skoglund, A.; Tronstad, L. Pulpal changes in replanted and autotransplanted immature teeth of dogs. *J. Endod.* **1981**, *7*, 309–316. [CrossRef] [PubMed]
38. Yamauchi, N.; Nagaoka, H.; Yamauchi, S.; Teixeira, F.B.; Miguez, P.; Yamauchi, M. Immunohistological characterization of newly formed tissues after regenerative procedure in immature dog teeth. *J. Endod.* **2011**, *37*, 1636–1641. [CrossRef]
39. Wang, X.; Thibodeau, B.; Trope, M.; Lin, L.M.; Huang, G.T.-J. Histologic characterization of regenerated tissues in canal space after the revitalization/revascularization procedure of immature dog teeth with apical periodontitis. *J. Endod.* **2010**, *36*, 56–63. [CrossRef]

Disclaimer/Publisher's Note: The statements, opinions and data contained in all publications are solely those of the individual author(s) and contributor(s) and not of MDPI and/or the editor(s). MDPI and/or the editor(s) disclaim responsibility for any injury to people or property resulting from any ideas, methods, instructions or products referred to in the content.

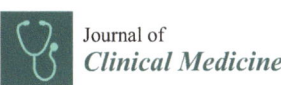

Article

Scattered Radiation Distribution Utilizing Three Different Cone-Beam Computed Tomography Devices for Maxillofacial Diagnostics: A Research Study

Sotirios Petsaros [1,†], Emmanouil Chatzipetros [1,†], Catherine Donta [1], Pantelis Karaiskos [2], Argiro Boziari [3], Evangelos Papadakis [1] and Christos Angelopoulos [1,*]

[1] Department of Oral Diagnosis and Radiology, Faculty of Dentistry, National and Kapodistrian University of Athens, 2 Thivon Street, Goudi, 11527 Athens, Greece; sotirios100@gmail.com (S.P.); e.chatzipetros@gmail.com (E.C.); edonta@dent.uoa.gr (C.D.); epapadak@dent.uoa.gr (E.P.)
[2] Medical Physics Laboratory, Faculty of Medicine, National and Kapodistrian University of Athens, 75 Mikras Asias Street, Goudi, 11527 Athens, Greece; pkaraisk@med.uoa.gr
[3] Greek Atomic Energy Commission, Agia Paraskevi, 15310 Attiki, Greece; argiro.boziari@eeae.gr
* Correspondence: angelopoulosc@gmail.com
† These authors contributed equally to this work.

Abstract: This study aimed to estimate scattered radiation and its spatial distribution around three cone-beam computed tomography (CBCT) devices, in order to determine potential positions for an operator to stand if they needed to be inside the CBCT room. The following devices were tested: Morita Accuitomo (CBCT1), Newtom Giano HR (CBCT2), Newtom VGi (CBCT3). Scattered radiation measurements were performed using different kVp, mA, and Field of View (FOV) options. An anthropomorphic phantom (NATHANIA) was placed inside the X-ray gantry to simulate clinical conditions. Scattered measurements were taken with the Inovision model 451P Victoreen ionization chamber once placed at fixed distances from each irradiation isocenter, away from the primary beam. A statistically significant ($p < 0.001$) difference was found in the mean value of the scattered radiation estimations between the CBCT devices. Scattered radiation was reduced with a different rate for each CBCT device as distance was increased. For CBCT1 the reduction was 0.047 µGy, for CBCT2 it was 0.036 µGy, and for CBCT3 it was 0.079 µGy, for every one meter from the X-ray gantry. Therefore, at certain distances from the central X-ray, the scattered radiation was below the critical level of 1 mGy, which is defined by the radiation protection guidelines as the exposure radiation limit of the general population. Consequently, an operator could stay inside the room accompanying the patient being scanned, if necessary.

Keywords: cone-beam computed tomography; dosimetry; radiation protection; scattered radiation

1. Introduction

Cone-beam computed tomography (CBCT) is one of the most important technological achievements in oral and maxillofacial radiology in the last forty years. In time, this has found numerous applications, from diagnostic applications to pre-implant assessment and surgical guidance using specialized software [1]. The main parameter that determines CBCT image quality is image resolution, which refers to the overall detail of the acquired image and is described by the maximum frequency that can be perceived [2]. Resolution is distinguished between spatial resolution and contrast resolution. Spatial resolution is a key intrinsic parameter that characterizes imaging systems and is widely used for their evaluation. It expresses the ability of the imaging system (in mm) to distinguish between two small objects that are very close to each other, in a high-contrast environment, and for this reason it is also called high-contrast discrimination ability [3,4]. Contrast resolution is the parameter that describes the ability of a system to distinguish between small differences in the intensity of the recorded signal and to be able to image anatomical structures with approximately linear attenuation coefficients. Factors affecting resolution are mA, kV, Field of View (FOV), and image reconstruction algorithms. Moreover, general image degradation factors such as noise, radiation scatter, and artifacts may compromise resolution [5].

The X-ray beam of the CBCT machine consists of primary radiation, which yields useful imaging information through the patient, and secondary radiation which is scattered radiation [1]. The primary radiation is produced within the X-ray tube, enters the patient, interacts with human tissues, and attenuates variably in the area under examination, conveying the useful information about the structures to be imaged [1,2]. Scattered radiation is a secondary radiation generated during the interaction of the primary beam with the patient tissues [6]. The scattered photons are of a lower energy and show an altered direction in comparison with that of the primary beam. Thus, scattered radiation has a negative effect on image quality [7] and essentially stands as the main factor contributing to reduced spatial resolution, reduced contrast resolution, and increased noise in CBCT [8–10].

The health risks associated with occupational radiation exposure are either of a deterministic or stochastic nature [11]. Stochastic effects occur by chance and include cancer risk. The stochastic effect risk is considered to increase with dose according to the linear-no-threshold model. The International Commission on Radiological Protection has recommended an annual occupational exposure limit of 20 mSv/year, averaged over 5 years, in both effective dose and equivalent eye lens dose [12,13]. These effects can develop independently of the radiation dose, and no threshold effect can be defined. Therefore, added exposures of the patient increase the chance of occurrence of a stochastic effect [14]. Although radiation doses are low during dental practice, there is always a concern in the dental community about radiation exposure [15–18]. Deterministic effects are limited to a certain threshold dose, and are thus unlikely to appear with a range of dental examination exposures [11].

Our hypothesis assumes that in some exceptional occasions the dentist or the staff (dental assistant, radiology technologist) may need to be present in the X-ray room during the CBCT examination, to visually and verbally direct and encourage the patient to place themselves correctly. Thus, we wanted to determine if there is a safe distance from the CBCT device to stand, so to receive the lowest possible scattered radiation [6,11].

This original research study specifically aims to estimate the patterns of scattered radiation and its spatial distribution around three CBCT devices, in order to determine potential positions for an operator to stand if they need to be present in the X-ray room during the CBCT examination for maxillofacial diagnostics.

2. Materials and Methods

2.1. Study Material

The following devices were tested in this research study: Morita Accuitomo (CBCT1) (J. Morita Corp., Osaka, Japan), Newtom Giano HR (CBCT2) (Cefla s.c., Bologna, Italy), and Newtom VGi (CBCT3) (Cefla s.c., Bologna, Italy). Exposure measurements were performed for different kVp, mA, and Field of View (FOV) values ((CBCT1; exposure time: 9 s, kVp: 90 kV, mA: 7 mA, voxel size: 0.125 mm), (CBCT2; exposure time: 3.6 s, kVp: 90 kV, mA: 3.66 mA, voxel size: 0.125 mm), (CBCT3; exposure time: 3.6 s, kVp: 110 kV, mA: 3.66 mA, voxel size: 0.3 mm)). An anthropomorphic phantom (NATHANIA) (Computerized Imaging Reference Systems, CIRS, Inc., Norfolk, VA, USA) was placed in the X-ray gantry to imitate clinical conditions (Figure 1).

In terms of ambient dose equivalent $H^*(10)$, scattered radiation measurements were taken with a Victoreen ionization chamber (Inovision 451P), with dimensions 10 cm $\times$ 20 cm $\times$ 15 cm (451P) (Fluke Biomedical Radiation Management Services, Cleveland, Ohio, USA). Calibration of ionization chambers provides traceability to Physikalisch-Technische Bundesanstalt (PTB) through the Ionizing Radiation Calibration Laboratory of the Greek Atomic Energy Commission (Secondary Standard Dosimetry Laboratory, (SSDL)). The survey meter was placed at fixed distances from each irradiation isocenter, away from the primary beam [11,19]. The ionization chamber (451P) exhibited a direct response for measuring scattered radiation dose and showed a high detection capability for very small radiation doses, including radiation present in the natural environment and stable energy dependence in the 40–100 keV range. Scattered radiation measurements were performed at the same distances from the CBCT devices (Figure 2).

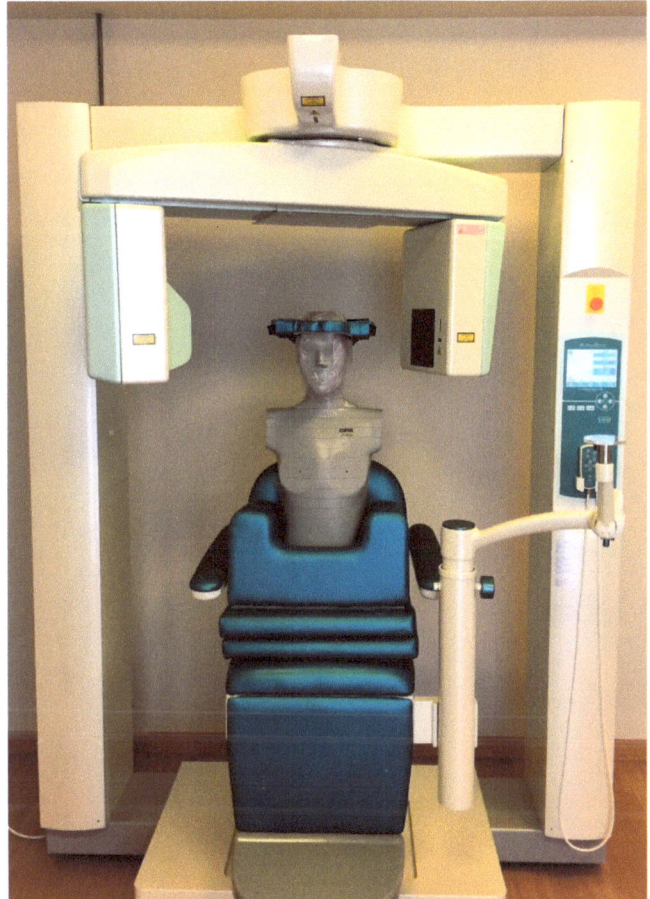

Figure 1. Anthropomorphic phantom (NATHANIA) was placed in the X-ray gantry of the cone-beam computed tomography (CBCT) device to imitate clinical conditions.

The placement positions of 451P were determined in each CBCT room based on point "0", which represented the fixed position of each CBCT device [20]. More specifically, two reference axes were drawn in the floor: the first (x-axis) represented the distance (in m) of the 451P to the right and left of the CBCT device, showing positive (right) and negative (left) values, respectively. The second (y-axis) represented the distance (in m) of the 451P from the CBCT device, in front of the CBCT device, perpendicular to the x-axis (Figure 2) [20].

A total of 191 (CBCT1) and 32 (CBCT2) measurements of scattered radiation at two different heights (1 m or 1.3 m from the floor) were carried out in the rooms of CBCT1 and CBCT2 devices at each point of intersection of the x and y axes (yellow points) (Figure 2). The measurement at the height of 1 m from the floor represented the anatomical location of the gonads and the height of 1.3 m from the floor represented the anatomical location of the thyroid gland [21]. It is of importance that in the CBCT3 room, all measurements

(36 measurements) were carried out at the same height (1.3 m) due to technical difficulties (room and device restrictions).

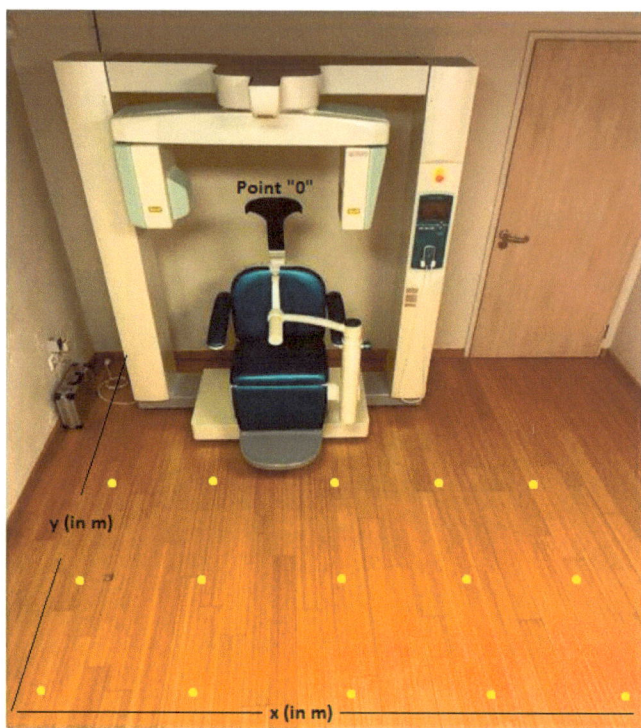

Figure 2. Topographic drawing of the placement positions of the Victoreen ionization chamber, Inovision model 451P (451P). Point "0" represented the fixed position of the cone-beam computed tomography (CBCT) device in each room. The x-axis (in m) (thin black horizontal line) represented the distance of the 451P to the right and left from the CBCT device. The y-axis (in m) (thin black vertical line) represented the distance of 451P from the CBCT device, in front of the CBCT device, perpendicular to the x-axis. The yellow points represented the fixed positions of the 451P at the same distances from the CBCT device (1 m or 1.3 m from the floor).

Measurements of scattered radiation from different Fields of View (FOVs) were also performed. More specifically, measurements of scattered radiation were carried out in the CBCT1 device in three different FOVs ((4 × 4), (6 × 6), (8 × 8)), in the CBCT2 device in two different FOVs ((8 × 8), (11 × 8)), and in the CBCT3 device in two different FOVs ((8 × 8), (15 × 15)).

2.2. Statistical Analysis

Data were described using mean values and standard deviation (SD) for the scattered radiation dose measurements (μGy) in the ionization chamber (451P) at three different rooms of CBCT devices (CBCT1, CBCT2, CBCT3). One-way analysis of variance (ANOVA) and independent samples *t*-test were used to assess the mean difference of 451P measurements between the three rooms and between the FOVs in each room. Then, Bonferroni tests for multiple comparison corrections were applied. In order to investigate whether the position of CBCT device, in the three rooms, was related to 451P, the Euclidean distance of each measurement point was calculated as the distance in meters (m). Generalized additive models (GAMs) were applied to assess the relationship between 451P (dependent variable) and distance (m) from the CBCT device (independent variable), in each room. Mixed effect linear regression models were used to assess the relationship between 451P and the FOV, in each room. All models were adjusted for the height (m) that the measurement was carried out and for the coordinates (x, y) of each measurement point, by including a bivariate smooth function (thin plate spline) of (x, y). The spatial distribution of scattered radiation in 451P was estimated through the rigging universal interpolation method. A test for trend was applied to investigate the trend of 451P in the FOVs of each room.

All statistical analysis was performed using R version 4.1.3 (10 March 2022), library (mgcv) and library (lme4). All spatial analysis was conducted using ArcGIS Desktop v.10.1. (Spatial Analyst Tools, Interpolation, Spline). Two-tailed p-values are reported. A p-value less than 0.05 was considered as statistically significant.

3. Results

Table 1 presents the number of points and measurements performed in each room, the height of the measurements performed, the distribution of 451P measurements, and the maximum distance value from point "0". It is worth noting that all measurements were carried out at the same height in room 3. A statistically significant difference was observed in mean 451P measurements ($p < 0.001$) between rooms. Specifically, after applying the Bonferroni test, differences in the mean 451P measurements were statistically significant between rooms 2 and 3 ($p < 0.001$), rooms 1 and 3 ($p < 0.001$), and between rooms 1 and 2 ($p < 0.001$). The maximum value of 451P measurements (9.03 µGy) was observed in CBCT1, in a distance of 100 cm from point "0", while in CBCT2 and CBCT3 the maximum values were 5.70 and 8.70 µGy at a distance of 50 cm and 55 cm from point "0", respectively (Table 1).

Table 1. Distribution of scattered radiation (451P) (µGy) measurements performed, by room.

			Scattered Radiation 451P Measurements (µGy)	
Room (CBCT)	Points/Measurements (n)	Height (m)	Mean (SD)	Maximum (Distance from point "0")
1	24/191	1/1.3	1.27 (±1.60)	9.03 (100 cm from point "0")
2	7/32	1/1.3	0.84 (±1.06)	5.70 (50 cm from point "0")
3	10/36	1.3	2.86 (±2.21)	8.70 (55 cm from point "0")

Room (CBCT): X-ray room during cone-beam computed tomography (CBCT). Points: The points represented the fixed positions of the Victoreen ionization chamber (Inovision 451P) at the same distances from the CBCT device; measurements (n): the number of measurements of scattered radiation that were carried out in the rooms (CBCT1, CBCT2, CBCT3). Height (m): The measurement at the height of 1 m from the floor represented the anatomical location of the gonads, and the height of 1.3 m from the floor represented the anatomical location of the thyroid gland. Scattered radiation 451P measurements (µGy): Scattered radiation measurements were taken with a Victoreen ionization chamber (Inovision 451P). Mean: mean value of scattered radiation (451P) (µGy) measurements. SD: standard deviation of scattered radiation (451P) (µGy) measurements. Maximum: maximum value of scattered radiation (451P) (µGy) measurements. Distance from point "0": Distance (cm) from CBCT device. Point "0" represented the fixed position of the CBCT device in each room.

Table 2 presents the distribution of 451P measurements, for different FOVs in each room. A statistically significant difference in 451P measurements according to FOV was found in room 1 ($p = 0.012$) and in room 3 ($p = 0.001$). Regarding room 1, a significant difference in 451P measurements was observed between FOVs 4 × 4 and 8 × 8 (Bonferroni multiple comparison $p = 0.010$). Moreover, as the FOV increased, a significant increasing trend in 451P measurements was shown in rooms 1 and 3 ($p < 0.001$). For example, in room 1, 451P measurements made at FOV 6 × 6, compared to FOV 4 × 4, were on average higher by 0.523 µGy (95% Confidence Interval (C.I.): 0.139 to 0.820) µGy). Moreover, 451P measurements performed at FOV 8 × 8, compared to 4 × 4, were on average higher by 0.776 µGy (95% C.I.: 0.365 to 1.053) µGy) (Table 2).

Table 2. Distribution of scattered radiation (451P) (μGy), by Field of View (FOV) and room.

Room (CBCT)	FOV	Scattered Radiation 451P Measurements (μGy) Mean (SD)	p-Value	p-Value Test for Trend
1	4 × 4	0.652 (±1.017)	0.012 *[1]	<0.001 **
	6 × 6	1.175 (±1.403)		
	8 × 8	1.428 (±1.696)		
2	8 × 8	0.948 (±1.362)	0.559 [2]	0.473
	11 × 8	0.723 (±0.581)		
3	8 × 8	1.521 (±0.818)	0.001 *[2]	<0.001 **
	15 × 15	3.924 (±2.395)		

Room (CBCT): X-ray room during cone-beam computed tomography (CBCT). FOV: Field of View; Scattered radiation 451P measurements (μGy): Scattered radiation measurements were taken with a Victoreen ionization chamber (Inovision 451P). Mean: mean value of scattered radiation (451P) (μGy) measurements. SD: standard deviation of scattered radiation (451P) (μGy) measurements. [1] One-way analysis of variance (ANOVA) [2] independent samples t-test * statistically significant, α = 5% ** statistically significant, α = 1‰.

Table 3 shows the results from applying generalized additive models, with 451P measurement as the dependent variable and distance of measurements as the independent variable, also adjusting for height of measurements made (only in rooms 1 and 2) and coordinates (x, y) of measurement points, in each room. In room 1, a 1 m increase in the distance from the CBCT device, resulted in a decrease in mean 451P by 0.047 μGy (95% C.I.: −0.057 to −0.037 μGy), adjusting for the other variables. In room 2, a 1 m increase in the distance from the CBCT device, resulted in a decrease in mean 451P by 0.036 μGy (95% C.I.: −0.062 to −0.010 μGy), taking into account the other variables. Note that in both rooms, the height of the measurements did not significantly predict 451P ($p = 0.956$ and $p = 0.323$, respectively). In room 3, a 1 m increase in the distance from the CBCT device resulted in a decrease in mean 451P by 0.079 μGy (95% C.I.: −0.115 to −0.043 μGy), adjusting for the other variables (Table 3).

Table 3. Beta coefficient (β) and corresponding 95% Confidence Interval (C.I.) from generalized additive models, with measurements of scattered radiation in ionization chamber (451P) as the dependent variable and distance of measurements as the independent variable, also adjusting for height of measurements [1] made and coordinates (x, y) of measurement points, by room.

Room (CBCT)	Distance (m)		
	β (μGy)	95% C.I. for β (μGy)	p-Value
1	−0.047	(−0.057 to −0.037)	<0.001 **
2	−0.036	(−0.062 to −0.010)	0.012 *
3	−0.079	(−0.115 to −0.043)	<0.001 **

[1] height of measurements varies only in rooms 1 and 2. Room (CBCT): X-ray room during cone-beam computed tomography (CBCT). Distance (m): 1 m increase in the distance (m) from CBCT device. C.I.: Confidence Interval; β: beta coefficient * statistically significant, α = 5% ** statistically significant, α = 1‰.

Table 4 presents the results from linear mixed effect regression models, with 451P measurement as the dependent variable and FOV as the independent variable, also adjusting for height of measurements made (only for room 1 and 2) and coordinates (x, y) of measurement points, in each room. A statistically significant effect between FOV and 451P was found in rooms 1 and 3. Specifically in room 1, FOV 6 × 6 and 8 × 8, compared to FOV 4 × 4, had on average a higher value of 451P by 0.480 (95% C.I.: 0.139 to 0.820 μGy) and 0.709 μGy (95% C.I.: 0.365 to 1.053 μGy), respectively. In room 3, FOV 15 × 15, compared to FOV 8 × 8, had a higher mean value of 451P by 2.005 μGy (95% C.I.: 1.453 to 2.558 μGy) (Table 4).

Table 4. Beta coefficient (β) and corresponding 95% Confidence Interval (C.I.) from linear mixed effect regression models, with scattered radiation measurements (451P) (µGy) as the dependent variable and Field of View (FOV) as the independent variable, also adjusting for height of measurements [1] made and coordinates (x, y) of measurement points, by room.

Room (CBCT)	FOV	β (µGy)	95% C.I. for β (µGy)	p-Value
1	4 × 4		Reference category	
	6 × 6	0.480	(0.139 to 0.820)	0.006 *
	8 × 8	0.709	(0.365 to 1.053)	<0.001 **
2	8 × 8		Reference category	
	11 × 8	−0.257	(−0.805 to 0.291)	0.358
3	8 × 8		Reference category	
	15 × 15	2.005	(1.453 to 2.558)	<0.001 **

[1] height of measurements varies only in rooms 1 and 2. Room (CBCT): X-ray room during cone-beam computed tomography (CBCT). FOV: Field of View. C.I.: Confidence Interval; β: beta coefficient * statistically significant, α = 5% ** statistically significant, α = 1‰.

The spatial distribution of scattered radiation in 451P was estimated through the rigging universal interpolation method. Color maps of dose distributions were drawn for horizontal and vertical planes. Scattered radiation dose mapping in the ionization chamber (451P) was depicted per room (CBCT1, CBCT2, CBCT3) on the scattered radiation dose distributions color maps (Figures 3–5). It is worth noting that color maps in rooms 1 and 2 appeared to be uniform (CBCT1, CBCT2), regardless of the measurement height. Measurement height did not statistically significantly differentiate the measurement of scattered radiation in the ionization chamber.

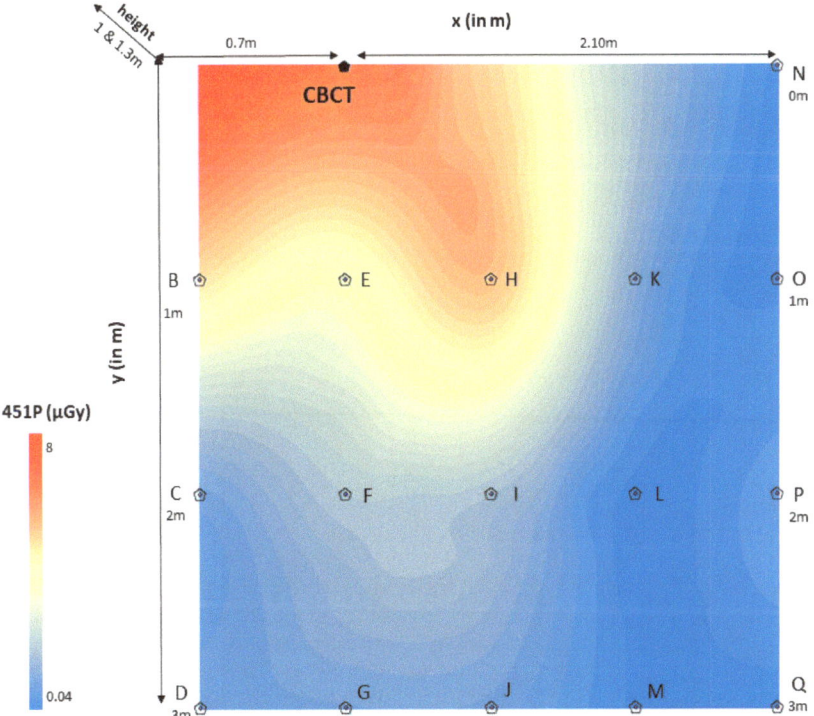

Figure 3. Color map of spatial distribution of scattered radiation (µGy) in room 1 (2.8 × 3 m).

- CBCT: Cone-beam computed tomography device 1 (CBCT1); point "0".
- x (in m): x-axis defined the distance (in m) of the ionization chamber (451P) to the right and left of the CBCT1 device (point "0"), showing sometimes positive (right) and sometimes negative (left) values. In this color map, the absolute values are displayed in order to avoid confusion ((point A − point "0" = 0.7 m), (point "0" − point N = 2.10 m)).
- y (in m): y-axis defined the distance (in m) of the ionization chamber (451P) from the CBCT1 device in an anterior position, perpendicular to the x-axis ((point A − point D = 3 m), (point N − point Q = 3 m)).
- 451P (μGy): Scattered radiation measurements (μGy) were taken with the Inovision model 451P Victoreen ionization chamber (0.04–8μGy). Red color means very high scattered radiation dose, while blue color means very low scattered radiation dose.
- Height (1 and 1.3 m): The measurement carried out at a height of 1 m from the floor represented the anatomical location of the gonads. The measurement carried out at a height of 1.3 m from the floor represented the anatomical location of the thyroid gland.

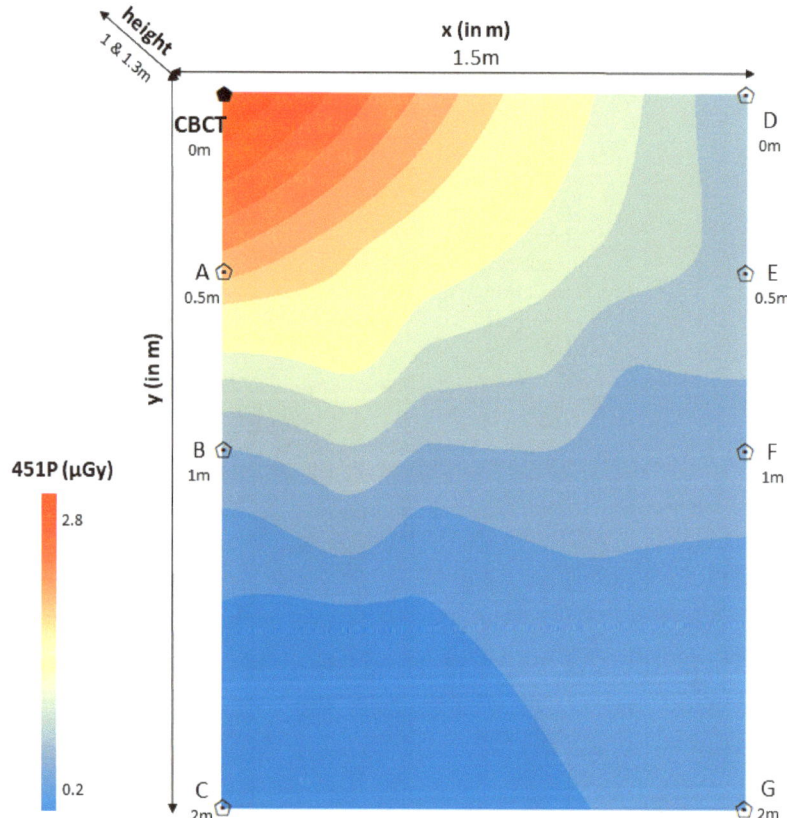

Figure 4. Color map of spatial distribution of scattered radiation (μGy) in room 2 (1.5 × 2 m).

- CBCT: Cone-beam computed tomography device 2 (CBCT2); point "0".
- x (in m): x-axis defined the distance (in m) of the ionization chamber (451P) to the right of the CBCT2 device (point "0"), showing positive values (point "0" − point D = 1.5 m).
- y (in m): y-axis defined the distance (in m) of the ionization chamber (451P) from the CBCT2 device in an anterior position, perpendicular to the x-axis ((point "0" − point C = 2 m), (point D − point G = 2 m)).

- 451P (μGy): Scattered radiation measurements (μGy) were taken with the Inovision model 451P Victoreen ionization chamber (0.2–2.8 μGy). Red color means very high scattered radiation dose, while blue color means very low scattered radiation dose.
- Height (1 and 1.3 m): The measurement carried out at a height of 1 m from the floor represented the anatomical location of the gonads. The measurement carried out at a height of 1.3 m from the floor represented the anatomical location of the thyroid gland.

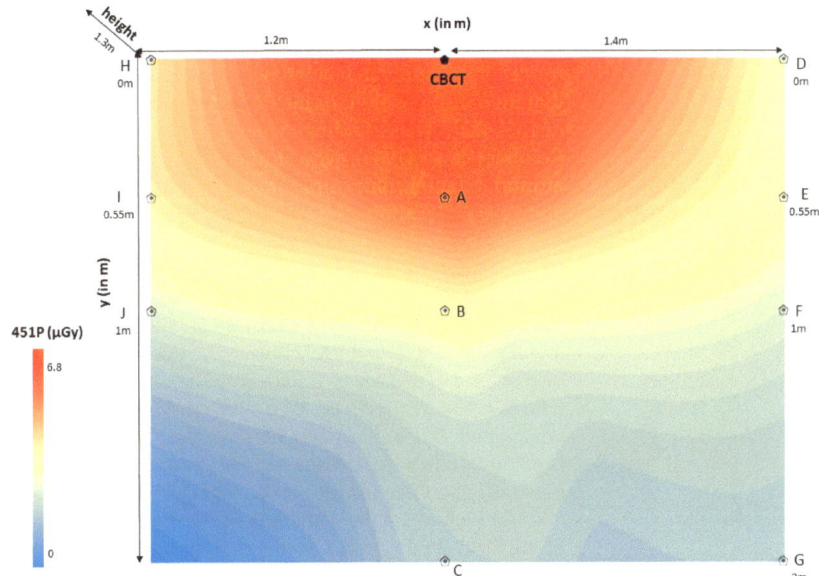

Figure 5. Color map of spatial distribution of scattered radiation (μGy) in room 3 (2 × 2.6 m).

- CBCT: Cone-beam computed tomography device 3 (CBCT3); point "0".
- x (in m): x-axis defined the distance (in m) of the ionization chamber (451P) to the right and left of the CBCT3 device (point "0"), showing sometimes positive (right) and sometimes negative (left) values. In this color map, the absolute values are displayed in order to avoid confusion ((point H − point "0" = 1.2 m), (point "0" − point D = 1.4 m)).
- y (in m): y-axis defined the distance (in m) of the ionization chamber (451P) from the CBCT3 device in an anterior position, perpendicular to the x-axis ((point H − point J = 0.55 m), (point D − point G = 2 m)).
- 451P (μGy): Scattered radiation measurements (μGy) were taken with the Inovision model 451P Victoreen ionization chamber (0–6.8μGy). Red color means very high scattered radiation dose, while blue color means very low scattered radiation dose.
- height (1.3 m): The measurement carried out at a height of 1.3 m from the floor represented the anatomical location of the thyroid gland.

4. Discussion

In this research study, measurements of the scattered radiation dose were collected inside rooms with CBCT installations. The spatial distribution of scattered radiation measured with ionization chamber (451P) was estimated through the rigging universal interpolation method and the safest locations of the people who could be present inside the X-ray room were determined (>100 cm from CBCT1, >50 cm from CBCT2, and >55 cm from CBCT3).

The protection against scattered radiation is a perennial concern of the scientific community, even when the radiation dose is quite low, such as during intraoral radiography [20,22,23]. A research study showed that occupationally exposed individuals presented a higher incidence of thyroid cancer, especially in the past when the radiation protection measurements were not as strict [21]. A similar epidemiological study in Canada argued that repeated exposure to low doses by occupation was limited to long-term harmful effects and cancer incidence [24]. Cewe et al. (2022) demonstrated that staff can use freestanding radiation protection shields instead of heavy aprons during intraoperative CBCT imaging, to achieve effective whole body dose reduction with improved comfort [11].

Alcaraz et al. (2006) measured the scattered radiation at various distances from the patient, who was lying supine, 48 cm from the floor. The measurements were carried out at distances of 60, 90, 120, 150, and 180 cm, and at an angle of 0°, 135°, and 180°. The results of this study in relation with dose reduction of intraoral dental radiography showed that the safest position for the dentist was behind and right of the X-ray beam at an angle of 135° [22]. These findings were in agreement with the results of a previous study by Rolofson et al. (1969), who studied radiation isoexposure curves of scattered radiation around a dental chair during radiography. Rolofson et al. (1969) reported that the most appropriate location with the lowest absorbed radiation dose to the gonadal anatomical region was directly behind the X-ray beam or to the side of the patient's head, opposite the X-ray beam [23]. Yamaji et al. (2021) noticed that if a physician or staff member needs to observe the patient near the table, it would be recommended to stand in the back of the base CBCT device. With the use of a ceiling-mounted transparent lead-acryl screen and a table suspended lead curtain, the doses were reduced 45–92% at a direction of 210° degrees and a distance of 120 cm [19]. In our study, the safest positions of people within the CBCT area were proposed to be >100 cm from the CBCT1 device, >50 cm from the CBCT2 device, and >55 cm from the CBCT3 device. Therefore, our findings were in agreement with previous studies. A limitation of our study was that we did not use angle measurements when placing the ionization chamber (451P) in the three rooms with the CBCT devices.

An increase in the scattered radiation at a height of 100 cm from the floor, at the level of the X-ray gantry, and a decrease in the absorbed dose of radiation near the gantry, were observed by other researchers [6]. Conversely, an increase in scattered radiation behind the gantry was observed during head imaging with computed tomography (General Electric Hi Speed Advantage CT) [25]. Various research studies showed that scattered radiation decreases as we move away from the X-ray beam. More specifically, at a distance of 10 and 20 cm from the X-ray beam in a third-generation computed tomography device, the scattered radiation was detected at high levels of 10 and 18 mSv, while it was greatly reduced, to 2 mSv, at a distance of 30 cm from the X-ray beam [26]. In the present study, it was observed to a statistically significant extent that, in room 1, a 1 m increase in the distance from the CBCT device resulted in a decrease in mean 451P by 0.047 µGy (95% C.I.: −0.057 to −0.037 µGy), adjusting for the other variables. Moreover, in room 2, a 1 m increase in the distance from the CBCT device resulted in a decrease in mean 451P by 0.036 µGy (95% C.I.: −0.062 to −0.010 µGy), taking into account the other variables. Furthermore, in room 3, a 1 m increase in the distance from the CBCT device resulted in a decrease in mean 451P by 0.079 µGy (95% C.I.: −0.115 to −0.043 µGy), adjusting for the other variables. These findings were in agreement with the results of previous studies. However, this by no means implies that our results suggest that radio protection rooms with shielding of the walls are unnecessary.

Yamaji et al. (2021) measured the distribution of scattered radiation by C-arm conebeam computed tomography (CBCT) in the angiographic suite. In this study, the measurements showed the highest radiation dose over 600 µGy by a single CBCT image acquisition at a distance of 60 cm from the beam entry site and a height of 90 cm from the floor [19]. In the present study, the safest positions of the people who can be found within the CBCT area were proposed to be >100 cm from the CBCT1 device, >50 cm from the CBCT2 device, and >55 cm from the CBCT3 device. However, the values obtained from the measurements were overall much lower than 1 mGy, which is defined by the radiation protection guidelines as the exposure radiation limit of the general population [27]. A comparative advantage of our study was that the measurement of the scattered radiation was carried out in three different

CBCT devices and numerous measurements of the scattered radiation were carried out at two different heights. The measurement made at a height of 1 m represented the anatomical region of the gonads. The measurement carried out at a height of 1.3 m represented the anatomical region of the thyroid gland. It was noted, however, that the height of the measurements did not appear to statistically significantly differentiate the measurement of the scattered radiation in the ionization chamber (451P) ($p > 0.05$). In addition, due to technical difficulties, a limitation of the present study was that in room 3 (CBCT3) all measurements were made at the same height (1.3 m). The present study provides future prospects for further investigation of scattered radiation distribution with more CBCT devices for maxillofacial diagnostics.

5. Conclusions

In all CBCT devices that were tested in this study, the scattered radiation that an individual may be exposed significantly decreased with distance. The Newtom VGi CBCT showed the greatest decrease with distance. In all instances the measured scattered radiation was below 1 mGy, which is defined by the radiation protection guidelines as the exposure radiation limit of the general population. Nevertheless, the scattered radiation is significantly reduced, as long as the dentist, radiology technologist, or other occupationally exposed individual stands at a safe distance and position from the patient (as determined by our results) in the X-ray room during the CBCT examination for maxillofacial diagnostics.

Author Contributions: Conceptualization: S.P., E.C., C.D., P.K., A.B., E.P. and C.A.; methodology: S.P., E.C. and C.D.; software: S.P. and E.C.; validation: S.P., E.C., C.D., P.K, A.B., E.P. and C.A.; formal analysis: S.P., E.C., C.D., P.K. and C.A.; investigation: S.P., E.C., C.D., P.K., A.B., E.P. and C.A.; resources: S.P., E.C., C.D. and C.A.; data curation: E.C., C.D. and C.A.; writing—original draft preparation: E.C.; writing—review and editing: S.P., E.C., C.D., P.K., A.B., E.P. and C.A.; visualization: S.P., E.C., C.D., E.P. and C.A.; supervision: C.D., P.K, A.B., E.P. and C.A.; project administration: S.P., E.C., C.D., P.K., A.B., E.P. and C.A.; funding acquisition: S.P., E.C., C.D., E.P. and C.A. All authors have read and agreed to the published version of the manuscript.

Funding: This research received no external funding.

Institutional Review Board Statement: Not applicable.

Informed Consent Statement: Not applicable.

Data Availability Statement: The datasets used and/or analyzed during the current study are available from the corresponding author upon reasonable request.

Conflicts of Interest: The authors of this manuscript declare no relevant conflict of interest and no relationship with any companies whose products or services may be related to the subject matter of the article.

References

1. Scarfe, W.C.; Farman, A. What is Cone-Beam CT and How Does it Work? *Dent. Clin. N. Am.* **2008**, *52*, 707–730. [CrossRef]
2. Scarfe, W.C.; Angelopoulos, C. *Maxillofacial Cone Beam Computed Tomography, Principles, Techniques and Clinical Applications*, 1st ed.; Springer International Publishing AG: Cham, Switzerland, 2018; pp. 43–95.
3. Liao, C.W.; Lih-Jyh, F.; Yen-Wen, S.; Heng-Li, H.; ChiH-Wei, K.; Ming-Tzu, T.; Jui-Ting, H. Self-Assembled Micro-Computed Tomography for Dental Education. *PLoS ONE* **2018**, *13*, e0209698. [CrossRef] [PubMed]
4. Pauwels, R.; Beinsberger, J.; Stamatakis, H.; Tsiklakis, K.; Walker, A.; Bosmans, H.; Bogaerts, R.; Jacobs, R.; Horner, K.; SEDENTEXCT Project Consortium. Comparison of spatial and contrast resolution for cone-beam computed tomography scanners. *Oral Surg. Oral Med. Oral Pathol. Oral Radiol.* **2012**, *114*, 127–135. [CrossRef] [PubMed]
5. Honey, O.B.; Scarfe, W.C.; Hilgers, M.J.; Klueber, K.; Silveira, A.M.; Haskell, B.S.; Farman, A.G. Accuracy of cone-beam computed tomography imaging of the temporomandibular joint: Comparisons with panoramic radiology and linear tomography. *Am. J. Orthod. Dentofacial Orthop.* **2007**, *132*, 429–438. [CrossRef] [PubMed]
6. Mellenberg, D.E.; Sato, Y.; Thompson, B.H.; Warnock, N.G. Personnel exposure rates during simulated biopsies with a real-time CT scanner. *Acad. Radiol.* **1999**, *6*, 687–690. [CrossRef] [PubMed]
7. Siewerdsen, J.H.; Jaffray, D.A. Cone-beam computed tomography with a flat-panel imager: Magnitude and effects of X-ray scatter. *Med. Phys.* **2001**, *28*, 220–231. [CrossRef] [PubMed]

8. Graham, S.A.; Moseley, D.J.; Siewerdsen, J.H.; Jaffray, D.A. Compensators for dose and scatter management in cone-beam computed tomography. *Med. Phys.* **2007**, *34*, 2691–2703. [CrossRef]
9. Thanasupsombat, C.; Thongvigitmanee, S.S.; Aootaphao, S.; Thajchayapong, P. A Simple Scatter Reduction Method in Cone-Beam Computed Tomography for Dental and Maxillofacial Applications Based on Monte Carlo Simulation. *Biomed. Res. Int.* **2018**, *2018*, 5748281. [CrossRef]
10. Gonçalves, O.D.; Boldt, S.; Nadaes, M.; Devito, K.L. Evaluating the scattered radiation intensity in CBCT. *Radiat. Phys. Chem.* **2018**, *144*, 159–164. [CrossRef]
11. Cewe, P.; Vorbau, R.; Omar, A.; Elmi-Terander, A.; Edström, E. Radiation distribution in a hybrid operating room, utilizing different X-ray imaging systems: Investigations to minimize occupational exposure. *J. Neurointerv. Surg.* **2022**, *14*, 1139–1144. [CrossRef]
12. The 2007 Recommendations of the International Commission on Radiological Protection. ICRP publication 103. *Ann ICRP.* **2007**, *37*, 1–332.
13. Stewart, F.A.; Akleyev, A.V.; Hauer-Jensen, M.; Hendry, J.H.; Kleiman, N.J.; Macvittie, T.J.; Aleman, B.M.; Edgar, A.B.; Mabuchi, K.; Muirhead, C.R.; et al. ICRP publication 118: ICRP statement on tissue reactions and early and late effects of radiation in normal tissues and organs–threshold doses for tissue reactions in a radiation protection context. *Ann. ICRP* **2012**, *41*, 1–322. [CrossRef] [PubMed]
14. Engel, H.P. Radiation protection in medical imaging. *Radiography* **2006**, *12*, 153–160. [CrossRef]
15. Longstreth, W.T., Jr.; Dennis, L.K.; McGuire, V.M.; Drangsholt, M.T.; Koepsell, T.D. Epidemiology of intracranial meningioma. *Cancer* **1993**, *72*, 639–648. [CrossRef]
16. Preston-Martin, S.; White, S.C. Brain and salivary gland tumors related to prior dental radiography: Implications for current practice. *J. Am. Dent. Assoc.* **1990**, *120*, 151–158. [CrossRef]
17. Horn-Ross, P.L.; Ljung, B.M.; Morrow, M. Environmental factors and the risk of salivary gland cancer. *Epidemiology* **1997**, *8*, 414–419. [CrossRef]
18. Hallquist, A.; Hardell, L.; Degerman, A.; Wingren, G.; Boquist, L. Medical diagnostic and therapeutic ionizing radiation and the risk for thyroid cancer: A case-control study. *Eur. J. Cancer Prev.* **1994**, *3*, 259–267. [CrossRef]
19. Yamaji, M.; Ishiguchi, T.; Koyama, S.; Ikeda, S.; Kitagawa, A.; Hagihara, Y.; Itoh, Y.; Nakamura, M.; Ota, T.; Suzuki, K. Distribution of scatter radiation by C-arm cone-beam computed tomography in angiographic suite: Measurement of doses and effectiveness of protection devices. *Nagoya J. Med. Sci.* **2021**, *83*, 277–286.
20. Hoogeveen, R.C.; van Beest, D.; Berkhout, E. Ambient dose during intraoral radiography with current techniques: Part 3: Effect of tube voltage. *Dentomaxillofac. Radiol.* **2021**, *50*, 20190362. [CrossRef]
21. Lope, V.; Pérez-Gómez, B.; Aragonés, N.; López-Abente, G.; Gustavsson, P.; Floderus, B.; Dosemeci, M.; Silva, A.; Pollán, M. Occupational exposure to ionizing radiation and electromagnetic fields in relation to the risk of thyroid cancer in Sweden. *Scand. J. Work. Environ. Health* **2006**, *32*, 276–284. [CrossRef]
22. Alcaraz, M.; Navarro, C.; Vicente, V.; Canteras, M. Dose reduction of intraoral dental radiography in Spain. *Dentomaxillofac. Radiol.* **2006**, *35*, 295–298. [CrossRef]
23. Rolofson, J.W.; Hamel, A.; Stewart, H.F. Radiation isoexposure curves about a dental chair during radiography. *J. Am. Dent. Assoc.* **1969**, *78*, 310–319. [CrossRef]
24. Sont, W.N.; Zielinski, J.M.; Ashmore, J.P.; Jiang, H.; Krewski, D.; Fair, M.E.; Band, P.R.; Létourneau, E.G. First analysis of cancer incidence and occupational radiation exposure based on the National Dose Registry of Canada. *Am. J. Epidemiol.* **2001**, *153*, 309–318. [CrossRef]
25. Langer, S.G.; Gray, J.E. Radiation shielding implications of computed tomography scatter exposure to the floor. *Health Phys.* **1998**, *75*, 193–196. [CrossRef]
26. Chan, C.B.; Chan, L.K.; Lam, H.S. Scattered radiation level during videofluoroscopy for swallowing study. *Clin. Radiol.* **2002**, *57*, 614–616. [CrossRef]
27. Horner, K.; Equipment HPAWPODCBCT. *Guidance on the Safe Use of Dental Cone Beam CT (Computed Tomography) Equipment*, 1st ed.; Health Protection Agency (HPA CRCE scientific and technical report series): Chilton, Didcot, Oxfordshire, UK, 2010; pp. 1–64.

Disclaimer/Publisher's Note: The statements, opinions and data contained in all publications are solely those of the individual author(s) and contributor(s) and not of MDPI and/or the editor(s). MDPI and/or the editor(s) disclaim responsibility for any injury to people or property resulting from any ideas, methods, instructions or products referred to in the content.

Article

Correlation Analysis of Nasal Septum Deviation and Results of AI-Driven Automated 3D Cephalometric Analysis

Natalia Kazimierczak [1], Wojciech Kazimierczak [1,2,*], Zbigniew Serafin [2], Paweł Nowicki [1], Adam Lemanowicz [2], Katarzyna Nadolska [2] and Joanna Janiszewska-Olszowska [3]

1. Kazimierczak Private Dental Practice, Dworcowa 13/u6a, 85-009 Bydgoszcz, Poland
2. Collegium Medicum, Nicolaus Copernicus University in Torun, Jagiellońska 13-15, 85-067 Bydgoszcz, Poland; serafin@cm.umk.pl (Z.S.)
3. Department of Interdisciplinary Dentistry, Pomeranian Medical University in Szczecin, 70-111 Szczecin, Poland; jjo@pum.edu.pl or joanna.janiszewska.olszowska@pum.edu.pl
* Correspondence: wojtek.kazimierczak@gmail.com; Tel.: +48-606670881

Abstract: The nasal septum is believed to play a crucial role in the development of the craniofacial skeleton. Nasal septum deviation (NSD) is a common condition, affecting 18–65% of individuals. This study aimed to assess the prevalence of NSD and its potential association with abnormalities detected through cephalometric analysis using artificial intelligence (AI) algorithms. The study included CT scans of 120 consecutive, post-traumatic patients aged 18–30. Cephalometric analysis was performed using an AI web-based software, CephX. The automatic analysis comprised all the available cephalometric analyses. NSD was assessed using two methods: maximum deviation from an ideal non-deviated septum and septal deviation angle (SDA). The concordance of repeated manual measurements and automatic analyses was assessed. Of the 120 cases, 90 met the inclusion criteria. The AI-based cephalometric analysis provided comprehensive reports with over 100 measurements. Only the hinge axis angle (HAA) and SDA showed significant ($p = 0.039$) negative correlations. The rest of the cephalometric analyses showed no correlation with the NSD indicators. The analysis of the agreement between repeated manual measurements and automatic analyses showed good-to-excellent concordance, except in the case of two angular measurements: LI-N-B and Pr-N-A. The CephX AI platform showed high repeatability in automatic cephalometric analyses, demonstrating the reliability of the AI model for most cephalometric analyses.

Keywords: artificial intelligence; nasal septum deviation; cephalometric analysis; orthodontics

1. Introduction

The nasal septum is a key factor in the development of the craniofacial skeleton during ontogeny [1–6]. Research conducted on animal models has shown that the mechanical forces generated by the growing nasal septum have a crucial impact on the surrounding sutural growth sites [7–9]. It is believed that the development of the nasal septum and the forces it exerts on surrounding tissues are responsible for the development of midface, sagittal, and vertical maxillary growth [8,10,11].

Numerous studies have demonstrated that, depending on the criteria applied and the populations examined, 18–65% of individuals exhibit nasal septum deviation (NSD), with a significantly higher prevalence observed in the European population [12–16]. The impact of NSD on the development of facial and cranial asymmetry remains a subject of ongoing research. Apart from the obvious correlations, such as nasal asymmetry and unilateral nasal turbinate hypertrophy [17–19], more distant correlations, such as facial and palatal asymmetries, have been demonstrated [20–23]. NSD and subsequent altered respiratory functions are linked to disrupted growth of the maxilla and mandible [24–26]. This suggests that NSD may have far-reaching effects on craniofacial development and highlights the importance of further investigation into the potential consequences of this condition. Considering the well-documented influence of the growing nasal septum on the anatomical proportions of the developing craniofacial structure, it is therefore pertinent to explore potential correlations between nasal septum abnormalities and the anatomical proportions of the craniofacial region.

Since its introduction in 1931, cephalometric analysis has been a fundamental technique used in orthodontics and craniofacial research to assess skeletal and dental relationships in the craniofacial complex [27]. It involves the use of X-ray lateral cephalograms of the head and face to obtain precise linear and angular measurements between predefined lanmarks. These measurements are then compared to established norms, allowing us to evaluate growth patterns, diagnose malocclusions, and plan orthodontic treatment. The obtained results provide valuable insights into the relationship between the maxilla, mandible, and cranial base, contributing to the diagnosis and treatment planning process. The advancement of technology has enabled the replacement of manual measurements with digital cephalometric analysis software, facilitating quicker measurements and the automatic presentation of analysis results. In recent years, there has been a growing interest in the application of artificial intelligence (AI) in the medical sciences, particularly in the field of medical imaging. This technology has seen rapid implementation in orthodontics, specifically in the analysis of X-ray images for pre-orthodontic treatment and cephalometric analysis. Manual analysis of cephalometric X-ray images is highly operator-dependent and prone to significant variability in landmark identification [28–31]. However, the results of automatic cephalometric analysis using AI have been shown to be relatively stable and repeatable compared to manual analysis. Several studies have reported the accuracy and reliability of AI software in cephalometric analysis, demonstrating potential for improving diagnostic accuracy and reducing variability and analysis time [32–38]. In addition to automated cephalometric analysis, AI has already proven its effectiveness in other orthodontic pre-treatment assessments. Lo Giudice et al. have demonstrated that automated segmentation of the upper airway and hard tissues (mandible) in CBCT scans, based on convolutional neural networks (CNNs), is as accurate as an experienced reader [39,40]. This efficiency can lead to improved workflow and productivity in dental practices.

The integration of AI and cone-beam computed tomography (CBCT) in dental diagnostics has paved the way for the development of AI-based programs such as WebCeph, WeDoCeph, and CephX. These programs automate the identification of anatomical measurement points, evaluate landmarks, calculate angles and distances, and generate automated analysis reports with significant findings. The primary advantage of such software is the ability to automatically perform measurements and analyses based on craniofacial CT scans, potentially reducing the need for additional cephalometric images for patients prior to orthodontic treatment. Studies conducted thus far have demonstrated a high degree of agreement between measurements and analyses performed with CephX software and those obtained through digital cephalometric analysis [35,36,41].

The first objective of our study was to perform cephalometric analysis on computed tomography (CT) scans of our sample population using AI-based algorithms. The second aim of our research was to evaluate the correlation between NSD and the results of the cephalometric analyses of our subjects.

2. Materials and Methods

2.1. Patient Selection

This study has been approved by the bioethical committee of our institution (decision reference No. KB 227/2023).

The study material comprised CT scans performed on 120 consecutive patients aged 18 to 30 admitted to the Emergency Department of our institution between 1 January 2020, and 31 December 2022. All the CT scans were performed on the same 64-slice CT scanner (Discovery 750HD; GE Health Care; Waukesha, WI, USA) using 64×0.625 mm collimation, 32 cm scan FOV, 260-mA tube current, 120 kVp tube voltage, 0.625 mm slice thickness, 0.8 s per gantry rotation, and a pitch of 0.531. CT scans were acquired in the range from the vertex to the lower levels of the cervical spine, covering the whole craniofacial area.

The indications for CT scans included post-traumatic assessments in patients who experienced generalized trauma or trauma to the craniofacial area.

The inclusion criteria were as follows:

1. CT scan covering the region from the chin to the vertex;
2. Age 18–30 years, to exclude multiple missing teeth and acquired craniofacial deformations from the measurements conducted;
3. Centric occlusion of the patient's teeth.

The exclusion criteria were as follows:

1. Fractures of the craniofacial bones;
2. Severe motion artifacts;
3. >4 teeth missing per dental arch;
4. Tumors in the craniofacial area;
5. Severe metal artifacts.

2.2. Cephalometric Analysis

CT scans were manually uploaded into a cloud-based AI software database—CephX (ORCA Dental AI, Las Vegas, NV, USA). The software automatically performed all the available cephalometric analyses and provided a report for each patient. Supplementary Table S1 summarizes all the automatically performed analyses. The major reference points are summarized in Table 1 and presented in Figure 1.

Table 1. Cephalometric landmarks used in analyses (part of).

	Landmark	Definition
S	Sella	Midpoint of the sella turcica
Co	Condylion	The extreme superior point on the condylar head
ANS	Anterior Nasal Spine	Tip of the bony anterior nasal spine in the midline
N	Nasion	The most anterior point of the frontonasal suture
A	Point A	The innermost point on the contour of the maxilla between the anterior nasal spine and the alveolar crest
B	Point B	The most posterior point in the concavity along the anterior border of the symphysis
Go	Gonion	The most prominent point on the angle of the mandible formed by the junction of the ramus and the body of the mandible
Gn	Gnathion	The most inferior bony point of the mandible
Ll	Lower Lip	The most anterior point of the lower lip
Me	Menton	The most inferior point of the mandibular symphysis in the midline
N	Nasion	The most anterior point of the frontonasal suture
Or	Orbitale	The lowest point on the inferior margin of the orbit
P	Porion	The central point on the upper margin of the external auditory meatus
Pr	Prosthion	The point of alveolar contact with the upper central incisor
Pg	Pogonion	The most anterior point on the contour of the bony chin

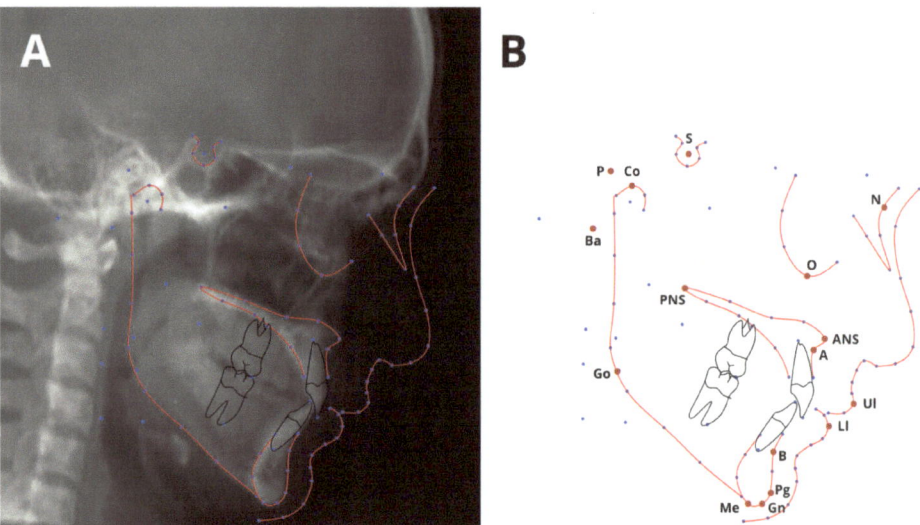

Figure 1. Cephalogram annotation example (**A**), showing major landmarks used in this study (**B**).

2.3. NSD Analysis

The NSD was assessed using a method that measures the maximum deviation from an "ideal" non-deviated septum. This hypothetical, non-deviated septum was determined based on multiplanar reconstructions (MPR), drawing a straight line between the perpendicular plate of the ethmoid bone and the midline palatine suture. The deviation measurement was obtained by calculating the maximum horizontal distance from the line representing the ideal, non-deviated septum to the most outer, bony, deviated septal contour. Previous studies have demonstrated the usefulness of the perpendicular plate–vomer suture (PPV) in assessing the maximum deviation of the nasal septum in computed tomography (CT) images [5,42]. The septal deviation angle (SDA) was measured in coronal CT sections using the criteria presented in papers by Orhan and Kajan [19,43]. Figure 2 presents both types of measurements.

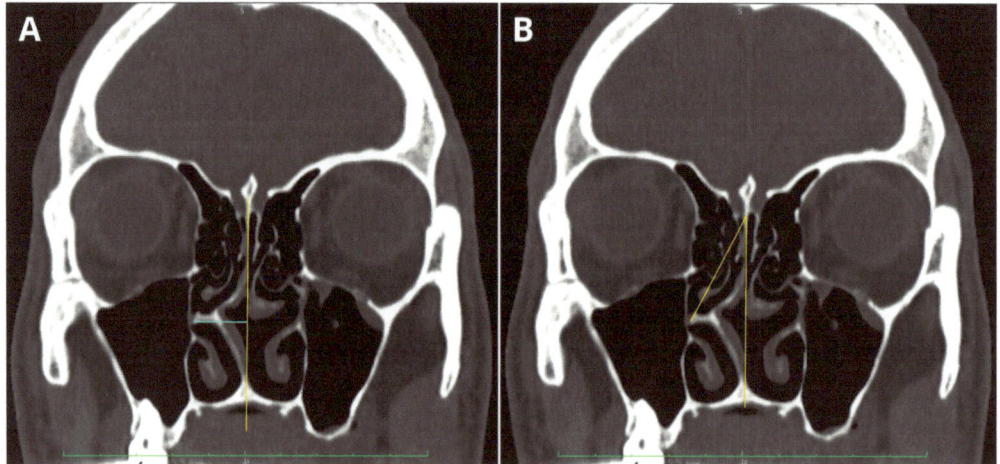

Figure 2. Sample of NSD measurements conducted in one patient: (**A**) perpendicular plate–vomer (PPV) measurement; (**B**) septal deviation angle (SDA) measurement.

Due to high variability, the thickness of the nasal septum mucous membrane was not considered in the measurements. All manual measurements were performed using the OsiriX MD v. 13.1 software (Pixmeo SARL; Geneva, Switzerland).

2.4. Error Study

Twenty randomly selected subjects were re-examined by the same author 1 month after initial tracings. PPV and SDA measurements were repeated 1 month later by the same investigator in 20 randomly selected CT scans to calculate the intraobserver repeatability. The repeatability of measurements was assessed using a one-sided Wilcoxon test. The intraclass correlation coefficient (ICC) regarding AR calculations was calculated to assess the agreement between examinations.

Twenty randomly selected subjects were re-uploaded to the AI-software database in order to assess the repeatability of automatic measurements. The ICC regarding the results of repeated automatic analyses was calculated to assess the agreement between examinations.

2.5. Statistical Evaluation

Sample size was verified using an online sample size calculator (https://clincalc.com (accessed on 10 January 2023)). Clinical significance was set at the level of 1 mm in linear measurements and $1°$ in angular measurements. The correlations between quantitative variables were analyzed using Spearman's correlation coefficient. The agreement between manual measurements and automatic analysis for quantitative variables was assessed using the intraclass correlation coefficient (ICC) of type 2, according to the classification by Shrout and Fleiss. The significance level for all statistical tests was set to 0.05. R 4.2.3. statistical software was used for computations.

3. Results

3.1. Population

The authors reviewed the CT scans of 120 cases. Thirty cases were excluded as they failed to meet our inclusion criteria. Measurements from 90 patients were included. The mean age of all participants was 23.9 years (SD 3.81; median 24; range 18–30). This constituted 66 males with a mean age of 23.7 (SD 3.18; range 18–30) and 24 females with a mean age of 21.15 (SD 4.03; range 18–29).

3.2. Automatic Cephalometric Analysis

The results of automated cephalometric analyses conducted by AI were primarily provided in the form of reports containing >100 measurements (linear and angular), with the established range, normal values, and comments on potential clinical implications. Part of the sample report is shown in Figure 3.

3.3. NSD Analysis

The findings from the two methods employed for assessing NSD, namely SSD and PPV, demonstrated a significant ($p < 0.001$) and positive correlation, with Spearman's correlation coefficient equating to 0.967. This suggests that as the deviation in millimeters increases, so does the angle of deviation. A graphical representation of the results from this analysis can be found in Figure 4.

Gender:	Male							
Age:	18							
Growth at N:	1							
Growth at Gn:	3							

Ricketts

Descriptor	Meas.	Type	Mean	Sd	Patient	Graph	Comment
*****cephxSubTitleField*****	MAX. POSITION						
MAX DEPTH	FH to N-A	Deg	95.0	5.0	90.89	-(*)+	
MAX HEIGHT	N-PTV to A pt	Deg	54.0	5.0	53.76	-(*)+	
SN TO PALATAL PLANE		Deg	3.0	5.0	5.28	-(*)+	
*****cephxSubTitleField*****	MAND. POSITION						
FACIAL DEPTH	FH to N-Pog	Deg	90.0	4.0	95.36	-(|*)+	Prognathic mandible
FACIAL AXIS	Na-Ba to PTV-Gn	Deg	90.0	4.0	95.97	-(|*)+	Forward growth
FACIAL TAPER	Na-Gn-Go	Deg	67.0	4.0	67.67	-(*)+	
MAND. PLANE	FH-GoGn	Deg	28.0	3.0	17.63	-(* |)+	Low Mandibular Plane
CORPUS LENGTH	Xi to Pm	mm	70.0	5.0	81.27	-(|*)+	Large corpus length
MAND. ARC	DC-Xi to Xi-Pm	Deg	27.0	5.0	20.86	-(*|)+	Closed Arc
*****cephxSubTitleField*****	MAX.TO MAND RELATIONSHIP						
A pt. CONVEXITY	A to N-Pog	mm	3.0	2.0	-4.87	-(* |)+	Class III Skeletal tendency
LOW.FACE.HEIGHT	ANS-Xi-Pog	Deg	47.0	5.0	39.03	-(*|)+	Short Lower face height
*****cephxSubTitleField*****	DENTURE RELATIONSHIP						
MAX.1 to APo		mm	6.0	3.0	3.59	-(*)+	
MAX.6 to PTV		mm	21.0		-0.55	-( )+	
MAND. 1 to APo		mm	1.0	2.0	-0.91	-(*)+	
HINGE AXIS ANGLE	DC - Go - Ll	Deg	90.0	3.0	98.01	-(|*)+	Open bite tendency
MAX.1 to MAND.1		Deg	131.0	5.0	138.2	-(|*)+	Incisors too vertical
OVERJET		mm	2.5	2.0	2.75	-(*)+	
OVERBITE		mm	2.5	2.0	5.63	-(|*)+	
*****cephxSubTitleField*****	ESTHETICS						
UPPER LIP to E-LINE		mm	-4.0	2.0	-4.11	-(*)+	
LOWER LIP to E-LINE		mm	-2.0	2.0	-5.96	-(*|)+	Lower lip retruded

Figure 3. Part of sample, automatic, AI-derived cephalometric report. Patient: 18-year-old male with class III malocclusion, with graphical representations of the results regarding to norm range (column "Graph") and clinical comments.

Out of multiple correlations between NSD measurements and the results of the cephalometric analyses, only the hinge axis angle (HAA) and SDA showed a significant negative correlation ($p < 0.05$, $r < 0$). However, no significant correlation was found between HAA and PPV. See Figure 5 for a visual representation and Table 2 for the sample results of the correlation analysis.

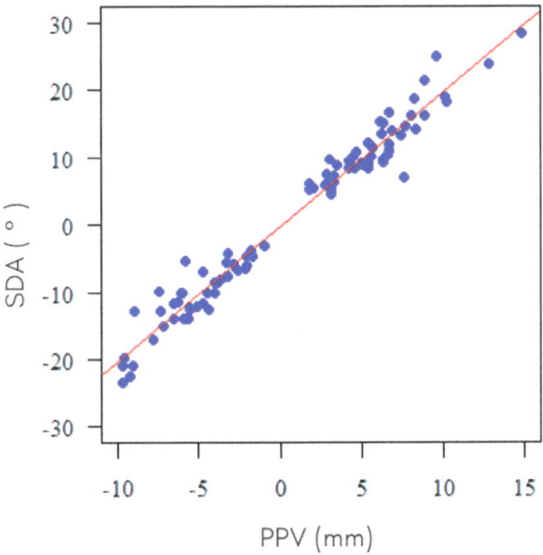

Figure 4. Plot displaying the correlation between SDA and PPV measurements.

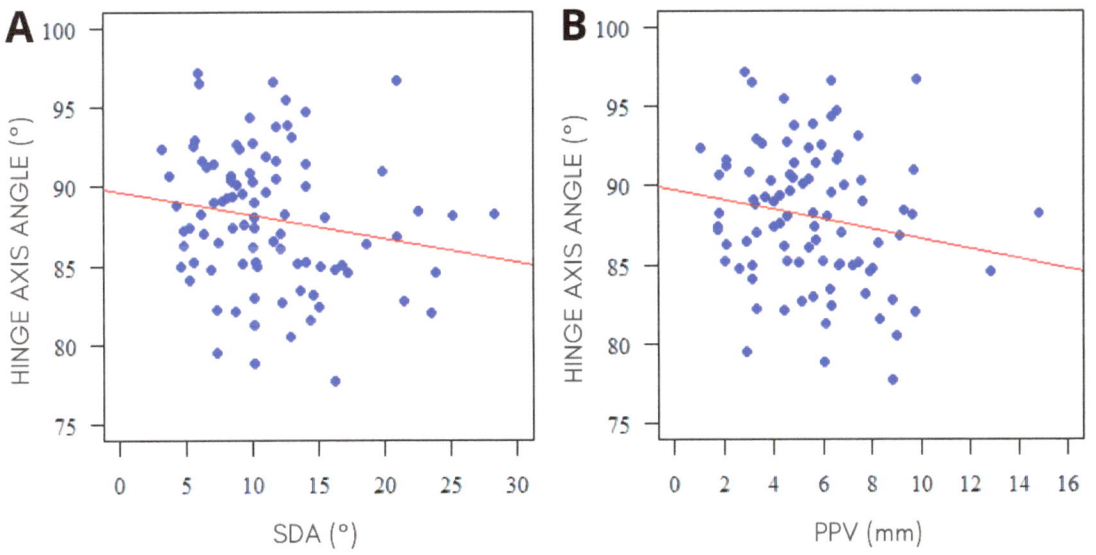

Figure 5. Plot displaying the correlations between HAA and NSD parameters: (**A**) SDA (r = −0.218, p = 0.039); (**B**) PPV (r = −0.186, p = 0.079).

Table 2. Sample of correlation analysis performed: NSD/HAA, and NSD/results of Björk–Jarabak cephalometric analysis.

Parameter	SDA (°) Spearman's Rank Correlation Coefficient	PPV (mm) Spearman's Rank Correlation Coefficient
HINGE AXIS ANGLE (°)	r = −0.218, p = 0.039 *	r = −0.186, p = 0.079
Björk–Jarabak cephalometric analysis		
SADDLE ANGLE (°)	r = 0.017, p = 0.875	r = −0.02, p = 0.853
ARTICULAR ANGLE (°)	r = 0.103, p = 0.335	r = 0.104, p = 0.329
GONIAL ANGLE (°)	r = −0.154, p = 0.148	r = −0.129, p = 0.226
SUM OF ANGLES (°)	r = 0.044, p = 0.679	r = 0.03, p = 0.782
UPPER GONIAL ANGLE (°)	r = −0.175, p = 0,099	r = −0.183, p = 0.084
LOWER GONIAL ANGLE (°)	r = −0.002, p = 0.984	r = 0.023, p = 0.826
ANT. CRANIAL BASE (mm)	r = −0.011, p = 0.915	r = 0.018, p = 0.67
POST. CRANIAL BASE (mm)	r = 0.018, p = 0.866	r = 0.052, p = 0.626
RAMUS HEIGHT (mm)	r = 0.024, p = 0.825	r = 0.099, p = 0.353
MANDIBULAR BODY (mm)	r = −0.02, p = 0.851	r = −0.004, p = 0.972
POST. FACE HEIGHT (mm)	r = 0.031, p = 0.77	r = 0.096, p = 0.368
ANT. FACE HEIGHT (mm)	r = −0.016, p = 0.879	r = 0.043, p = 0.69
PFH:AFH (%)	r = 0.023, p = 0.832	r = 0.053, p = 0.623
ACB:MAND.BODY (%)	r = 0.004, p = 0.97	r = −0.023, p = 0.832
UI to SN (°)	r = −0.096, p = 0.37	r = −0.094, p = 0.376
UI to FH (°)	r = −0.073, p = 0.497	r = −0.074, p = 0.486
UPPER FACE HEIGHT (%)	r = −0.127, p = 0.233	r = −0.057, p = 0.596
LOWER FACE HEIGHT (%)	r = 0.125, p = 0.24	r = 0.065, p = 0.544

*—statistically significant relationship ($p < 0.05$). Abbreviations: SDA—septal deviation angle; PPV—perpendicular plate–vomer measurement.

3.4. Error Study

The analysis of the repeatability of PPV and SDA measurements carried out by the reader demonstrated excellent concordance (data summarized in Table 3).

Table 3. Results of repeatability of manual measurements.

Parameter	Measurement I (Mean ± SD)	Measurement II (Mean ± SD)	ICC	95% CI		Agreement (Cicchetti)	Agreement (Koo and Li)
PPV (mm)	5.19 ± 2.6	5.28 ± 2.49	0.974	0.937	0.990	Excellent	PPV (mm)
SDA (°)	10.78 ± 5.69	10.85 ± 5.73	0.972	0.931	0.989	Excellent	SDA (°)

Abbreviations: PPV—perpendicular plate–vomer measurement; SDA—septal deviation angle.

The results of the repeatability of automatic cephalometric measurements showed excellent concordance in the majority of measurements. A list of parameters with poor concordance of repeated measurements is shown in Table 4. A full list of the conducted repeatability analyses is provided in the Supplementary Material—Table S2.

Table 4. List of parameters with low agreement in repeated measurements.

Parameter	Measurement 1 (Mean ± SD)	Measurement 2 (Mean ± SD)	ICC	95% CI		Agreement (Cicchetti)	Agreement (Koo and Li)
LI-N-B	21.73 ± 8.41	36.67 ± 45.54	0.000	−0.536	0.548	Poor	Poor
Pr-N-A	1.76 ± 0.66	1.85 ± 0.54	0.302	−0.287	0.730	Poor	Poor

Abbreviations: SD—Standard Deviation; I—Incisor; NB—Nasion–B-Point; Pr—Prosthion; A—A-Point; ICC—Interclass Correlation Coefficient; CI—Confidence Interval.

4. Discussion

Our study revealed no significant correlations between NSD parameters (SDA and PPV) and the majority of cephalometric measurements, with the exception of a weak correlation between SDA and HAA ($p = 0.039$). No significant correlation was found between PPV and HAA. The concordance of repeated manual reader measurements demonstrated excellent repeatability, while the majority of parameters in the repeated automatic analysis displayed good-to-excellent concordance, excluding two angular measurements: Lower Incisor–Nasion–B-Point (LI-N-B) and Prosthion–Nasion–A-Point (Pr-N-A). The latter indicates the need for the correction of algorithms determining single cephalometric points. Good, and in most cases excellent, concordance of the repeated analysis results indicates the high effectiveness of the tested AI algorithms in determining cephalometric landmarks.

The results of our study align with earlier published research, demonstrating the potential of AI cephalometric analysis, with varying degrees of success. A study by Lee et al. (2018) developed an AI system for automatic cephalometric landmark detection. The system was found to be highly accurate, with a mean landmark error of 1.53 ± 1.74 mm and an error of less than 2 mm for 82% of landmarks. However, the study also highlighted that the performance of the AI system varied depending on the specific landmark, suggesting the need for further refinement and training of the AI algorithm [44]. Similar results were achieved by other research teams, demonstrating a superior AI success classification rate compared to humans in some cephalometric analysis measures [30,31,45]. An interesting study by Bao et al. (2023) evaluated the accuracy of AI in the automated cephalometric analysis of reconstructed lateral cephalograms from CBCTs for 85 patients. The mean radial error for 19 chosen landmarks was 2.07 ± 1.35 mm and an error of less than 3 mm in 71.7% with the automatic program. The authors concluded that automatic analysis is almost effective enough to be acceptable in clinical work, but is not currently capable of completely replacing manual tracing [46]. Some minor inaccuracies have also been found in previously published papers regarding the reliability of CephX cephalometric analysis. Despite these issues, the authors unanimously concluded that the software is reliable for cephalometric analysis [35,36,41].

The hinge axis (HA) remains an integral part of dental assessments, especially orthognathic and orthodontic assessments, regardless of disputes over the existence of pure rotational movement in temporo-mandibular joints [47]. The HAA has emerged as a critical parameter in cephalometric analysis, providing invaluable insights into craniofacial morphology and growth patterns. The HAA refers to the angle formed by the intersection of the Frankfort horizontal (FH) plane and a line passing through the anatomical HA of the mandible [48]. The HAA in our study was defined as the angle between three cephalometric landmarks, Dc–Go–LI (distobuccal cusp of the first permanent upper molar–gonion–lower lip). Studies have shown that a larger HAA indicates a more vertical growth pattern, while a smaller HAA suggests a more horizontal growth pattern [48]. However, it is crucial to recognize that the HAA is influenced by several factors, including cranial base flexure, facial height, and the position of the mandible [48–50]. Our analysis revealed only a slight, negative correlation between HAA and SDA, and no correlation with PPV. This means that as the deviation angle of the nasal septum increases, the HAA decreases. Contrary to expectations, no significant correlation between HAA and PPV was found. A review of the scientific literature did not reveal any articles convincingly demonstrating a correlation between HAA and NSD. Therefore, we assume that the correlation between HAA and SDA might be coincidental. Further studies with a larger patient sample are necessary to clarify this issue.

NSD is associated with a range of direct disorders, such as headaches, rhinosinusitis, gastroesophageal reflux, and sleep apnea [51–54]. Understanding the full extent of NSD's impact on facial and cranial asymmetry will be crucial in developing effective treatment strategies and improving patient outcomes. Among the factors influencing NSD, midfacial trauma, septal abscess, and craniofacial anomalies (e.g., cleft lip and palate) have been identified [11,23,55,56]. In some cases, a more subtle influence of the anatomical relationships of the surrounding nasofacial skeleton, including developmental constraints and morphological details of the nasal septum, has been suggested to contribute to the development of NSD [57]. A number of studies have demonstrated that a smaller volume of the nasal cavity is associated with a higher percentage of NSD, indicating a mutual influence between these phenomena [12,43,57,58]. More distant correlations between NSD and facial structures have also been found. A study published by Kim et al. [22] revealed a relationship between NSD and horizontal facial asymmetries. Additionally, Gray et al. found a high correlation between septal and palatal asymmetries and dental malocclusion [20,21,23]. A study conducted in 2015, involving 55 patients, demonstrated a correlation between NSD and asymmetries in the nasal and palatal regions [4]. However, it did not establish a correlation between these asymmetries and those of the lateral facial region.

Doubts about the generally accepted norms of cephalometric analysis results and prevailing beauty standards have been present for some time [59,60]. Additionally, the issues of beauty and attractiveness can be perceived differently by orthodontists and patients. Furthermore, apart from skeletal scaffolding, the assessment of soft facial tissues, which greatly influence the matter, is significantly limited in 2D cephalometric assessment, leading to an increasing trend of including 3D scans of the face and intraoral tissues (such as 3D dental models, 2D or 3D X-ray images, and photographs) in the standard set of examinations [60–62]. Such a multimodal, diverse dataset could later be used to create a more complete representation, display, and perception of the relevant structures [63]. It could also be used to create a "virtual patient" for discussing the expected treatment outcomes with the patient [64]. The issue of treatment planning, visualization of its results, and the integration of large-scale, multimodal datasets is a problem that hinders the implementation of these concepts. Therefore, there is an increasing focus on the use of AI in the analysis of 3D faces and in further treatment outcome planning [65–67]. Studies that assessed the accuracy of three-dimensional soft tissue prediction for Le Fort I osteotomy and orthognathic cases using Dolphin 3D software showed a limited reliability of the software [66,67]. However, in a 2022 study, Tanikawa attempted to develop AI systems that predict the 3D facial morphology after orthodontic treatment and orthognathic surgery [65]. The authors utilized lateral cephalograms, 3D facial images, and two AI systems to predict facial morphology after dental treatment. The AI systems proved to sufficiently predict facial morphology after treatment and were considered clinically acceptable. Such integration of AI, multimodal facial morphology assessment, treatment planning, and advanced visualization appears to be the future of orthodontics.

Our study evaluated lateral cephalograms, assessing the correlation of NSD mainly using vertical facial morphology. Considering the results of our work and existing data from the literature, the strongest potential connection appears to be between NSD and horizontal facial asymmetries. Taking into account the previously cited studies based on animal models, narrowing down the study group to patients with nasal septum damage at an early stage of development would likely reveal correlations not present in our group of consecutive, post-traumatic patients admitted to the Emergency Department. Furthermore, although we consider the AI-driven cephalometric analysis to be highly efficient and cost-effective in modern orthodontic practices, we believe that further studies regarding its performance must be conducted. Issues related to the influence of study quality on cephalometric analysis results, the repeatability of analysis results, and refinements and reliability of the algorithms are certainly areas that should be further explored. It should also be noted that our study is one of the initial analyses of selected morphological parameters using AI. An exciting future prospect is the ability of AI to automatically analyze large databases of imaging studies available on PACS servers at large institutions. This will certainly enable the discovery of subtle, previously unnoticed correlations between distant morphological parameters. It will undoubtedly have a significant impact on the development of fields as "hoary" and seemingly explored as anatomy.

The potential limitations of this study could be attributed to the relatively small sample size of patients included, potentially limiting the ability to detect subtle correlations between the studied parameters, which might only become apparent when analyzing larger groups. A geographic limitation was also present, as all radiographs were obtained from the same research center. Attention should also be given to the potential influence of errors in AI algorithms when determining cephalometric landmarks in the analysis results. It should also be noted that our study analyzed one of the commercially available solutions, and the obtained results should not be generalized to other AI software.

5. Conclusions

In conclusion, the results of the multiparametric cephalometric analysis were not correlated with the degree of nasal septum deviation in patients in our study group, except for a weak, negative correlation between HAA and SDA. The results of automatic cephalometric analyses performed by the CephX AI platform showed excellent repeatability, except for two types of angular measurements, LI-N-B and Pr-N-A, indicating the high reproductivity of the tested AI model in most cephalometric analyses.

Supplementary Materials: The following supporting information can be downloaded at: https://www.mdpi.com/article/10.3390/jcm12206621/s1; Table S1: List of performed automatic cephalometric analyses; Table S2: Results of repeatability analysis of automatic AI cephalometric analyses.

Author Contributions: Conceptualization, N.K., W.K. and J.J.-O.; methodology, N.K. and W.K.; software, W.K.; validation, Z.S. and J.J.-O.; formal analysis, P.N.; investigation, N.K. and P.N.; resources, W.K.; data curation, P.N.; writing—original draft preparation, N.K. and W.K.; writing—review and editing, N.K., W.K., A.L. and K.N.; visualization, W.K.; supervision, Z.S. and J.J.-O.; project administration, N.K. and W.K. All authors have read and agreed to the published version of the manuscript.

Funding: This research received no external funding. The APC was funded by the authors.

Institutional Review Board Statement: The study was conducted in accordance with the Declaration of Helsinki, and approved by the Ethics Committee of Collegium Medicum, Nicolaus Copernicus University in Torun, Poland (protocol No. KB 227/2023, 10.04.20223) for studies involving humans.

Informed Consent Statement: Patient consent was waived due to the retrospective nature of the study and patients' data anonymization.

Data Availability Statement: Data are available on request.

Acknowledgments: LD, a statistician, was involved in data analysis.

Conflicts of Interest: The authors declare no conflict of interest.

References

1. Latham, R.A. Maxillary Development and Growth: The Septo-Premaxillary Ligament. *J. Anat.* **1970**, *107*, 471–478.
2. Goergen, M.J.; Holton, N.E.; Grünheid, T. Morphological Interaction between the Nasal Septum and Nasofacial Skeleton during Human Ontogeny. *J. Anat.* **2017**, *230*, 689–700. [CrossRef]
3. Pirsig, W. Growth of the Deviated Septum and Its Influence on Midfacial Development. *Facial Plast. Surg.* **1992**, *8*, 224–232. [CrossRef]
4. Hartman, C.; Holton, N.; Miller, S.; Yokley, T.; Marshall, S.; Srinivasan, S.; Southard, T. Nasal Septal Deviation and Facial Skeletal Asymmetries. *Anat. Rec.* **2015**, *299*, 295–306. [CrossRef] [PubMed]
5. Denour, E.; Roussel, L.O.; Woo, A.S.; Boyajian, M.; Crozier, J. Quantification of Nasal Septal Deviation with Computed Tomography Data. *J. Craniofacial Surg.* **2020**, *31*, 1659–1663. [CrossRef]
6. Rönning, O.; Kantomaa, T. Experimental Nasal Septum Deviation in the Rat. *Eur. J. Orthod.* **1985**, *7*, 248–254. [CrossRef] [PubMed]
7. Lieberman, D.E.; Hallgrímsson, B.; Liu, W.; Parsons, T.E.; Jamniczky, H.A. Spatial Packing, Cranial Base Angulation, and Craniofacial Shape Variation in the Mammalian Skull: Testing a New Model Using Mice. *J. Anat.* **2008**, *212*, 720–735. [CrossRef] [PubMed]
8. Baddam, P.; Kung, T.; Adesida, A.B.; Graf, D. Histological and Molecular Characterization of the Growing Nasal Septum in Mice. *J. Anat.* **2020**, *238*, 751–764. [CrossRef] [PubMed]
9. Parsons, T.E.; Downey, C.M.; Jirik, F.R.; Hallgrimsson, B.; Jamniczky, H.A. Mind the Gap: Genetic Manipulation of Basicranial Growth within Synchondroses Modulates Calvarial and Facial Shape in Mice through Epigenetic Interactions. *PLoS ONE* **2015**, *10*, e0118355. [CrossRef]

10. Babula, W.J.; Smiley, G.R.; Dixon, A.D. The Role of the Cartilaginous Nasal Septum in Midfacial Growth. *Am. J. Orthod.* **1970**, *58*, 250–263. [CrossRef]
11. Hall, B.K.; Precious, D.S. Cleft Lip, Nose, and Palate: The Nasal Septum as the Pacemaker for Midfacial Growth. *Oral Surg. Oral Med. Oral Pathol. Oral Radiol.* **2013**, *115*, 442–447. [CrossRef] [PubMed]
12. Holton, N.E.; Yokley, T.R.; Figueroa, A. Nasal Septal and Craniofacial Form in European- and African-Derived Populations. *J. Anat.* **2012**, *221*, 263–274. [CrossRef] [PubMed]
13. Stallman, J.S.; Lobo, J.N.; Som, P.M. The Incidence of Concha Bullosa and Its Relationship to Nasal Septal Deviation and Paranasal Sinus Disease. *Am. J. Neuroradiol.* **2004**, *25*, 1613–1618.
14. Smith, K.D.; Edwards, P.C.; Saini, T.S.; Norton, N.S. The Prevalence of Concha Bullosa and Nasal Septal Deviation and Their Relationship to Maxillary Sinusitis by Volumetric Tomography. *Int. J. Dent.* **2010**, *2010*, 404982. [CrossRef]
15. Zielnik-Jurkiewicz, B.; Olszewska-Sosińska, O. The Nasal Septum Deformities in Children and Adolescents from Warsaw, Poland. *Int. J. Pediatr. Otorhinolaryngol.* **2006**, *70*, 731–736. [CrossRef] [PubMed]
16. Šubarić, M.; Mladina, R. Nasal Septum Deformities in Children and Adolescents: A Cross Sectional Study of Children from Zagreb, Croatia. *Int. J. Pediatr. Otorhinolaryngol.* **2002**, *63*, 41–48. [CrossRef]
17. Egeli, E.; Demirci, L.; Yazýcý, B.; Harputluoglu, U. Evaluation of the Inferior Turbinate in Patients with Deviated Nasal Septum by Using Computed Tomography. *Laryngoscope* **2004**, *114*, 113–117. [CrossRef]
18. Estomba, C.C.; Schmitz, T.R.; Echeverri, C.C.O.; Reinoso, F.A.B.R.; Velasquez, A.O.; Hidalgo, C.S. Compensatory Hypertrophy of the Contralateral Inferior Turbinate in Patients with Unilateral Nasal Septal Deviation. A Computed Tomography Study. *Otolaryngol. Polska* **2015**, *69*, 14–20. [CrossRef]
19. Orhan, I.; Aydin, S.; Ormeci, T.; Yilmaz, F. A Radiological Analysis of Inferior Turbinate in Patients with Deviated Nasal Septum by Using Computed Tomography. *Am. J. Rhinol. Allergy* **2014**, *28*, e68–e72. [CrossRef]
20. Gray, L.P.; Brogan, W.F. Septal Deformity Malocclusion and Rapid Maxillary Expansion. *Orthodontist* **1972**, *4*, 2–14.
21. Gray, L.P. The Development and Significance of Septal and Dental Deformity from Birth to Eight Years. *Int. J. Pediatr. Otorhinolaryngol.* **1984**, *6*, 265–277. [CrossRef]
22. Kim, Y.M.; Rha, K.S.; Weissman, J.D.; Hwang, P.H.; Most, S.P. Correlation of Asymmetric Facial Growth with Deviated Nasal Septum. *Laryngoscope* **2011**, *121*, 1144–1148. [CrossRef]
23. Gray, L.P.; Dillon, P.I.; Brogan, W.F.; Henry, P.J. The Development of Septal and Dental Deformity from Birth. *Angle Orthod.* **1982**, *52*, 265–278.
24. Vig, K.W. Nasal Obstruction and Facial Growth: The Strength of Evidence for Clinical Assumptions. *Am. J. Orthod. Dentofac. Orthop.* **1998**, *113*, 603–611. [CrossRef]
25. D'Ascanio, L.; Lancione, C.; Pompa, G.; Rebuffini, E.; Mansi, N.; Manzini, M. Craniofacial Growth in Children with Nasal Septum Deviation: A Cephalometric Comparative Study. *Int. J. Pediatr. Otorhinolaryngol.* **2010**, *74*, 1180–1183. [CrossRef]
26. Freng, A.; Kvam, E.; Kramer, J. Facial Skeletal Dimensions in Patients with Nasal Septal Deviation. *Scand. J. Plast. Reconstr. Surg.* **1988**, *22*, 77–81. [CrossRef]
27. Leonardi, R.; Giordano, D.; Maiorana, F.; Spampinato, C. Automatic Cephalometric Analysis: A Systematic Review. *Angle Orthod.* **2008**, *78*, 145–151. [CrossRef] [PubMed]
28. Chen, Y.J.; Chen, S.K.; Yao, J.C.C.; Chang, H.F. The Effects of Differences in Landmark Identification on the Cephalometric Measurements in Traditional versus Digitized Cephalometry. *Angle Orthod.* **2004**, *74*, 155–161. [PubMed]
29. Dias Da Silveira, H.L.; Dias Silveira, H.E. Reproducibility of Cephalometric Measurements Made by Three Radiology Clinics. *Angle Orthod.* **2006**, *76*, 394–399.
30. Hwang, H.-W.; Moon, J.-H.; Kim, M.-G.; Donatelli, R.E.; Lee, S.J. Evaluation of Automated Cephalometric Analysis Based on the Latest Deep Learning Method. *Angle Orthod.* **2021**, *91*, 329–335. [CrossRef]
31. Hwang, H.W.; Park, J.H.; Moon, J.H.; Yu, Y.; Kim, H.; Her, S.B.; Srinivasan, G.; Aljanabi, M.N.A.; Donatelli, R.E.; Lee, S.J. Automated Identification of Cephalometric Landmarks: Part 2-Might It Be Better than Human? *Angle Orthod.* **2020**, *90*, 69–76. [CrossRef]
32. Nishimoto, S. Locating Cephalometric Landmarks with Multi-Phase Deep Learning. *J. Dent. Health Oral Res.* **2023**, *4*, 1–13. [CrossRef]
33. Kang, S.H.; Jeon, K.; Kang, S.H.; Lee, S.H. 3D Cephalometric Landmark Detection by Multiple Stage Deep Reinforcement Learning. *Sci. Rep.* **2021**, *11*, 17509. [CrossRef]
34. Chung, E.J.; Yang, B.E.; Park, I.Y.; Yi, S.; On, S.W.; Kim, Y.H.; Kang, S.H.; Byun, S.H. Effectiveness of Cone-Beam Computed Tomography-Generated Cephalograms Using Artificial Intelligence Cephalometric Analysis. *Sci. Rep.* **2022**, *12*, 20585. [CrossRef]
35. Meric, P.; Naoumova, J. Web-Based Fully Automated Cephalometric Analysis: Comparisons between App-Aided, Computerized, and Manual Tracings. *Turk. J. Orthod.* **2020**, *33*, 142–149. [CrossRef] [PubMed]
36. Alqahtani, H. Evaluation of an Online Website-Based Platform for Cephalometric Analysis. *J. Stomatol. Oral Maxillofac. Surg.* **2020**, *121*, 53–57. [CrossRef] [PubMed]
37. Bulatova, G.; Kusnoto, B.; Grace, V.; Tsay, T.P.; Avenetti, D.M.; Sanchez, F.J.C. Assessment of Automatic Cephalometric Landmark Identification Using Artificial Intelligence. *Orthod. Craniofac. Res.* **2021**, *24*, 37–42. [CrossRef] [PubMed]

38. Tsolakis, I.A.; Tsolakis, A.I.; Elshebiny, T.; Matthaios, S.; Palomo, J.M. Comparing a Fully Automated Cephalometric Tracing Method to a Manual Tracing Method for Orthodontic Diagnosis. *J. Clin. Med.* **2022**, *11*, 6854. [CrossRef]
39. Lo Giudice, A.; Ronsivalle, V.; Spampinato, C.; Leonardi, R. Fully Automatic Segmentation of the Mandible Based on Convolutional Neural Networks (CNNs). *Orthod. Craniofac. Res.* **2021**, *24*, 100–107. [CrossRef]
40. Lo Giudice, A.; Ronsivalle, V.; Gastaldi, G.; Leonardi, R. Assessment of the Accuracy of Imaging Software for 3D Rendering of the Upper Airway, Usable in Orthodontic and Craniofacial Clinical Settings. *Prog. Orthod.* **2022**, *23*, 22. [CrossRef] [PubMed]
41. Mosleh, M.A.A.; Baba, M.S.; Malek, S.; Almaktari, R.A. Ceph-X: Development and Evaluation of 2D Cephalometric System. *BMC Bioinform.* **2016**, *17*, 499. [CrossRef]
42. Lin, J.K.; Wheatley, F.C.; Handwerker, J.; Harris, N.J.; Wong, B.J.F. Analyzing Nasal Septal Deviations to Develop a New Classification System: A Computed Tomography Study Using MATLAB and OsiriX. *JAMA Facial Plast. Surg.* **2014**, *16*, 183–187. [CrossRef]
43. Dalili, K.Z.; Khademi, J.; Nemati, S.; Niksolat, E. The Effects of Septal Deviation, Concha Bullosa, and Their Combination on the Depth of Posterior Palatal Arch in Cone-Beam Computed Tomography. *J. Dent.* **2016**, *17*, 26–31.
44. Lee, J.H.; Yu, H.J.; Kim, M.J.; Kim, J.W.; Choi, J. Automated Cephalometric Landmark Detection with Confidence Regions Using Bayesian Convolutional Neural Networks. *BMC Oral Health* **2020**, *20*, 270. [CrossRef]
45. Song, Y.; Qiao, X.; Iwamoto, Y.; Chen, Y.W. Automatic Cephalometric Landmark Detection on X-Ray Images Using a Deep-Learning Method. *Appl. Sci.* **2020**, *10*, 2547. [CrossRef]
46. Bao, H.; Zhang, K.; Yu, C.; Li, H.; Cao, D.; Shu, H.; Liu, L.; Yan, B. Evaluating the Accuracy of Automated Cephalometric Analysis Based on Artificial Intelligence. *BMC Oral Health* **2023**, *23*, 191. [CrossRef] [PubMed]
47. Barretto, M.D.A.; Melhem-Elias, F.; Deboni, M.C.Z. Methods of Mandibular Condyle Position and Rotation Center Used for Orthognathic Surgery Planning: A Systematic Review. *J. Stomatol. Oral Maxillofac. Surg.* **2022**, *123*, 345–352.
48. Ricketts, R.M. Perspectives in the Clinical Application of Cephalometrics. The First Fifty Years. *Angle Orthod.* **1981**, *51*, 115–150. [PubMed]
49. Solow, B.; Tallgren, A. Natural Head Position in Standing Subjects. *Acta Odontol. Scand.* **1971**, *29*, 591–607. [CrossRef]
50. Billiaert, K.; Al-Yassary, M.; Antonarakis, G.S.; Kiliaridis, S. Measuring the Difference in Natural Head Position between the Standing and Sitting Positions Using an Inertial Measurement Unit. *J. Oral Rehabil.* **2021**, *48*, 1144–1149. [CrossRef] [PubMed]
51. Torre, C.; Capasso, R.; Zaghi, S.; Williams, R.; Liu, S.Y.-C. High Incidence of Posterior Nasal Cavity Obstruction in Obstructive Sleep Apnea Patients. *Sleep Sci. Pract.* **2017**, *1*, 286. [CrossRef]
52. Wong, E.; Deboever, N.; Sritharan, N.; Singh, N. Laryngopharyngeal Reflux Is Associated with Nasal Septal Deviation. *Eur. J. Rhinol. Allergy* **2020**, *3*, 1–3. [CrossRef]
53. Kwon, S.H.; Lee, E.J.; Yeo, C.D.; Kim, M.G.; Kim, J.S.; Noh, S.J.; Kim, E.J.; Kim, S.G.; Lee, J.-H.; Yoo, J.S.; et al. Is Septal Deviation Associated with Headache? *Medicine* **2020**, *99*, e20337. [CrossRef]
54. Orlandi, R.R. A Systematic Analysis of Septal Deviation Associated with Rhinosinusitis. *Laryngoscope* **2010**, *120*, 1687–1695. [CrossRef]
55. Grymer, L.F.; Bosch, C. The Nasal Septum and the Development of the Midface. A Longitudinal Study of a Pair of Monozygotic Twins. *Rhinology* **1997**, *35*, 6–10.
56. Pirsig, W. Historical Notes and Actual Observations on the Nasal Septal Abscess Especially in Children. *Int. J. Pediatr. Otorhinolaryngol.* **1984**, *8*, 43–54. [CrossRef] [PubMed]
57. Kim, J.; Kim, S.W.; Kim, S.W.; Cho, J.H.; Park, Y.J. Role of the Sphenoidal Process of the Septal Cartilage in the Development of Septal Deviation. *Otolaryngol. Head Neck Surg.* **2012**, *146*, 151–155. [CrossRef] [PubMed]
58. Mays, S. Nasal Septal Deviation in a Mediaeval Population. *Am. J. Phys. Anthropol.* **2012**, *148*, 319–326. [CrossRef] [PubMed]
59. Peck, H.; Peck, S. A Concept of Facial Esthetics. *Angle Orthod.* **1970**, *40*, 284–317.
60. Masoud, M.I.; Bansal, N.; Castillo, J.C.; Manosudprasit, A.; Allareddy, V.; Haghi, A.; Hawkins, H.C.; Otárola-Castillo, E. 3D Dentofacial Photogrammetry Reference Values: A Novel Approach to Orthodontic Diagnosis. *Eur. J. Orthod.* **2017**, *39*, 215–225. [CrossRef]
61. Tanikawa, C. Facial Morphospace: A Clinical Quantitative Analysis of the Three-Dimensional Face in Patients with Cleft Lip and Palate. *Plast. Aesthet. Res.* **2020**, *7*, 48. [CrossRef]
62. Tanikawa, C.; Akcam, M.O.; Takada, K. Quantifying Faces Three-Dimensionally in Orthodontic Practice. *J. Cranio Maxillofac. Surg.* **2019**, *47*, 867–875. [CrossRef]
63. Tomaka, A.A.; Luchowski, L.; Pojda, D.; Tarnawski, M.; Domino, K. The Dynamics of the Stomatognathic System from 4D Multimodal Data. In *Multiscale Locomotion: Its Active-Matter Addressing Physical Principles*; Gadomski, A., Ed.; Publishing Department of the UTP University of Science & Technology: Bydgoszcz, Poland, 2019.
64. Joda, T.; Gallucci, G.O. The Virtual Patient in Dental Medicine. *Clin. Oral Implants. Res.* **2015**, *26*, 725–726. [CrossRef] [PubMed]
65. Tanikawa, C.; Yamashiro, T. Development of Novel Artificial Intelligence Systems to Predict Facial Morphology after Orthognathic Surgery and Orthodontic Treatment in Japanese Patients. *Sci. Rep.* **2021**, *11*, 15853. [CrossRef] [PubMed]

66. Resnick, C.M.; Dang, R.R.; Glick, S.J.; Padwa, B.L. Accuracy of Three-Dimensional Soft Tissue Prediction for Le Fort I Osteotomy Using Dolphin 3D Software: A Pilot Study. *Int. J. Oral Maxillofac. Surg.* **2017**, *46*, 289–295. [CrossRef] [PubMed]
67. Elshebiny, T.; Morcos, S.; Mohammad, A.; Quereshy, F.; Valiathan, M. Accuracy of Three-Dimensional Soft Tissue Prediction in Orthognathic Cases Using Dolphin Three-Dimensional Software. *J. Craniofacial Surg.* **2019**, *30*, 525–528. [CrossRef]

Disclaimer/Publisher's Note: The statements, opinions and data contained in all publications are solely those of the individual author(s) and contributor(s) and not of MDPI and/or the editor(s). MDPI and/or the editor(s) disclaim responsibility for any injury to people or property resulting from any ideas, methods, instructions or products referred to in the content.

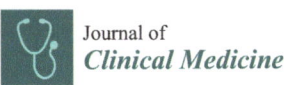

Journal of Clinical Medicine

Article

Accuracy of Palatal Orthodontic Mini-Implants Placed Using Fully Digital Planned Insertion Guides: A Cadaver Study

Lea Stursa [1,*], Brigitte Wendl [1], Norbert Jakse [1], Margit Pichelmayer [1], Frank Weiland [2], Veronica Antipova [3] and Barbara Kirnbauer [1]

1. Department of Dental Medicine and Oral Health, Division of Oral Surgery and Orthodontics, Medical University of Graz, Billrothgasse 4, 8010 Graz, Austria; brigitte.wendl@medunigraz.at (B.W.); norbert.jakse@medunigraz.at (N.J.); margit.pichelmayer@medunigraz.at (M.P.); barbara.kirnbauer@medunigraz.at (B.K.)
2. Private Practice, Untere Schmiedgasse 16, 8530 Deutschlandsberg, Austria; frank.weiland@medunigraz.at
3. Division of Macroscopic and Clinical Anatomy, Gottfried Schatz Research Center, Medical University of Graz, Auenbruggerplatz 25, 8036 Graz, Austria; veronica.antipova@medunigraz.at
* Correspondence: lea.stursa@stud.medunigraz.at; Tel.: +43-31638582248

Abstract: Digital workflows have become integral in orthodontic diagnosis and therapy, reducing risk factors and chair time with one-visit protocols. This study assessed the transfer accuracy of fully digital planned insertion guides for orthodontic mini-implants (OMIs) compared with freehanded insertion. Cone-beam computed tomography (CBCT) datasets and intraoral surface scans of 32 cadaver maxillae were used to place 64 miniscrews in the anterior palate. Three groups were formed, two using printed insertion guides (A and B) and one with freehand insertion (C). Group A used commercially available customized surgical templates and Group B in-house planned and fabricated insertion guides. Postoperative CBCT datasets were superimposed with the planning model, and accuracy measurements were performed using orthodontic software. Statistical differences were found for transverse angular deviations (4.81° in A vs. 12.66° in B and 5.02° in C, $p = 0.003$) and sagittal angular deviations (2.26° in A vs. 2.20° in B and 5.34° in C, $p = 0.007$). However, accurate insertion depth was not achieved in either guide group; Group A insertion was too shallow (−0.17 mm), whereas Group B insertion was deeper (+0.65 mm) than planned. Outsourcing the planning and fabrication of computer-aided design and computer-aided manufacturing insertion guides may be beneficial for certain indications; particularly, in this study, commercial templates demonstrated superior accuracy than our in-house–fabricated insertion guides.

Keywords: orthodontics; mini-implant; temporary anchorage device; guided surgery; surgical template; CBCT; intraoral scan; digital workflow; CAD/CAM; transfer accuracy

Citation: Stursa, L.; Wendl, B.; Jakse, N.; Pichelmayer, M.; Weiland, F.; Antipova, V.; Kirnbauer, B. Accuracy of Palatal Orthodontic Mini-Implants Placed Using Fully Digital Planned Insertion Guides: A Cadaver Study. *J. Clin. Med.* **2023**, *12*, 6782. https://doi.org/10.3390/jcm12216782

Academic Editor: Eiji Tanaka

Received: 21 September 2023
Revised: 20 October 2023
Accepted: 25 October 2023
Published: 26 October 2023

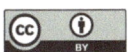

Copyright: © 2023 by the authors. Licensee MDPI, Basel, Switzerland. This article is an open access article distributed under the terms and conditions of the Creative Commons Attribution (CC BY) license (https://creativecommons.org/licenses/by/4.0/).

1. Introduction

Since their introduction by Gainsforth and Higley in 1945 [1], orthodontic mini-implants (OMIs) have expanded the treatment options in orthodontics, serving as temporary anchorage devices (TADs) for intraoral anchorage reinforcement and proving superior to conventional methods [2]. Their advantages include reduced need for patient compliance, improved anchorage, cost-effectiveness, and ease of insertion and removal, making them essential in modern orthodontics [3].

Despite these advantages, risks such as nerve involvement, bleeding from blood vessel trauma, and perforation into the nasal cavity or maxillary sinus persist [4]. Therefore, precise preoperative planning is crucial to minimize these risks and ensure accurate OMI placement [5].

The field of dentistry has shown increasing interest in three-dimensional (3D) technologies in recent years, revolutionizing the orthodontic treatment planning process [6]. Cone-beam computed tomography (CBCT) has enabled better preoperative planning by providing a 3D view of adjacent anatomical structures [7]. Dedicated software allows virtual implant position planning and the creation of corresponding surgical guides. With advancements in 3D technologies, insertion templates and digitally designed orthodontic appliances can be "computer-aided design and computer-aided manufacturing" (CAD/CAM)-fabricated without analog in-between steps [8]. Surgical templates aim to achieve a one-visit protocol, enhancing clinician precision and reducing chair time [9]. CBCT-based insertion guides are particularly beneficial for patients with challenging anatomical situations, such as cleft palate, impacted teeth, or minor palatal bone support [10]. Based on the virtual position of planned OMIs, an individual orthodontic appliance can be designed and CAD/CAM-printed, enabling the installation of miniscrews and orthodontic devices in a single appointment, thereby reducing patient chair time and costs [11]. In this context, some recent studies investigated the transfer accuracy of different insertion guides, although not all of them applied a solely digital workflow, as presented in this study [5,12–14]. Möhlhenrich et al.'s cadaveric study [12] showed that tooth-supported silicone guides were superior in terms of transfer precision compared to gingiva-supported guides, with sagittal angular deviations of 3.67° (SD 2.25) vs. 6.46° (SD 5.5). The study by Ludwig et al. [13] investigating "sterile" and "nonsterile" CAD/CAM insertion guides demonstrated that heat treatment during the sterilization process improved transfer accuracy and achieved a clinically acceptable mean deviation of 0.81% at the coronal distance of the mid-mini-implant head. Pozzan et al. [14] analyzed the influence of different steps of the digital workflow on the deviation of the OMI's axis of guided insertion and showed that the laboratory step resulted in significantly lower axial deviations ($2.12° \pm 1.62°$) than the clinical step ($6.23° \pm 3.75°$).

This anatomical study compares two different insertion guides, both fabricated within a purely digital workflow, and investigates their precision to determine if one method may be preferable. The data gathered during this study allow comparison with conventional freehand OMI insertion.

2. Materials and Methods

Ethical approval for this study was obtained from the ethics committee of the Medical University of Graz (EK 32-550 ex 19/20).

While alive, all body donors provided informed consent for the donation of their postmortem tissues for research. All body donors were bequeathed to the Division of Macroscopic and Clinical Anatomy of the Medical University of Graz under the approval of the Anatomical Donation Program of the Medical University of Graz and in accordance with Austrian laws concerning body donation.

This study examined 32 human cadaver heads, provided by the Division of Macroscopic and Clinical Anatomy of the Medical University of Graz, with intact palatal gingiva that were embalmed using a modified Thiel technique [15]. These body donor skulls were randomly divided into three groups for OMI insertion. In Group A (n = 12), a commercially available and individually prefabricated surgical guide (Accuguide®; Forestadent Bernhard Förster GmbH, Pforzheim, Germany) was used. In Group B (n = 12), self-designed, individually adapted 3D-printed insertion templates were used. In contrast, in Group C (n = 8), a surgical guide was not used, with the TADs being placed conventionally in a freehanded manner. In total, 64 orthodontic mini-implants (1.7×8.0 mm; OrthoEasy® Pal; Forestadent Bernhard Förster GmbH), with 2 OMIs (right and left OMIs) per body donor head, were inserted in the anterior palate, lateral to the palatal suture by an experienced oral surgeon.

2.1. Digital Planning and Clinical Procedure

The digital planning and clinical procedure involved obtaining a CBCT dataset (Planmeca Promax 3D Max®, Helsinki, Finland) with dimensions of 10.0×9.3 cm (diameter × height) and a voxel size of 200 µm, along with an intraoral scan of the upper jaw (Trios 3®; 3Shape, Copenhagen, Denmark) for each body donor head.

In Group A, digital imaging and communications in medicine (DICOM) data and a surface standard triangulation language (STL) file for each skull were uploaded to the encoded professional planning portal (Forestadent Bernhard Förster GmbH). OMI positioning was performed by an internationally renowned TAD expert and digital dentistry pioneer. After final approval of the positioning proposal, the printed insertion guide and a resin-printed 3D model were delivered.

For Group B, the DICOM data were uploaded into specific orthodontic planning software (Onyxceph; Image Instruments GmbH, Chemnitz, Germany) and matched with the corresponding STL file of the intraoral scan of the upper jaw (Figure 1).

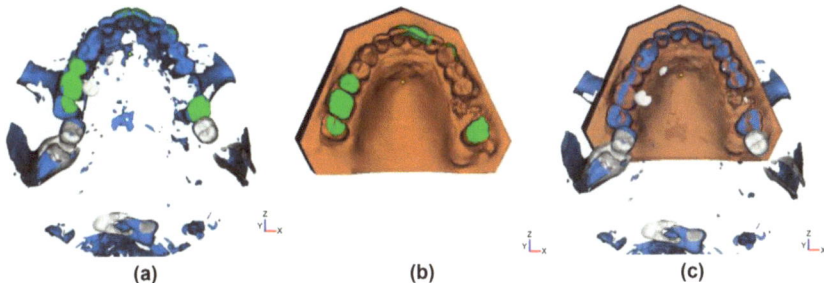

Figure 1. Preoperative superimposition using Onyxceph: (**a**) CBCT dataset; (**b**) intraoral surface scan model; (**c**) superimposition (based on green surfaces **a** + **b**) of both datasets.

After superimposition, screw positions were virtually planned using the TADmatch module of Onyxceph, selecting the same TADs from a virtual library used in the clinical procedure. The virtual OMIs were positioned based on the planned orthodontic device and adjacent anatomical structures. Two mini-implants (1.7 × 8 mm; OrthoEasy® Pal; Forestadent Bernhard Förster GmbH, Pforzheim, Germany) with a 6 or 7 mm interscrew distance were planned in a paramedian position at an angle of approximately 90° to the palatal plane. The STL file of the positioning model was exported to Appliance Designer® software (3Shape), where the dental technician virtually designed the surgical guides. The guides were then 3D-printed using a light processing technique (Asiga Pro2®; Dentona, Dortmund, Germany) and subjected to light hardening (Otoflash G171®; Dentona) with 2 × 2000 flashes in the presence of nitrogen (N_2) gas. The aim was to create a reduced-size template with a more skeletonized design compared with previous insertion guides.

During OMI insertion, the surgical guides were positioned on the teeth and held in place by an assistant, and the oral surgeon performed the insertion without predrilling.

In Group C, the oral surgeon examined the initial records and performed conventional freehanded manual insertion, as typically conducted during the clinical routine.

A contra-angle handpiece drive (Prosthodontic Implant Driver; W&H, Bürmoos, Ignaz-Glaser Str. 53, 5111 Bürmoos, Austria) with a corresponding screwdriver was used for screw insertion without predrilling in all groups. Torque was limited to 35 Ncm. Using the surgical templates, the insertion automatically stopped when the screwdriver contacted the top edge of the insertion guide (Figure 2).

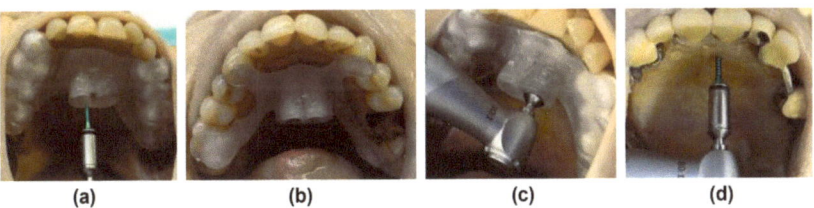

Figure 2. Insertion process of all groups: (**a**) Accuguide® and drill guide with OMI; (**b**) in-house–fabricated insertion guide; (**c**) integrated automatic stop; (**d**) conventional freehanded insertion.

2.2. Software Analysis and Accuracy Measurements

Postoperatively, CBCT scans (Planmeca Promax 3D Max®, Helsinki, Finland) were performed on each body donor head using the same settings applied preoperatively. The postoperative CBCT data were then matched with the corresponding preoperative planning data using the Register3D tool in Onyxceph. Dental reference points on each model were used for superimposition of the datasets. Once the pre- and postsurgical models were aligned, the actual OMI positions from the obtained postsurgical CBCTs were superimposed with the virtual OMIs using an iterative closest point algorithm for automatic surface registration (Figure 3).

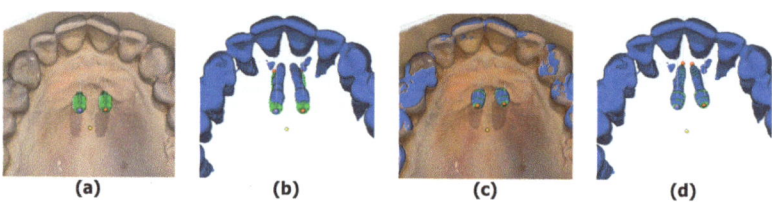

Figure 3. Postoperative superimposition and measurements (e.g., blue mark = "Point 1"): (**a**) presurgical planning model with digital OMIs; (**b**) digital OMIs and postoperative CBCT dataset; (**c**) postsurgical superimposition; (**d**) digital OMIs matched with the postsurgical CBCT dataset.

Linear measurements were conducted to evaluate the insertion depth and to measure deviations and interscrew distances at the head and tip of the screw. Angular measurements were performed to assess the parallelism of the OMIs and their deviations compared with the preoperatively planned positions. All superimposition and measurements were performed three times by a single experienced orthodontist.

In Group C, postoperative measurements were directly performed in the CBCT software (Planmeca Romexis®, Helsinki, Finland). The axes of the OMIs were defined, and sagittal and transversal angles were measured to examine OMI parallelism. These angular deviations between left and right miniscrews were compared with guided insertion.

2.3. Statistical Analysis

Statistical analysis was performed using the software package SPSS version 27.0 (IBM SPSS Statistics, IBM Corporation, Armonk, New York, NY, USA). Continuous variables were presented as means ± standard deviations. The independent Student's *t*-test was used to compare OMI position data, and analysis of variance was performed for comparison among the three groups. The significance level was set at $p \leq 0.05$.

With a sample size of 12 in each of the two main groups, the study had a power of 87.71% to detect a difference in means of −0.4 (the difference between a Group 1 mean, μ_1, of 0.56 and a Group 2 mean, μ_2, of 0.96), assuming a common standard deviation of 0.3, using a two-group *t*-test with a 5% two-sided significance level.

3. Results

Preoperatively, all cases exhibited parallelism between right and left OMIs, but postoperatively, none of the investigated miniscrew pairs were exactly parallel. The deviation from parallelism was measured as angles between both implant axes, and it was significantly smaller ($p = 0.030$) in Group A (5.19° ± 2.71°) than in Group B (10.41° ± 7.29°).

There were no significant differences between the left and right OMIs in both groups (right OMI: $p = 0.720$; left OMI: $p = 0.206$). However, in Group A, the angular deviation was higher for the right miniscrew (4.68° ± 1.77°), whereas in Group B, the left OMI exhibited higher deviations (6.66° ± 6.13°). When considering both groups together, no significant differences were found between the left and right mini-implants ($p = 0.698$).

Mean interscrew distances, measured at the implant tip and head, became smaller between the planned and actual positions in both groups, but these changes were not statistically significant (Figure 4; Table 1). The actual implant head positions in both groups were found to be closer to the median palatal suture (Group A: 0.30 ± 0.22 mm; Group B: 0.27 ± 0.18 mm) compared with the virtually planned implants.

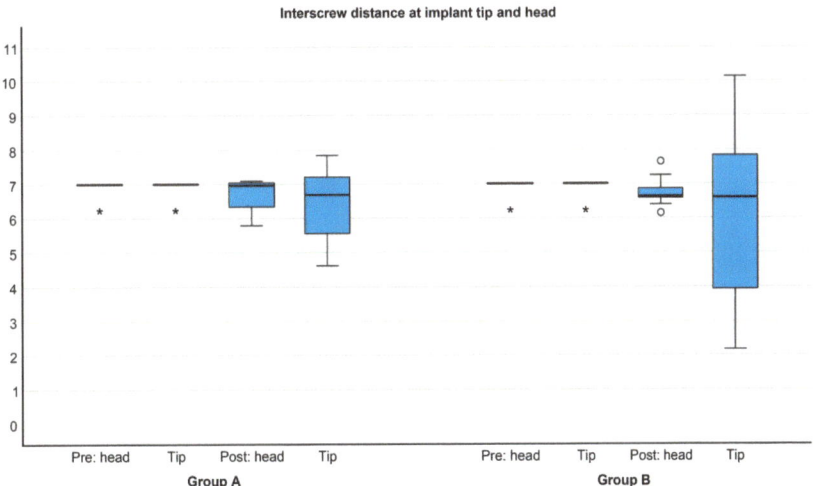

Figure 4. Interscrew distance (mm) measured at the implant tip and head levels pre- and postoperatively in Groups A and B. Preoperatively, in both groups, at least 50% had an interscrew distance of 7 mm, and all other measurements were detected as extreme outliers (*). The postoperative dispersion was larger and less symmetrical for tip measurements compared to measurements at the OMI head. Two mild outliers (°) were detected in the measurement group "post head".

Table 1. Interscrew distances (mm) measured at the implant head and implant tip pre- and postsurgically (*: t-test for independent samples).

Interscrew Distance		Min	Max	Mean	SD (+/−)	Sign. p *
Head pre	Group A	6.00	7.00	6.83	0.39	$p = 0.557$
	Group B	6.00	7.00	6.92	0.29	
Tip pre	Group A	6.00	7.00	6.83	0.39	$p = 0.557$
	Group B	6.00	7.00	6.92	0.29	
Head post	Group A	5.78	7.09	6.71	0.46	$p = 0.895$
	Group B	6.13	7.64	6.74	0.39	
Tip post	Group A	4.61	7.83	6.41	1.10	$p = 0.719$
	Group B	2.16	10.12	6.12	2.57	

As presented in Table 2, the mean deviations between virtual and actual implant positions were higher in Group B for both OMIs, both at the level of the implant tip and head. These differences were statistically significant for the right OMI at the level of the implant head (0.90 ± 0.37 mm) and for the left OMI, both at the head level (0.96 ± 0.46 mm) and the implant tip (1.43 ± 0.82 mm).

Table 2. Deviations (mm) between virtual and real implant positions measured at the implant head and implant tip (*: *t*-test for independent samples; significant differences are shown in bold text).

Deviation Pre–Post		Min	Max	Mean	SD (+/−)	Sign. *p* *
Right OMI head	Group A	0.05	1.11	0.60	0.31	*p* = 0.003
	Group B	0.25	1.59	0.90	0.37	
Right OMI tip	Group A	0.18	2.05	0.87	0.43	*p* = 0.091
	Group B	0.20	3.34	1.17	0.76	
Left OMI head	Group A	0.24	1.14	0.56	0.28	*p* = 0.001
	Group B	0.18	1.83	0.96	0.46	
Left OMI tip	Group A	0.27	2.22	0.87	0.55	*p* = 0.008
	Group B	0.56	3.96	1.43	0.82	

Significant statistical differences were also observed for vertical deviations measured at the implant head (right OMI: $p = 0.002$; left OMI: $p < 0.001$). In Group A, the planned insertion depth of the implants (−0.17 mm) could not be achieved, whereas in Group B, the performed insertion was deeper (+0.65 mm) than planned.

In terms of transverse angular deviations between right and left OMIs for Groups A and B, Group A demonstrated significantly higher implant axis accuracy (4.81° ± 4.09°; $p = 0.028$). However, no statistical difference was found for sagittal angular deviations ($p = 0.929$), with mean angular deviations of 6.42° ± 2.26° in Group A and 5.10° ± 2.20° in Group B.

Figure 5 illustrates the comparisons among Groups A, B, and C for sagittal and transverse angular deviations between right and left mini-implants. Transverse angular deviations were significantly less accurate in Group B than in the other groups ($p = 0.003$), whereas sagittal angular deviations were significantly higher in Group C than in the other groups ($p = 0.007$).

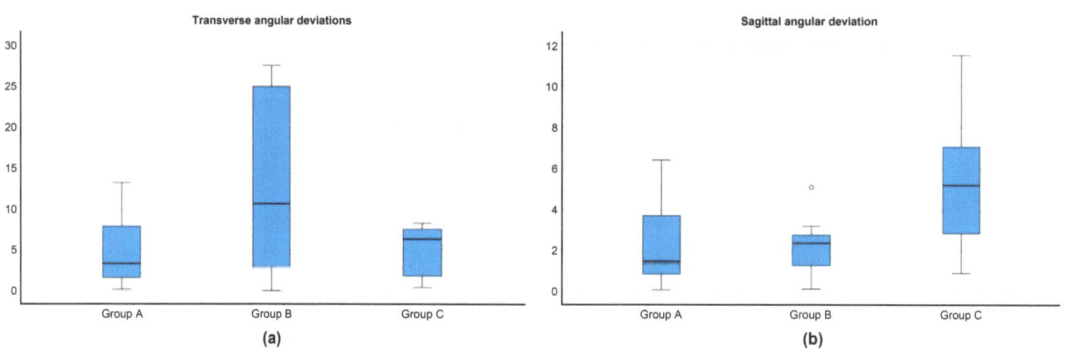

Figure 5. Comparison of transfer accuracy among Groups A, B, and C: (**a**) transverse angular deviations; (**b**) sagittal angular deviations. One mild outlier (°) was detected for sagittal angular deviations in Group B.

4. Discussion

The primary focus of this study was to compare guided miniscrew insertion using the applied digital workflow. The goal was to assess the accuracy and reliability of the virtual planning process with two different types of insertion guides and compare it to a control group with conventional freehand OMI insertion. Although Group A demonstrated better results, significant differences were found for all methods (Table 1; Figure 5). Deviations from the digitally planned positions were mostly within tenths of millimeters, and axial deviations were generally smaller than six degrees.

In contemporary dentistry, 3D imaging has become integral to various dental disciplines [16]. Intraoral surface scans have replaced conventional impressions owing to their increased precision, and CBCTs provide 3D radiologic information with lower radiation doses compared with computed tomographies [17]. The use of intraoral surface scans allows for the creation of precise surface models of teeth and gums, which streamline workflows. Research over recent years has shown that digital workflows in dentistry are at least as precise and effective as traditional methods [18].

CBCTs have become an essential diagnostic tool, especially in surgical dentistry, as they accurately display the 3D shape and position of teeth and jaw bones [19]. Cephalometric X-rays, routinely used in orthodontic practice, have limitations as they are two-dimensional (2D) projections of 3D anatomical structures, resulting in image distortion and overlapping of bilateral structures [20]. Owing to the low radiation dose and excellent spatial resolution of CBCTs, dentists can improve diagnosis and use the additional information for treatment planning.

The anterior palate has become a favored insertion site for OMIs owing to the abundance of cortical bone and available attached gingiva [21]. Studies, such as that of Jung et al. [22], have shown that lateral cephalometry provides a reliable assessment of the quantity of vertical bone for paramedian TAD insertion. In the present study, 3D imaging was used for accuracy measurements and to evaluate interferences with surrounding anatomical structures. However, in the clinical routine, an approach such as that of Maino et al. [23], which merges lateral cephalograms and digital dental models to plan and produce surgical guides, might be sufficient. Using lateral cephalograms comes with lower costs and reduced radiation exposure [23], and these 2D X-rays remain part of the basic radiological investigation and represent the gold standard of imaging in patients undergoing orthodontic therapy [22].

Previous studies have investigated various insertion guides, concluding that their use improves TAD insertion accuracy and stability while reducing the failure rate of mini-implants [5,10,12,13,24–29]. Tooth-supported guides, rigidly printed and supported on the edges of teeth, were found to ensure higher insertion precision compared with solely gingiva-supported templates [5,12]. Based on these findings, we chose to investigate only tooth-supported guides. Our measurements were performed following the approach of Casetta et al. [24], which involves comparing pre- and postsurgical CBCTs to calculate angular, coronal, and apical deviations between virtually planned and actual OMI positions.

CAD/CAM appliance design relies on virtually planned TAD positions provided by insertion guides, leading to a simplified and improved collaboration with the laboratory, a faster workflow, and more predictable appliances. The simultaneous digital manufacturing of the insertion guide and the superstructure enables a one-visit protocol for the insertion of mini-implants and orthodontic appliances [30,31]. However, achieving accurate TAD insertion is crucial for a successful one-visit protocol [32], particularly when an increased number of miniscrews and a more rigid orthodontic appliance are required. Exceeding a certain tolerance level for angular deviations may necessitate a two-step protocol [33]. Minor errors in the digital workflow or during clinical implementation can accumulate and result in deviations of the mini-implants, potentially leading to misfit of the prepared appliance. Factors such as the coronal distance of the OMIs, insertion depth, apical distance, and the angle between the two TADs are relevant in this context [13]. The direction of the deviation may also play a role, as TAD deviations can potentially compensate for each other in some favorable cases [14]. A systematic review investigating the accuracy of surgical guides for dental implantology found mean angular deviations of 3.5° and mean vertical deviations of 1.2 and 1.4 mm at the implant head and implant tip, respectively, which were deemed clinically acceptable [34].

Although freehand insertion is generally safe and accurate [35], when planning a TAD-supported orthodontic appliance, a second visit becomes necessary because the exact positions of the OMIs cannot be predefined.

Comparing workflows with and without surgical templates, similar interscrew parallelism can be achieved. It has been shown that OMIs may not remain absolutely stationary and can experience angular displacements up to 11° per OMI due to orthodontic loading [36]. Thus, even if TADs were initially parallel, they may not remain parallel throughout the entire treatment.

The deviation in insertion depth found in our study aligns with the findings of Kniha et al. [5], who attributed this effect to the resilient properties of silicone. The vertical inaccuracies observed in our study may be related to the difference in rigidity between the surgical guides in Group B and those in Group A. The in-house-produced guides in Group B might have been less rigid, resulting in deeper insertion, whereas the other guides were more rigid, making it impossible to reach the final insertion depth. Different printing settings and offsets between the two groups could also contribute to these variations. Tissue rigidity is unlikely to have been relevant in this study, as all guides were designed to be tooth-supported. The fit of the insertion guides in Group A appeared superior, possibly due to their more pronounced extension to the buccal tooth surface compared with Group B, whereas the in-house-produced guides sometimes appeared to lack reliable stability and did not stay in place without the assistance of fixation.

Comparing our study to others is challenging owing to the heterogeneity of reference points and measurement methods among published studies. Differences in anatomical areas, study protocols, and measurement techniques make direct comparisons difficult [9,10,12,14,37].

Despite promising results, this study has limitations. First, the use of embalmed cadaver heads with preserved tissue may not fully represent the real clinical situation, as blood perfusion is lacking, tissue quality and properties change after preservation [5], and bone remodeling is absent [38]. Second, the age difference between the body donors, elderly individuals with multiple missing or filled teeth and even dental implants or prostheses, and the typical orthodontic clientele, mostly adolescents or young adults with complete dentition, is also a limitation [39]. Third, artefacts caused by prosthetic restorations in the cadavers' CBCT datasets could have influenced superimposition accuracy. The sample size is another limitation of this study, as n = 12 would have been ideal for all three investigation groups. Unfortunately, insufficient appropriate body donors were available at the time of this study. Hence, we opted for n = 8 for Group C, viewing it as an additional group, with groups A and B as the main investigation groups. Finally, hard and soft tissue behavior in the body donors might differ from that in a real clinical situation.

To date, few studies have investigated the transfer accuracy of guided OMI insertion using postoperative CBCTs. To the best of our knowledge, only two such studies have been conducted in a clinical setting. Casetta et al. [24] performed a clinical study comparing presurgical and postsurgical CBCTs of five patients receiving palatal OMIs, whereas Liu et al. [40] investigated surgical guides for interradicular OMI insertion using CT scans. Kniha et al. [5] used presurgical lateral cephalograms and postoperative CBCTs in a body donor study. Bae et al. [10] conducted another cadaver study to examine the transfer accuracy of insertion guides for interradicular OMI placement using CBCTs. To avoid possible sequelae of radiation exposure to living participants, the current study followed this precedent and limited the analysis to embalmed specimens. The next step would be a clinical study examining the precision of surgical guides, ideally incorporating alternative imaging methodologies with reduced radiation exposure. CBCT-based investigations of transfer accuracy are clinically relevant as scanbody measurements focus on the oral portion, which may lead to incomplete data regarding the orientation of the implant tip. Precise visualization of the implant tip is crucial for avoiding damage to adjacent anatomical structures in clinical settings.

Although many studies have investigated the accuracy of guided OMI insertion and deemed deviations clinically acceptable, no maximum tolerance level has been defined for deviations in one-visit protocols. Further studies are needed to investigate the required accuracy for simultaneous installation of OMIs and TAD-based appliances and to establish clear tolerance limits for individually manufactured appliance insertion.

5. Conclusions

CBCT has become a vital imaging tool in dentistry. Although guided OMI insertion shows slight deviations, it remains an accurate and safe method that is widely used in daily clinical practice. The ability to apply a one-visit protocol is a major advantage of digitally planned insertion guides over freehanded TAD insertion. However, achieving 100% accuracy in delivering the planned TAD position is not always possible. Our study found that treatment results were more reliable using commercially available insertion guides compared with in-house self-fabricated insertion guides, making the former the recommended choice when insertion guides are indicated.

Author Contributions: L.S.: Conceptualization, Methodology, Investigation, Data curation, Formal analysis, Writing—original draft preparation, Visualization, Project Administration. B.K.: Conceptualization, Methodology, Investigation, Data curation, Formal analysis, Writing—review and editing, Supervision, Visualization. B.W.: Conceptualization, Methodology, Investigation, Writing—review and editing, Supervision, Project administration. N.J.: Conceptualization, Methodology, Writing—review and editing, Supervision. M.P.: Conceptualization, Methodology, Writing—review and editing, Supervision. F.W.: Conceptualization, Methodology, Writing—review and editing, Supervision. V.A.: Conceptualization, Methodology, Writing—review and editing. All authors have read and agreed to the published version of the manuscript.

Funding: This research received no external funding, but Forestadent Bernhard Förster GmbH (Pforzheim, Germany) provided all TADs (n = 64; 1.7 × 8 mm; OrthoEasy® Pal) and surgical templates (n = 12; Accuguides®).

Institutional Review Board Statement: The current study was conducted according to the guidelines of the Declaration of Helsinki. Ethical approval was obtained from the ethics committee of the Medical University of Graz (Review Board Number: 32-550 ex 19/20).

Informed Consent Statement: During their lifetime, the donors provided permission for their bodies to be used for research and educational purposes.

Data Availability Statement: The data that support the findings of this study are available from the corresponding author upon reasonable request. The data are not publicly available owing to ethical restrictions.

Acknowledgments: The authors would like to thank Irene Mischak for the statistical analysis and Niels Hammer (Division of Macroscopic and Clinical Anatomy, Medical University of Graz) for his collaboration.

Conflicts of Interest: The authors declare no conflict of interest.

References

1. Gainsforth, B.L.; Higley, L.B. A study of orthodontic anchorage possibilities in basal bone. *Am. J. Orthod. Oral Surg.* **1945**, *31*, 406–417. [CrossRef]
2. Antoszewska-Smith, J.; Sarul, M.; Łyczek, J.; Konopka, T.; Kawala, B. Effectiveness of orthodontic miniscrew implants in anchorage reinforcement during en-masse retraction: A systematic review and meta-analysis. *Am. J. Orthod. Dentofac. Orthop.* **2017**, *151*, 440–455. [CrossRef] [PubMed]
3. Baumgaertel, S. Temporary skeletal anchorage devices: The case for miniscrews. *Am. J. Orthod. Dentofac. Orthop.* **2014**, *145*, 558–564. [CrossRef] [PubMed]
4. Kravitz, N.D.; Kusnoto, B. Risks and complications of orthodontic miniscrews. *Am. J. Orthod. Dentofac. Orthop.* **2007**, *131*, 43–51. [CrossRef] [PubMed]
5. Kniha, K.; Brandt, M.; Bock, A.; Modabber, A.; Prescher, A.; Hölzle, F.; Danesh, G.; Möhlhenrich, S.C. Accuracy of fully guided orthodontic mini-implant placement evaluated by cone-beam computed tomography: A study involving human cadaver heads. *Clin. Oral Investig.* **2021**, *25*, 1299–1306. [CrossRef] [PubMed]
6. Francisco, I.; Ribeiro, M.P.; Marques, F.; Travassos, R.; Nunes, C.; Pereira, F.; Caramelo, F.; Paula, A.B.; Vale, F. Application of three-dimensional digital technology in orthodontics: The state of the art. *Biomimetics* **2022**, *7*, 23. [CrossRef] [PubMed]
7. Buser, D.; Sennerby, L.; De Bruyn, H. Modern implant dentistry based on osseointegration: 50 years of progress, current trends and open questions. *Periodontol. 2000* **2017**, *73*, 7–21. [CrossRef] [PubMed]
8. Willmann, J.H.; Wilmes, B.; Chhatwani, S.; Drescher, D. Klinische Anwendung des digitalen Workflows am Beispiel von Mini-Implantaten. *Inf. Aus Orthod. Kieferorthopädie* **2020**, *52*, 121–127. [CrossRef]

9. Iodice, G.; Nanda, R.; Drago, S.; Repetto, L.; Tonoli, G.; Silvestrini-Biavati, A.; Migliorati, M. Accuracy of direct insertion of TADs in the anterior palate with respect to a 3D-assisted digital insertion virtual planning. *Orthod. Craniofac. Res.* **2021**, *25*, 192–198. [CrossRef]
10. Bae, M.-J.; Kim, J.-Y.; Park, J.-T.; Cha, J.-Y.; Kim, H.-J.; Yu, H.-S.; Hwang, C.-J. Accuracy of miniscrew surgical guides assessed from cone-beam computed tomography and digital models. *Am. J. Orthod. Dentofac. Orthop.* **2013**, *143*, 893–901. [CrossRef]
11. Wilmes, B.; Vasudavan, S.; Drescher, D. CAD–CAM-fabricated mini-implant insertion guides for the delivery of a distalization appliance in a single appointment. *Am. J. Orthod. Dentofac. Orthop.* **2019**, *156*, 148–156. [CrossRef] [PubMed]
12. Möhlhenrich, S.C.; Brandt, M.; Kniha, K.; Prescher, A.; Hölzle, F.; Modabber, A.; Wolf, M.; Peters, F. Accuracy of orthodontic mini-implants placed at the anterior palate by tooth-borne or gingiva-borne guide support: A cadaveric study. *Clin. Oral Investig.* **2019**, *23*, 4425–4431. [CrossRef] [PubMed]
13. Ludwig, B.; Krause, L.; Venugopal, A. Accuracy of sterile and nonsterile CAD/CAM insertion guides for orthodontic mini-implants. *Front. Dent. Med.* **2022**, *3*, 768103. [CrossRef]
14. Pozzan, L.; Migliorati, M.; Dinelli, L.; Riatti, R.; Torelli, L.; Di Lenarda, R.; Contardo, L. Accuracy of the digital workflow for guided insertion of orthodontic palatal TADs: A step-by-step 3D analysis. *Prog. Orthod.* **2022**, *23*, 27. [CrossRef] [PubMed]
15. Thiel, W. Supplement to the conservation of an entire cadaver according to W. Thiel. *Ann. Anat.* **2002**, *184*, 267–269. [CrossRef] [PubMed]
16. Costalos, P.A.; Sarraf, K.; Cangialosi, T.J.; Efstratiadis, S. Evaluation of the accuracy of digital model analysis for the American Board of Orthodontics objective grading system for dental casts. *Am. J. Orthod. Dentofac. Orthop.* **2005**, *128*, 624–629. [CrossRef] [PubMed]
17. Qiu, L.; Haruyama, N.; Suzuki, S.; Yamada, D.; Obayashi, N.; Kurabayashi, T.; Moriyama, K. Accuracy of orthodontic miniscrew implantation guided by stereolithographic surgical stent based on cone-beam CT-derived 3D images. *Angle Orthod.* **2012**, *82*, 284–293. [CrossRef] [PubMed]
18. Vandenberghe, B. The crucial role of imaging in digital dentistry. *Dent. Mater.* **2020**, *36*, 581–591. [CrossRef]
19. Lin, H.H.; Chiang, W.C.; Lo, L.J.; Hsu, S.S.; Wang, C.H.; Wan, S.Y. Artifact-resistant superimposition of digital dental models and cone-beam computed tomography images. *J. Oral Maxillofac. Surg.* **2013**, *71*, 1933–1947. [CrossRef]
20. Dot, G.; Rafflenbeul, F.; Salmon, B. Voxel-based superimposition of cone beam CT scans for orthodontic and craniofacial follow-up: Overview and clinical implementation. *Int. Orthod.* **2020**, *18*, 739–748. [CrossRef]
21. Ludwig, B.; Glasl, B.; Bowman, S.J.; Wilmes, B.; Kinzinger, G.S.; Lisson, J.A. Anatomical guidelines for miniscrew insertion: Palatal sites. *J. Clin. Orthod.* **2011**, *45*, 433–441; quiz 467. [PubMed]
22. Jung, B.A.; Wehrbein, H.; Heuser, L.; Kunkel, M. Vertical palatal bone dimensions on lateral cephalometry and cone-beam computed tomography: Implications for palatal implant placement. *Clin. Oral. Implant. Res.* **2011**, *22*, 664–668. [CrossRef] [PubMed]
23. Maino, B.G.; Paoletto, E.; Lombardo, L., 3rd; Siciliani, G. A three-dimensional digital insertion guide for palatal miniscrew placement. *J. Clin. Orthod.* **2016**, *50*, 12–22. [PubMed]
24. Cassetta, M.; Altieri, F.; Di Giorgio, R.; Barbato, E. Palatal orthodontic miniscrew insertion using a CAD-CAM surgical guide: Description of a technique. *Int. J. Oral Maxillofac. Surg.* **2018**, *47*, 1195–1198. [CrossRef] [PubMed]
25. Kirnbauer, B.; Rugani, P.; Santigli, E.; Tepesch, P.; Ali, K.; Jakse, N. Fully guided placement of orthodontic miniscrews—A technical report. *Australas. Orthod. J.* **2019**, *35*, 71–74. [CrossRef]
26. Suzuki, E.Y.; Suzuki, B. Accuracy of miniscrew implant placement with a 3-dimensional surgical guide. *J. Oral Maxillofac. Surg.* **2008**, *66*, 1245–1252. [CrossRef]
27. Miyazawa, K.; Kawaguchi, M.; Tabuchi, M.; Goto, S. Accurate pre-surgical determination for self-drilling miniscrew implant placement using surgical guides and cone-beam computed tomography. *Eur. J. Orthod.* **2010**, *32*, 735–740. [CrossRef] [PubMed]
28. Su, L.; Song, H.; Huang, X. Accuracy of two orthodontic mini-implant templates in the infrazygomatic crest zone: A prospective cohort study. *BMC Oral Health* **2022**, *22*, 252. [CrossRef]
29. Jedliński, M.; Janiszewska-Olszowska, J.; Mazur, M.; Ottolenghi, L.; Grocholewicz, K.; Galluccio, G. Guided insertion of temporary anchorage device in form of orthodontic titanium miniscrews with customized 3d templates—A systematic review with meta-analysis of clinical studies. *Coatings* **2021**, *11*, 1488. [CrossRef]
30. Graf, S.; Cornelis, M.A.; Hauber Gameiro, G.; Cattaneo, P.M. Computer-aided design and manufacture of hyrax devices: Can we really go digital? *Am. J. Orthod. Dentofac. Orthop.* **2017**, *152*, 870–874. [CrossRef]
31. Wilhelmy, L.; Willmann, J.H.; Tarraf, N.E.; Wilmes, B.; Drescher, D. Maxillary space closure using a digital manufactured Mesialslider in a single appointment workflow. *Korean J. Orthod.* **2022**, *52*, 236–245. [CrossRef] [PubMed]
32. Wilmes, B.; Vasudavan, S.; Drescher, D. Maxillary molar mesialization with the use of palatal mini-implants for direct anchorage in an adolescent patient. *Am. J. Orthod. Dentofac. Orthop.* **2019**, *155*, 725–732. [CrossRef] [PubMed]
33. Perinetti, G.; Tonini, P.; Bruno, A. Inserzione guidata di miniviti ortodontiche: Il sistema di pianificazione 'REPLICA'. *Il Nuovo Lab Odontotec.* **2020**, *5*, 23–33.
34. Tahmaseb, A.; Wu, V.; Wismeijer, D.; Coucke, W.; Evans, C. The accuracy of static computer-aided implant surgery: A systematic review and meta-analysis. *Clin. Oral Implant. Res.* **2018**, *29*, 416–435. [CrossRef] [PubMed]
35. Wilmes, B.; Ludwig, B.; Vasudavan, S.; Nienkemper, M.; Drescher, D. The t-zone: Median vs. paramedian insertion of palatal mini-implants. *J. Clin. Orthod.* **2016**, *50*, 543–551. [PubMed]

36. Migliorati, M.; De Mari, A.; Annarumma, F.; Aghazada, H.; Battista, G.; Campobasso, A.; Menini, M.; Giudice, A.L.; Cevidanes, L.H.S.; Drago, S. Three-dimensional analysis of miniscrew position changes during bone-borne expansion in young and late adolescent patients. *Prog. Orthod.* **2023**, *24*, 20. [CrossRef] [PubMed]
37. Vasoglou, G.; Stefanidaki, I.; Apostolopoulos, K.; Fotakidou, E.; Vasoglou, M. Accuracy of mini-implant placement using a computer-aided designed surgical guide, with information of intraoral scan and the use of a cone-beam CT. *Dent. J.* **2022**, *10*, 104. [CrossRef]
38. Bourassa, C.; Hosein, Y.K.; Pollmann, S.I.; Galil, K.; Bohay, R.N.; Holdsworth, D.W.; Tassi, A. In-vitro comparison of different palatal sites for orthodontic miniscrew insertion: Effect of bone quality and quantity on primary stability. *Am. J. Orthod. Dentofac. Orthop.* **2018**, *154*, 809–819. [CrossRef]
39. Budsabong, C.; Trachoo, V.; Pittayapat, P.; Chantarawaratit, P.O. The association between thread pitch and cortical bone thickness influences the primary stability of orthodontic miniscrew implants: A study in human cadaver palates. *J. World Fed. Orthod.* **2022**, *11*, 68–73. [CrossRef]
40. Liu, H.; Liu, D.X.; Wang, G.; Wang, C.L.; Zhao, Z. Accuracy of surgical positioning of orthodontic miniscrews with a computer-aided design and manufacturing template. *Am. J. Orthod. Dentofac. Orthop.* **2010**, *137*, 728–729. [CrossRef]

Disclaimer/Publisher's Note: The statements, opinions and data contained in all publications are solely those of the individual author(s) and contributor(s) and not of MDPI and/or the editor(s). MDPI and/or the editor(s) disclaim responsibility for any injury to people or property resulting from any ideas, methods, instructions or products referred to in the content.

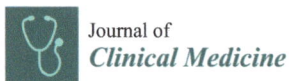 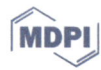

Article

Neurosensory Deficits of the Mandibular Nerve Following Extraction of Impacted Lower Third Molars—A Retrospective Study

Marcus Rieder [1], Bernhard Remschmidt [1,*], Vera Schrempf [2], Matthäus Schwaiger [2], Norbert Jakse [2] and Barbara Kirnbauer [2]

[1] Division of Oral and Maxillofacial Surgery, Department of Dental Medicine and Oral Health, Medical University of Graz, 8036 Graz, Austria; marcus.rieder@medunigraz.at

[2] Division of Oral Surgery and Orthodontics, Department of Dental Medicine and Oral Health, Medical University of Graz, 8010 Graz, Austria; matthaeus.schwaiger@medunigraz.at (M.S.); norbert.jakse@medunigraz.at (N.J.); barbara.kirnbauer@medunigraz.at (B.K.)

* Correspondence: bernhard.remschmidt@medunigraz.at

Abstract: Background: Neurosensory deficits are one of the major complications after impacted lower third molar extraction leading to an impaired patient's quality of life. This study aimed to evaluate the incidence of neurosensory deficits after lower third molar extraction and compare it radiologically to the corresponding position of the inferior alveolar nerve. Methods: In a retrospective study, all patients who underwent impacted lower third molar extraction between January and December 2019 were compiled. Therefore, clinical data as well as preoperative radiological imaging were assessed. Results: In total, 418 patients who underwent lower third molar extractions ($n = 555$) were included in this study. Of these, 33 (5.9%) had short-term (i.e., within the initial 7 postoperative days) and 12 (1.3%) long-term (i.e., persisting after 12 months) neurosensory deficits documented. The inferior alveolar nerve position in relation to the tooth roots showed apical position in 27%, buccal position in 30.8%, lingual position in 35.4%, and interradicular position in 6.9%. Conclusions: A statistically significant increased incidence of neurosensory deficits occurs when the inferior alveolar nerve is directly positioned lingually to the tooth roots ($p = 0.01$).

Keywords: third molar extraction; neurosensory disturbance; wisdom tooth removal; oral surgery; mandibular nerve; inferior alveolar nerve; lingual nerve; neurosensory deficit

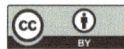

1. Introduction

The prevalence of individuals harboring at least one impacted tooth is documented to range between 18.8% and 40.5%, with lower third molars (LTMs) demonstrating the highest propensity for impaction [1–5]. Especially in people with a reduced gonial angle, and, consequently, a reduced retromolar space, there is a higher frequency of deeply impacted, horizontally positioned LTMs [6–8]. The extraction of LTMs represents one of the most frequently conducted procedures in the field of oral and maxillofacial surgery [9–13]. The indications for LTM removal encompass both therapeutic reasons, such as acute or chronic pericoronitis, cyst formation, non-restorable caries lesions, and prophylactic considerations [2,14]. Although there are rare complications, surgical site infections, pain, trismus, and three-dimensional measurable facial swelling are observed after LTM extraction [15]. However, by far the severest complication is postoperative neurosensory deficits. The anatomical variability and the position of LTMs in the posterior region of the alveolar crest near the inferior alveolar nerve (IAN) and the lingual nerve (LN) may result in a higher probability of complication occurrence compared to conventional tooth extractions, where these nerves are not in close proximity [16]. Damage to these structures is a substantial and quality-of-life-impacting complication that can arise after LTM removal [11,17]. This damage may occur due to a variety of factors, including injury to the neurovascular bundle during local anesthesia administration, as well as pressure exerted during tooth elevation or direct mechanical trauma to the nerve itself [18,19]. IAN deficits after LTM removal may manifest as hypesthesia, paresthesia, dysesthesia, or anesthesia affecting the lower lip, chin, buccal gingivae, and teeth on the affected side [20]. The documented incidence of complications to the IAN after LTM extraction exhibits a spectrum, ranging from 0.26% to 8.4% [11,21–34]. An injury to the LN, characterized by sensory deficits affecting the anterior two-thirds of the ipsilateral tongue and concurrent taste impairments, is reported with an incidence spanning from 0.1% to 22% [11,16,21,24–33,35]. However, it is imperative to distinguish between short-term and enduring sensory disturbances. Beyond the clinical evaluation of LTM, the incorporation of preoperative radiographic image analysis along with a careful surgical strategy is crucial and beneficial to prevent or minimize the aforementioned complications [36–40].

The aim of the current investigation was to ascertain the incidence of neurosensory deficits affecting the mandibular nerve (MN) after impacted LTM surgery, conducted at the Division of Oral Surgery and Orthodontics, Department of Dental Medicine and Oral Health, Medical University of Graz. In this study, particular attention was paid to assessing the relationship between the IAN and adjacent LTMs and distinguishing between short-term (7 days postoperatively) and long-term (at least 12 months postoperatively) sensory deficits.

2. Materials and Methods

First, a retrospective analysis was conducted based on preoperative radiological datasets and medical records of patients who underwent extraction of at least one impacted LTM in 2019 at the Department of Dental Medicine and Oral Health, Division of Oral Surgery and Orthodontics, Medical University of Graz. Exclusion criteria included preexisting neurosensory deficits of the MN prior to surgery and inadequate documentation. Second, a prospective evaluation of patients with postoperative neurosensory deficits was continued afterward.

The study was approved by the local ethics committee (IRB00002556, re: 33-093 ex 2012 and 33-575 ex 20/21). Patient consent was given from all participants of the clinical investigation.

All surgical procedures were executed following a standardized protocol at the University Clinic of Dental Medicine and Oral Health, Medical University Graz. First, local anesthesia was performed by a nerve block directed at the inferior alveolar nerve and the lingual nerve. In addition, depots were administered on the ascending mandible to anesthetize the buccal nerve, and submucosal depots were performed in the buccal region corresponding to teeth 37 and 47, respectively. The surgical access was made through an incision at the marginal gingiva of teeth 46 to 47, during which the dental papilla was detached. The incision was then extended from the distobuccal side of tooth 47 on the ascending mandible into the vestibule. Afterward, a freer was used to raise a full-thickness envelope flap. The retractor was employed to hold off the buccal portion of the flap, while a curved raspatorium was carefully inserted subperiosteal on the lingual side to ensure the preservation of the lingual nerve. The osteotomy was carried out with a rose bur until the crown of the tooth was completely exposed, and, if needed, the tooth was divided into pieces using a Lindemann bur. The removal of the tooth or the individual pieces was performed by means of a lever according to the leg or with surgical clamps. The wound was closed using non-absorbable sutures.

Data were analyzed from patient records and dental radiographs using the in-house computer systems Medocs (SAP, Walldorf, Germany) and Sidexis (version 4, Sirona Dentsply, Charlotte, NC, USA). All patients were examined one week after surgery, on the day of suture removal. Objective assessments including tests such as the light touch test, two-point discrimination threshold, pin-prick test, and vitality test of ipsilateral mandibular teeth were performed if subjective neurosensory deficits were reported by patients. The tests were conducted to evaluate the quality of neurosensory deficits (e.g., hypesthesia: light touch test, negative; two-point discrimination: negative; pin-prick test: positive; vitality test: positive). In cases of neurosensory deficits, follow-up examinations were conducted for a duration of 12 months after the suture removal. Incomplete recovery or persistent neurosensory deficits beyond 12 months of review were considered permanent. In cases where permanent deficits were observed, the Visual Analog Scale (VAS) ranging from zero to ten was employed to assess the pain impacting the quality of life.

Demographic data included age and sex. Radiological analysis was performed on the 2D panoramic radiographs (PR) datasets, as well as the standard dose 3D cone beam computed tomography (CBCT) datasets. PR scans were conducted using the Orthophos XG device (Dentsply Sirona, Bensheim, Germany). CBCT scans were conducted using either the Orthophos CBCT scanner (Dentsply Sirona, Bensheim, Germany) with the following parameters: 96 kV, 4.0 mA, an exposure time of 4.081 s, a field of view (FOV) of 10×5.9 cm, and a voxel size of 0.200 mm. Alternatively, the Planmeca ProMax 3D Max (Planmeca, Helsinki, Finland) with a field of view of 10.0×5.9 cm or 10.0×9.3 cm, covering a minimum of one complete dental arch, with a 200-mm voxel size (96 kV, 5.6–9.0 mA, 12 s) was employed.

The PR was used to evaluate the type of impaction (i.e., mesioangular, horizontal, distoangular, or vertical). CBCT scans were utilized to assess the positional alignment of the IAN in relation to the LTMs and to analyze their contact interactions. The position and the contact relation of the IAN relative to the roots of the LTM were defined according to Gu et al. and are provided below [36].

Class I: the mandibular canal is located on the apical side (apical position).
Class II: the mandibular canal is located on the buccal side (buccal position).
Class III: the mandibular canal is located on the lingual side (lingual position).
Class IV: the mandibular canal is located between the roots (interradicular position).

1. The mandibular third molar has no contact with the mandibular canal.
2. The mandibular third molar contacts with the mandibular canal with a complete white line.
3. The mandibular third molar contacts with the mandibular canal with a defective white line.
4. The mandibular third molar penetrates the mandibular canal.

Statistical analyses were performed using SPSS software (IBM SPSS statistics, version 27.0, IBM Corporation, Armonk, New York, NY, USA) with a 5% significance level. Chi-square tests were used for quantitative analyses. Fisher's exact tests and Chi-square tests were used to analyze categorical data. Independent Student's t-tests were applied to continuous variables.

3. Results

3.1. Incidence of Neurosensory Deficits

A total of 418 patients ($n = 418$) who underwent the surgical removal of their LTMs ($n = 555$) were included. Of these patients, 58% were female ($n = 241$), and 42% were male ($n = 177$). The age of the participants ranged from 15 to 93 years, with a mean age of 29.1 ± 11.2 years. In 51.2% of cases, the left LTM was extracted, while in 48.8% of cases, the right LTM was removed. A majority of the surgeries ($n = 399$, 70.1%) were carried out by postgraduate dentists or maxillofacial surgeons, while dentistry students conducted the remaining 29.9% of the operations ($n = 166$).

The overall incidence of acute neurosensory deficits of the MN (inferior alveolar nerve and/or lingual nerve) within the first 7 days after extraction of the LTM amounted to 5.9% (33/555). Among these cases, the inferior alveolar nerve (IAN) was affected in 2.9% ($n = 16$), while the lingual nerve (LN) was impaired in 2.2% ($n = 12$), with 0.5% ($n = 3$) experiencing combined deficits. Additionally, 0.4% of cases had an unknown area of affection. The predominant neurosensory deficit was an IAN impairment, constituting 48.5% of cases

(n = 16), closely followed by isolated LN deficits at 36.4% (n = 12). The occurrence of a simultaneous IAN and LN disturbance was rare and observed in only 9.1% of cases (n = 3). In two instances (n = 2), a neurosensory deficit was recorded in our electronic database; however, detailed information regarding the specific location of the affected nerve was lacking.

The documented characteristics of nerve deficits encompassed hypesthesia (45.4%; n = 15), paresthesia (27.3%; n = 9), anesthesia (15.1%; n = 5), and hyperesthesia (6.1%; n = 2) (Figure 1). As previously noted, detailed information on the nature of neurosensory deficits was absent in two cases. Notably, dysesthesia was not observed in any of the cases. The presence of hyperesthetic disturbances displayed statistical significance (p = 0.006, df = 3, χ^2 = 12.3).

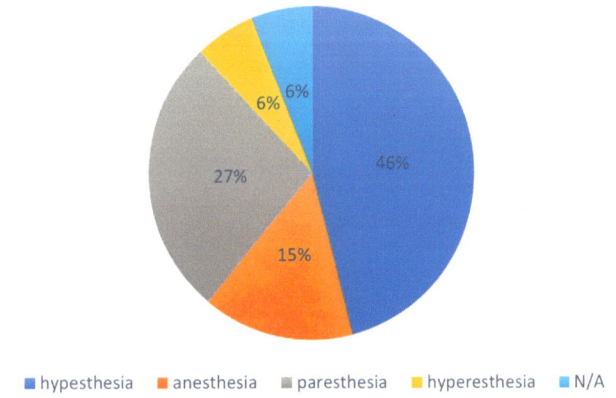

Figure 1. Quality of nerve disorder.

3.2. Type of Impaction

Using the standardized PRs, it was observed that 14.4% (n = 80) of the LTMs exhibited no angulation (vertical position). Mesioangular orientation was prevalent in 39.1% (n = 217) of cases, while 18.2% (n = 101) displayed a distoangular orientation. Furthermore, horizontal angulation was documented in 26.7% (n = 148) of the studied cases (Table 1). No statistical significance was observed concerning the association between the pattern of impaction and neurosensory deficits (p = 0.613, df = 3, χ^2 = 1.72).

Table 1. Pattern of impaction.

Angulation	n	Neurosensory Deficits
vertical	80 (14.4%)	5 (6.3%)
mesioangular	217 (39.1%)	14 (6.5%)
distoangular	101 (18.2%)	8 (7.9%)
horizontal	148 (26.7%)	6 (4.1%)

3.3. Position of the Mandibular Canal Relative to the Apex

The routine practice in our clinic does not involve the standard performance of a CBCT scan prior to LTM removal. Rather, we employ such scans selectively, guided by radiographic indicators within the PR suggesting an elevated risk of nerve injury during the extraction of the corresponding tooth. These indicators include instances of suspected contact or overlapping of structures between the LTM and the mandibular canal, alongside instances involving complex tooth anatomy or cystic lesions.

A preoperative CBCT scan was conducted in 47.2% of the surgical procedures (n = 263). Within this subset of images, the position of the IAN in relation to the tooth roots was assessed. The IAN showed an apical position relative to the tooth roots in 27% of cases (*n* = 71), a buccal position in 30.8% of cases (*n* = 81), a lingual position in 35.4% of cases (*n* = 93), and an interradicular position in 6.9% of cases (*n* = 18).

There was a notable predominance of LTM having direct contact with the IAN (84%, *n* = 221), whereas 16% (*n* = 42) of the third molars did not demonstrate this direct contact. In 21.7% (*n* = 57) the lower third molar contacted with the mandibular canal with a complete radiopaque boundary, in 32.3% (*n* = 85) with an interrupted radiopaque boundary, and in 30.4% (*n* = 80) the wisdom tooth penetrated the nerve canal (Figures 2 and 3).

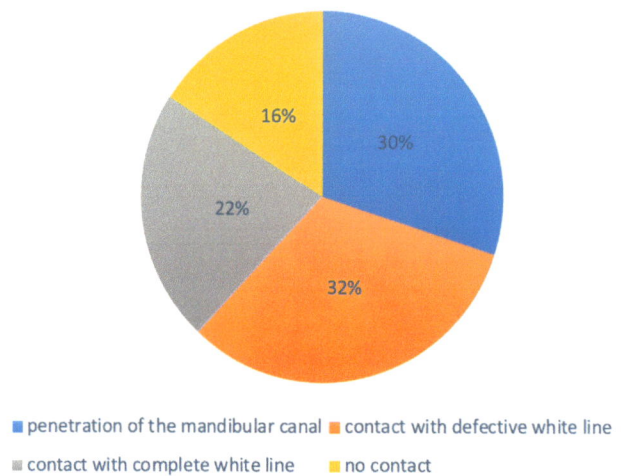

Figure 2. Contact relation of the inferior alveolar nerve canal with the wisdom tooth roots.

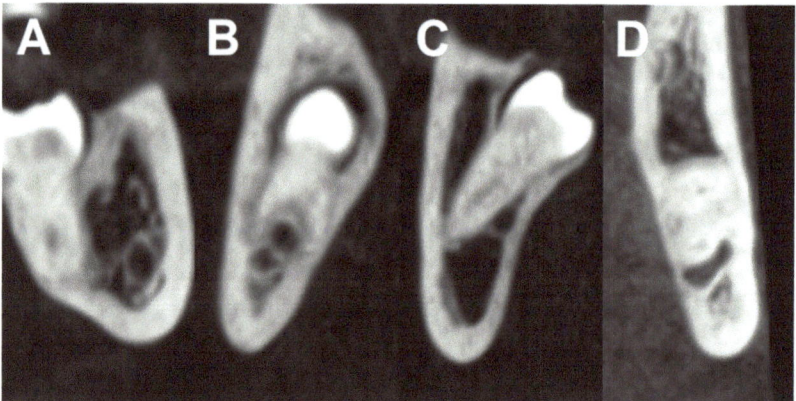

Figure 3. CBCT images illustrate the anatomical relationship between the mandibular canal and the roots of a lower third molar. (**A**) Class II/buccal: No contact; (**B**) Class IV/interradicular: Contact with a complete white line; (**C**) Class III/lingual: Contact with a defective white line; (**D**) Class I/apical: Penetration of the mandibular canal.

The incidence of IAN neurosensory deficits and the associated position of the roots of LTMs relative to the IAN were analyzed in LTMs with an available CBCT scan (16/263). It was found that those IANs having an apical position relative to the roots of LTMs, had an incidence of 0% of postoperative neurosensory disturbances. Buccal position resulted in 3.7% (3/81), interradicular position in 5.6% (1/18), and lingual position in 12.9% (12/93) in an acute postoperative neurosensory deficit. Nerve disturbance was significantly more frequent in the IANs having a lingual position relative to the roots of LTMs ($p = 0.01$, df = 4, $\chi^2 = 13.1$) (Figure 4).

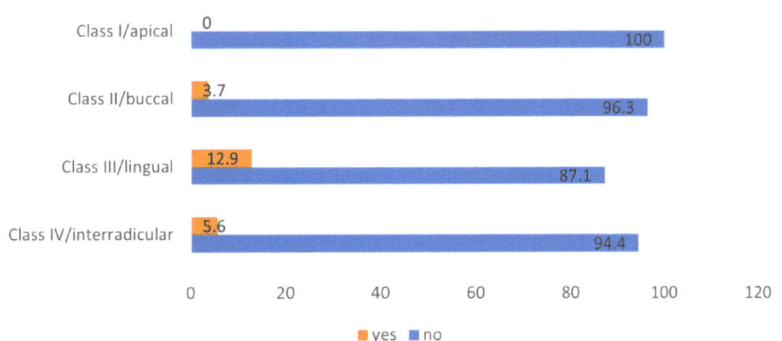

Figure 4. Relationship between the inferior alveolar nerve position and the lower third molar roots, and the occurrence of neurosensory deficits.

There was no case of neurosensory deficit when there was no contact between the LTM and the IAN (0/42) and an occurrence of 7.2% (16/221) when there was contact. However, no statistical significance could be found ($p = 0.061$, df = 1, $\chi^2 = 3.15$). Analyzing the exact contact relationships, it was noted that among the cases of nerve injuries observed, 3.5% ($n = 2$) involved the IAN making direct contact with the apex with a complete radiopaque boundary. In 5.9% ($n = 5$) of instances there was a contact with a defective radiopaque boundary and in 11.3% ($n = 9$) of the cases, the LTM exhibited a penetration of the mandibular canal. However, there was no statistically significant difference between the contact relation and the occurrence of neurosensory deficits ($p = 0.070$, df = 3; $\chi^2 = 7.06$) (Figure 5).

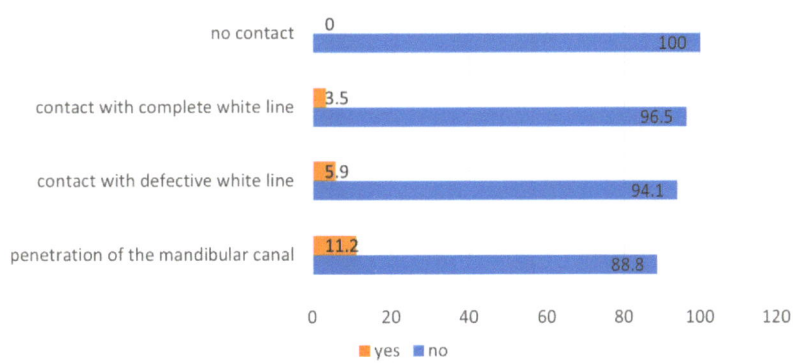

Figure 5. Contact relation and occurrence of neurosensory disorders (%).

3.4. Sex and Age

The incidence of acute postoperative neurosensory deficit of the MN in males and females was 4.6% (10/218) and 6.8% (23/337), respectively. No statistically significant difference in gender distribution was observed with respect to nerve disturbances ($p = 0.183$, df = 1, χ^2 = 1.85). The mean ages of patients who experienced MN injury were 29 ± 6.9 years old, and this was not significantly different from the mean age of 29.1 ± 11.4 years in patients who showed uneventful healing (p = 0.967, mean diff = −0.08; 95% CI [−4.94; 3.87]).

3.5. Experience of Operators

Among the surgical procedures executed by postgraduate dentists or maxillofacial surgeons, 5.9% (23/389) resulted in postoperative neurosensory deficits. Conversely, in the surgeries conducted by dental students, the occurrence rate was 6% (10/166). There was no statistically significant difference in the incidence of neurosensory deficits between the patients operated on by students and postgraduate doctors/maxillofacial surgeons (p = 0.548, df = 1, χ^2 = 0.003).

3.6. Recovery Patterns

A total of 14 out of 33 patients who experienced IAN or LN deficits within the initial seven postoperative days did not attend any follow-up appointments after the first postoperative review. This resulted in a drop-out rate of 42.4%. The follow-up period extended over 12 months, with the number of visits varying according to the performed therapy regime and therapy response.

In this study, the incidence of persisting neurosensory deficits of the mandibular nerve stood at 1.3% out of 555 removed teeth. Specifically, the IAN was affected in 0.8% of cases (n = 5) and the LN was affected in 0.5% of cases (n = 3), with no statistically significant difference detected (p = 0.705, df = 1, χ^2 = 0.14). In the cohort of patients with enduring nerve deficits, 71.4% (n = 5) exhibited hypoesthesia in the affected area, while 28.6% (n = 2) experienced paresthesia. No other sensory qualities were identified, and this outcome did not demonstrate statistical significance (p = 0.257, df = 1, χ^2 = 1.29). Employing a VAS, it was observed that none of the affected patients (0/7) exhibited permanent pain reducing their quality of life.

Therapy Regime

Five different therapeutic regimens were employed to treat acute postoperative neurosensory deficits, and the process of recovery was evaluated through objective assessments, including the light touch test, pin-prick test, and vitality test of the teeth on the affected side:

1. The combination of cortisone (prednisolone 5mg), vitamin B-complex, and low-level laser therapy was used in 26.3% (n = 5) of the cases and had a complete recovery in 60% (3/5).
2. The combination of vitamin B-complex and low-level laser therapy in 21.1% (n = 4) with a recovery rate of 50% (2/4).
3. Only low-level laser therapy in 15.8% (n = 3) with a recovery rate of 100% (3/3).
4. The combination of cortisone and vitamin B-complex in 5.3% (n = 1) with a recovery rate of 0% (0/1).
5. Only vitamin-b-complex in 21.1% (n = 4) with a recovery rate of 75% (3/4).

4. Discussion

According to the literature, the frequency of acute MN neurosensory deficit after removal of the LTM ranges from 1% to 16.3% [10–12,16,41–46]. In our study, the incidence of acute nerve deficits was 5.9% and is thereby consistent with results reported in the literature. According to Akashi et al., the majority of the affected patients suffer from hyperesthesia [10]. Concerning nerve deficits among the included patients, the IAN was affected in 2.9%, the LN in 2.2%, and a combination of both in 0.5%. The incidence of permanent neurosensory disorders of the MN after LTM surgery is reported to be approximately 1% in the majority of studies found in the literature [11,42,44,46–49]. Our study is also consistent with these findings, showing an incidence of 1.3%. Breaking down the permanent nerve deficits, the IAN was damaged in 0.8% of cases and the LN in 0.5% of cases.

Several authors found a correlation between age and a higher susceptibility to nerve disturbances following impacted LTM extractions. Bruce et al. demonstrated a significantly elevated risk of nerve deficits in patients aged 35 years or older compared to younger patients [25]. This result corresponds with the observations made by Blondeau et Daniel, who proposed that this association might be attributed to increased bone density, reduced bone elasticity, diminished healing capacity, and the completion of root formation [9]. Nevertheless, some studies refute a link between age and the risk of neurosensory deficits [11,24,28,50–52]. The findings of the current study also do not provide evidence to support the hypothesis that age elevates the risk of MN deficits ($p = 0.967$). Furthermore, as with most studies in the literature, we found no association between the gender of the participants and the incidence of nerve deficits.

The level of the surgeon's experience performing the removal of the impacted LTM has often been considered a potential risk factor for nerve deficits. Sisk et al. postulated that the likelihood of developing neurosensory deficits increases with the surgeon's lack of experience [34]. Similarly, Cheung et al. observed and reported 33 of 45 mandibular nerve deficits when a dental student performed the surgeries [11]. In contrast to the aforementioned results, our study did not find a significant association between surgeon experience and the risk of neurosensory deficits. However, this lack of association could possibly be due to the fact that more challenging cases in our department were assigned to dentists with more experience. Furthermore, students were at the operations under the strict supervision of experienced surgeons.

Analysis of the standardized PRs of all LTMs with reference to the angulation found a mesioangular impaction in 39.1% being the most frequent angulation, followed by a horizontal angulation in 26.7%. Our results report the highest incidence of nerve deficits in mesial angulated LTMs (42.4%). However, no statistical significance was found. Barry et al. showed a similar frequency distribution regarding angulation in their study but could not present a significant result of the association between angulation and nerve deficits [43]. Shiratori et al. found horizontal angulation to be the most common and described horizontally angulated LTM as having the highest risk of nerve deficits. However, no statistically significant result was found, which is in accordance with the current study [53].

In the case of 263 LTMs, we obtained a CBCT scan preoperatively. Analyzing the scans, we found the lingual position of the IAN relative to the roots to be the most frequent one (35.4%). This finding is contrary to the results of the study by Gu et al., where an apical position was observed in 88.1% of cases [36]. The difference and nearly uniform distribution of the IAN position to the root in our study may be due to the fact that when the PR showed apical root positions without contact with the IAN, no routine CBCT scans were performed.

Despite the lack of statistical significance, our study revealed a pattern in which acute postoperative neurosensory deficits manifested exclusively in patients whose LTMs were in direct contact with the IAN ($p = 0.061$). Lingually located nerves had a significantly higher risk of postoperative deficits, with a statistically significant result ($p = 0.011$). While Shiratori et al. reported comparable results, Barry et al., conversely, found an increased risk of neurosensory deficits when the nerve was located buccal or interradicular to the roots of LTMs [43,53]. According to several authors, the contact relation of the LTM and the IAN seems to be a more important nerve deficit risk predictor than the position itself [41,45,53]. It needs to be mentioned that our investigation did not identify a statistically significant difference in the incidence of IAN deficits, regardless of whether the contact between the roots and the IAN was demarcated by a complete radiopaque boundary, a defective radiopaque boundary, or a penetrating nerve ($p = 0.07$).

As mentioned, there were short-term neurosensory deficits at the LN in 2.2% and long-term deficits in 0.5% of the cases. In our department, a lingually inserted raspatorium is used to enhance visibility and protect the soft tissue. According to a meta-analysis, the incidence of transient nerve damage to the LN varies depending on the surgical technique, namely without lingual flap (1.24%), with lingual flap (2.39%), and with lingual split technique (2.44%). With regard to permanent damage, the study could not find any advantage for the use of lingual flaps or the lingual split technique [54].

Usually, neurosensory deficits recover spontaneously within the first 6 months after surgery [11,19,55–58]. However, a major challenge in the management of these neurosensory deficits is the lack of standardized treatment protocols [19]. Interestingly, it was observed that none of the patients with persistent neurosensory deficits (i.e., 12 deficits after 12 months) reported a decreased quality of life. It can be assumed that this phenomenon is due to a possible habituation effect.

Several limitations must be acknowledged in this study. First, the retrospective study design inherently carries the risk of selection bias and uncontrolled variables. Second, the absence of a standardized treatment regimen may introduce variability in patient outcomes. For example, the administration of drugs such as glucocorticoids before and after surgery could have affected the development of sensorimotor disorders. Third, the lack of standardized follow-up procedures hinders our ability to comprehensively assess the efficacy of individual treatments. Additionally, the high drop-out rate during follow-up, accounting for 42.4% of the initial cohort, poses challenges in drawing firm conclusions. In addition, there is a possibility that the MN was injured preoperatively during the administration of the nerve block. Unfortunately, the removal of LMTs near the nerve without a nerve block seems clinically impossible. To address these limitations, future studies should consider adopting a multicenter approach with well-defined and standardized treatment and follow-up regimens, thereby enhancing the reliability and generalizability of the findings.

5. Conclusions

The occurrence of neurosensory deficits at the MN after LTM surgery is relatively rare. Our results are consistent with the majority of published studies found. A lingual position of the IAN in close proximity to the LTM significantly increases the risk of nerve deficits. In this context, the use of CBCT scans appears promising as it can improve risk assessment and provide comprehensive preoperative patient information. It is noteworthy that in our study no decreased quality of life was observed in patients with persistent nerve deficits.

Author Contributions: Conceptualization, B.K., V.S. and M.S.; methodology, B.K. and M.S.; software, M.R.; validation, M.R., B.R., B.K., V.S., N.J. and M.S.; formal analysis, M.R., V.S. and B.R.; investigation, M.S., N.J. and B.K.; resources, M.R., B.R., B.K., V.S. and M.S.; data curation, M.S. and V.S.; writing—original draft preparation, M.R., B.R. and M.S.; writing—review and editing, M.R. and B.R.; visualization, M.S.; supervision, B.K. and N.J.; project administration, M.S.; funding acquisition, none. All authors have read and agreed to the published version of the manuscript.

Funding: This research received no external funding.

Institutional Review Board Statement: This study was conducted in accordance with the Declaration of Helsinki and approved by the Ethics Committee of the Medical University of Graz (IRB00002556, re: 33-093 ex 20/21 and 33-575 ex 20/21).

Informed Consent Statement: Patient consent was given from all participants of the clinical investigation.

Data Availability Statement: The data presented in this study are available on request from the corresponding author. The data are not publicly available due to privacy restrictions.

Acknowledgments: The authors would like to express their gratitude to Irene Mischak for her support in conducting the statistical analyses.

Conflicts of Interest: The authors declare no conflict of interest.

References

1. Hassan, A.H. Pattern of third molar impaction in a Saudi population. *Clin. Cosmet. Investig. Dent.* **2010**, *2*, 109–113. [CrossRef]
2. Alfadil, L.; Almajed, E. Prevalence of impacted third molars and the reason for extraction in Saudi Arabia. *Saudi Dent. J.* **2020**, *32*, 262–268. [CrossRef] [PubMed]

3. Dachi, S.F.; Howell, F.V. A survey of 3874 routine full-mouth radiographs. I. A study of retained roots and teeth. *Oral Surg. Oral Med. Oral Pathol.* **1961**, *14*, 916–924. [CrossRef] [PubMed]
4. Grover, P.S.; Lorton, L. The incidence of unerupted permanent teeth and related clinical cases. *Oral Surg. Oral Med. Oral Pathol.* **1985**, *59*, 420–425. [CrossRef] [PubMed]
5. Chu, F.C.; Li, T.K.; Lui, V.K.; Newsome, P.R.; Chow, R.L.; Cheung, L.K. Prevalence of impacted teeth and associated pathologies—A radiographic study of the Hong Kong Chinese population. *Hong Kong Med. J.* **2003**, *9*, 158–163. [PubMed]
6. Behbehani, F.; Artun, J.; Thalib, L. Prediction of mandibular third-molar impaction in adolescent orthodontic patients. *Am. J. Orthod. Dentofac. Orthop.* **2006**, *130*, 47–55. [CrossRef]
7. Barone, S.; Antonelli, A.; Averta, F.; Diodati, F.; Muraca, D.; Bennardo, F.; Giudice, A. Does Mandibular Gonial Angle Influence the Eruption Pattern of the Lower Third Molar? A Three-Dimensional Study. *J. Clin. Med.* **2021**, *10*, 4057. [CrossRef]
8. Gümrükçü, Z.; Balaban, E.; Karabağ, M. Is there a relationship between third-molar impaction types and the dimensional/angular measurement values of posterior mandible according to Pell & Gregory/Winter Classification? *Oral Radiol.* **2021**, *37*, 29–35. [CrossRef]
9. Blondeau, F.; Daniel, N.G. Extraction of impacted mandibular third molars: Postoperative complications and their risk factors. *J. Can. Dent. Assoc.* **2007**, *73*, 325.
10. Akashi, M.; Hiraoka, Y.; Hasegawa, T.; Komori, T. Temporal Evaluation of Neurosensory Complications after Mandibular Third Molar Extraction: Current Problems for Diagnosis and Treatment. *Open Dent. J.* **2016**, *10*, 728–732. [CrossRef]
11. Cheung, L.K.; Leung, Y.Y.; Chow, L.K.; Wong, M.C.; Chan, E.K.; Fok, Y.H. Incidence of neurosensory deficits and recovery after lower third molar surgery: A prospective clinical study of 4338 cases. *Int. J. Oral Maxillofac. Surg.* **2010**, *39*, 320–326. [CrossRef] [PubMed]
12. Sigron, G.R.; Pourmand, P.P.; Mache, B.; Stadlinger, B.; Locher, M.C. The most common complications after wisdom-tooth removal: Part 1: A retrospective study of 1199 cases in the mandible. *Swiss. Dent. J.* **2014**, *124*, 1042–1046, 1052–1056. [PubMed]
13. Bouloux, G.F.; Steed, M.B.; Perciaccante, V.J. Complications of third molar surgery. *Oral Maxillofac. Surg. Clin. N. Am.* **2007**, *19*, 117–128. [CrossRef] [PubMed]
14. Kunkel, M.; Becker, J.; Boehme, P.; Engel, P.; Göz, G.; Haessler, D.; Heidemann, D.; Hellwig, E.; Kopp, I.; Kreusser, B.; et al. Surgical extraction of wisdom teeth. *Mund. Kiefer Gesichtschir.* **2006**, *10*, 205–211. [CrossRef]
15. Antonelli, A.; Barone, S.; Bennardo, F.; Giudice, A. Three-dimensional facial swelling evaluation of pre-operative single-dose of prednisone in third molar surgery: A split-mouth randomized controlled trial. *BMC Oral Health* **2023**, *23*, 614. [CrossRef]
16. Kiencało, A.; Jamka-Kasprzyk, M.; Panaś, M.; Wyszyńska-Pawelec, G. Analysis of complications after the removal of 339 third molars. *Dent. Med. Probl.* **2021**, *58*, 75–80. [CrossRef]
17. Gargallo-Albiol, J.; Buenechea-Imaz, R.; Gay-Escoda, C. Lingual nerve protection during surgical removal of lower third molars: A prospective randomised study. *Int. J. Oral Maxillofac. Surg.* **2000**, *29*, 268–271. [CrossRef]
18. Krafft, T.C.; Hickel, R. Clinical investigation into the incidence of direct damage to the lingual nerve caused by local anaesthesia. *J. Cranio-Maxillofac. Surg.* **1994**, *22*, 294–296. [CrossRef]
19. Leung, Y.Y. Management and prevention of third molar surgery-related trigeminal nerve injury: Time for a rethink. *J. Korean Assoc. Oral Maxillofac. Surg.* **2019**, *45*, 233–240. [CrossRef]
20. Kqiku, L.; Weiglein, A.H.; Pertl, C.; Biblekaj, R.; Städtler, P. Histology and intramandibular course of the inferior alveolar nerve. *Clin. Oral Investig.* **2011**, *15*, 1013–1016. [CrossRef]
21. Bataineh, A.B. Sensory nerve impairment following mandibular third molar surgery. *J. Oral Maxillofac. Surg.* **2001**, *59*, 1012–1017; discussion 1017. [CrossRef] [PubMed]
22. Benediktsdóttir, I.S.; Wenzel, A.; Petersen, J.K.; Hintze, H. Mandibular third molar removal: Risk indicators for extended operation time, postoperative pain, and complications. *Oral Surg. Oral Med. Oral Pathol. Oral Radiol. Endodontol.* **2004**, *97*, 438–446. [CrossRef] [PubMed]
23. Berge, T.I.; Bøe, O.E. Predictor evaluation of postoperative morbidity after surgical removal of mandibular third molars. *Acta Odontol. Scand.* **1994**, *52*, 162–169. [CrossRef] [PubMed]
24. Brann, C.R.; Brickley, M.R.; Shepherd, J.P. Factors influencing nerve damage during lower third molar surgery. *Br. Dent. J.* **1999**, *186*, 514–516. [CrossRef] [PubMed]
25. Bruce, R.A.; Frederickson, G.C.; Small, G.S. Age of patients and morbidity associated with mandibular third molar surgery. *J. Am. Dent. Assoc.* **1980**, *101*, 240–245. [CrossRef]
26. Hochwald, D.A.; Davis, W.H.; Martinoff, J. Modified distolingual splitting technique for removal of impacted mandibular third molars: Incidence of postoperative sequelae. *Oral Surg. Oral Med. Oral Pathol.* **1983**, *56*, 9–11. [CrossRef] [PubMed]
27. Kipp, D.P.; Goldstein, B.H.; Weiss, W.W., Jr. Dysesthesia after mandibular third molar surgery: A retrospective study and analysis of 1,377 surgical procedures. *J. Am. Dent. Assoc.* **1980**, *100*, 185–192. [CrossRef]
28. Lopes, V.; Mumenya, R.; Feinmann, C.; Harris, M. Third molar surgery: An audit of the indications for surgery, post-operative complaints and patient satisfaction. *Br. J. Oral Maxillofac. Surg.* **1995**, *33*, 33–35. [CrossRef]
29. Miura, K.; Kino, K.; Shibuya, T.; Hirata, Y.; Shibuya, T.; Sasaki, E.; Komiyama, T.; Yoshimasu, H.; Amagasa, T. Nerve paralysis after third molar extraction. *Kokubyo Gakkai Zasshi* **1998**, *65*, 1–5. [CrossRef]

30. Queral-Godoy, E.; Valmaseda-Castellón, E.; Berini-Aytés, L.; Gay-Escoda, C. Incidence and evolution of inferior alveolar nerve lesions following lower third molar extraction. *Oral Surg. Oral Med. Oral Pathol. Oral Radiol. Endodontol.* **2005**, *99*, 259–264. [CrossRef]
31. Rood, J.P. Permanent damage to inferior alveolar and lingual nerves during the removal of impacted mandibular third molars. Comparison of two methods of bone removal. *Br. Dent. J.* **1992**, *172*, 108–110. [CrossRef] [PubMed]
32. Rud, J. The split-bone technic for removal of impacted mandibular third molars. *J. Oral Surg.* **1970**, *28*, 416–421. [PubMed]
33. Schultze-Mosgau, S.; Reich, R.H. Assessment of inferior alveolar and lingual nerve disturbances after dentoalveolar surgery, and of recovery of sensitivity. *Int. J. Oral Maxillofac. Surg.* **1993**, *22*, 214–217. [CrossRef] [PubMed]
34. Sisk, A.L.; Hammer, W.B.; Shelton, D.W.; Joy, E.D., Jr. Complications following removal of impacted third molars: The role of the experience of the surgeon. *J. Oral Maxillofac. Surg.* **1986**, *44*, 855–859. [CrossRef] [PubMed]
35. Valmaseda-Castellón, E.; Berini-Aytés, L.; Gay-Escoda, C. Lingual nerve damage after third lower molar surgical extraction. *Oral Surg. Oral Med. Oral Pathol. Oral Radiol. Endodontol.* **2000**, *90*, 567–573. [CrossRef] [PubMed]
36. Gu, L.; Zhu, C.; Chen, K.; Liu, X.; Tang, Z. Anatomic study of the position of the mandibular canal and corresponding mandibular third molar on cone-beam computed tomography images. *Surg. Radiol. Anat.* **2018**, *40*, 609–614. [CrossRef] [PubMed]
37. Rugani, P.; Kirnbauer, B.; Arnetzl, G.V.; Jakse, N. Cone beam computerized tomography: Basics for digital planning in oral surgery and implantology. *Int. J. Comput. Dent.* **2009**, *12*, 131–145. [PubMed]
38. Baumann, P.; Widek, T.; Merkens, H.; Boldt, J.; Petrovic, A.; Urschler, M.; Kirnbauer, B.; Jakse, N.; Scheurer, E. Dental age estimation of living persons: Comparison of MRI with OPG. *Forensic Sci. Int.* **2015**, *253*, 76–80. [CrossRef]
39. Kirnbauer, B.; Jakse, N.; Rugani, P.; Schwaiger, M.; Magyar, M. Assessment of impacted and partially impacted lower third molars with panoramic radiography compared to MRI-a proof of principle study. *Dentomaxillofac. Radiol.* **2018**, *47*, 20170371. [CrossRef]
40. Ghaeminia, H.; Meijer, G.J.; Soehardi, A.; Borstlap, W.A.; Mulder, J.; Bergé, S.J. Position of the impacted third molar in relation to the mandibular canal. Diagnostic accuracy of cone beam computed tomography compared with panoramic radiography. *Int. J. Oral Maxillofac. Surg.* **2009**, *38*, 964–971. [CrossRef]
41. Wang, D.; Lin, T.; Wang, Y.; Sun, C.; Yang, L.; Jiang, H.; Cheng, J. Radiographic features of anatomic relationship between impacted third molar and inferior alveolar canal on coronal CBCT images: Risk factors for nerve injury after tooth extraction. *Arch. Med. Sci.* **2018**, *14*, 532–540. [CrossRef]
42. Sayed, N.; Bakathir, A.; Pasha, M.; Al-Sudairy, S. Complications of Third Molar Extraction: A retrospective study from a tertiary healthcare centre in Oman. *Sultan Qaboos Univ. Med. J.* **2019**, *19*, e230–e235. [CrossRef] [PubMed]
43. Barry, E.; Ball, R.; Patel, J.; Obisesan, O.; Shah, A.; Manoharan, A. Retrospective evaluation of sensory neuropathies after extraction of mandibular third molars with confirmed "high-risk" features on cone beam computed topography scans. *Oral Surg. Oral Med. Oral Pathol. Oral Radiol.* **2022**, *134*, e1–e7. [CrossRef] [PubMed]
44. Kubota, S.; Imai, T.; Nakazawa, M.; Uzawa, N. Risk stratification against inferior alveolar nerve injury after lower third molar extraction by scoring on cone-beam computed tomography image. *Odontology* **2020**, *108*, 124–132. [CrossRef] [PubMed]
45. Ueda, M.; Nakamori, K.; Shiratori, K.; Igarashi, T.; Sasaki, T.; Anbo, N.; Kaneko, T.; Suzuki, N.; Dehari, H.; Sonoda, T.; et al. Clinical significance of computed tomographic assessment and anatomic features of the inferior alveolar canal as risk factors for injury of the inferior alveolar nerve at third molar surgery. *J. Oral Maxillofac. Surg.* **2012**, *70*, 514–520. [CrossRef]
46. Sklavos, A.; Delpachitra, S.; Jaunay, T.; Kumar, R.; Chandu, A. Degree of Compression of the Inferior Alveolar Canal on Cone-Beam Computed Tomography and Outcomes of Postoperative Nerve Injury in Mandibular Third Molar Surgery. *J. Oral Maxillofac. Surg.* **2021**, *79*, 974–980. [CrossRef] [PubMed]
47. Ghai, S.; Choudhury, S. Role of Panoramic Imaging and Cone Beam CT for Assessment of Inferior Alveolar Nerve Exposure and Subsequent Paresthesia Following Removal of Impacted Mandibular Third Molar. *J. Maxillofac. Oral Surg.* **2018**, *17*, 242–247. [CrossRef]
48. Sarikov, R.; Juodzbalys, G. Inferior alveolar nerve injury after mandibular third molar extraction: A literature review. *J. Oral Maxillofac. Res.* **2014**, *5*, e1. [CrossRef]
49. Xu, G.Z.; Yang, C.; Fan, X.D.; Yu, C.Q.; Cai, X.Y.; Wang, Y.; He, D. Anatomic relationship between impacted third mandibular molar and the mandibular canal as the risk factor of inferior alveolar nerve injury. *Br. J. Oral Maxillofac. Surg.* **2013**, *51*, e215–e219. [CrossRef]
50. Fielding, A.F.; Rachiele, D.P.; Frazier, G. Lingual nerve paresthesia following third molar surgery: A retrospective clinical study. *Oral Surg. Oral Med. Oral Pathol. Oral Radiol. Endodontol.* **1997**, *84*, 345–348. [CrossRef]
51. Middlehurst, R.J.; Barker, G.R.; Rood, J.P. Postoperative morbidity with mandibular third molar surgery: A comparison of two techniques. *J. Oral Maxillofac. Surg.* **1988**, *46*, 474–476. [CrossRef] [PubMed]
52. Valmaseda-Castellón, E.; Berini-Aytés, L.; Gay-Escoda, C. Inferior alveolar nerve damage after lower third molar surgical extraction: A prospective study of 1117 surgical extractions. *Oral Surg. Oral Med. Oral Pathol. Oral Radiol. Endodontol.* **2001**, *92*, 377–383. [CrossRef] [PubMed]
53. Shiratori, K.; Nakamori, K.; Ueda, M.; Sonoda, T.; Dehari, H. Assessment of the shape of the inferior alveolar canal as a marker for increased risk of injury to the inferior alveolar nerve at third molar surgery: A prospective study. *J. Oral Maxillofac. Surg.* **2013**, *71*, 2012–2019. [CrossRef] [PubMed]
54. Lee, J.; Feng, B.; Park, J.S.; Foo, M.; Kruger, E. Incidence of lingual nerve damage following surgical extraction of mandibular third molars with lingual flap retraction: A systematic review and meta-analysis. *PLoS ONE* **2023**, *18*, e0282185. [CrossRef] [PubMed]

55. Alling, C.C., 3rd. Dysesthesia of the lingual and inferior alveolar nerves following third molar surgery. *J. Oral Maxillofac. Surg.* **1986**, *44*, 454–457. [CrossRef]
56. Blackburn, C.W.; Bramley, P.A. Lingual nerve damage associated with the removal of lower third molars. *Br. Dent. J.* **1989**, *167*, 103–107. [CrossRef]
57. Jerjes, W.; Swinson, B.; Moles, D.R.; El-Maaytah, M.; Banu, B.; Upile, T.; Kumar, M.; Al Khawalde, M.; Vourvachis, M.; Hadi, H.; et al. Permanent sensory nerve impairment following third molar surgery: A prospective study. *Oral Surg. Oral Med. Oral Pathol. Oral Radiol. Endodontol.* **2006**, *102*, e1–e7. [CrossRef]
58. Wofford, D.T.; Miller, R.I. Prospective study of dysesthesia following odontectomy of impacted mandibular third molars. *J. Oral Maxillofac. Surg.* **1987**, *45*, 15–19. [CrossRef]

Disclaimer/Publisher's Note: The statements, opinions and data contained in all publications are solely those of the individual author(s) and contributor(s) and not of MDPI and/or the editor(s). MDPI and/or the editor(s) disclaim responsibility for any injury to people or property resulting from any ideas, methods, instructions or products referred to in the content.

Article

Relationship between the Status of Third Molars and the Occurrence of Dental and Periodontal Lesions in Adjacent Second Molars in the Polish Population: A Radiological Retrospective Observational Study

Daniel Poszytek * and Bartłomiej Górski

Department of Periodontology and Oral Mucosa Diseases, Medical University of Warsaw, 02-097 Warsaw, Poland; bartlomiej.gorski@wum.edu.pl
* Correspondence: daniel.poszytek@wum.edu.pl

Abstract: The aim of this study was to evaluate the effect of third molars on caries, external root resorption, and alveolar bone loss on the distal surface of adjacent second molars. A total of 2488 panoramic radiographs of adult Poles were evaluated. Third molars were classified, according to eruption status, into non-impacted, partially, or completely impacted, and according to angulation into horizontal, mesioangular, vertical, and distoangular. Completely impacted third molars were assigned as reference group. The odds ratios (ORs) and 95% confidence intervals for the occurrence of the above-mentioned pathologies were 1.39 (1.09–2.21), 6.51 (3.72–10.11), and 2.42 (1.22–4.09), respectively, for second molars with adjacent erupted third molars and 1.54 (1.11–2.82), 10.65 (7.81–20.19), and 5.21 (3.38–10.81), respectively, when partially impacted third molars were next to second molars. The ORs of lesions were significantly higher for horizontally and mesioangularly impacted third molars. Within the limitation of a radiological study, it might be concluded that the presence of erupted third molars is a risk factor for caries, while the presence of impacted third molars increases the risk of root resorption and bone loss on the distal surface of second molars.

Keywords: alveolar bone loss; dental caries; root resorption; molar; third; tooth; unerupted

1. Introduction

Tooth impaction is a phenomenon in which a tooth does not erupt through the gingival mucosa within the expected timeframe, specific to a given tooth group. [1] Based on radiological examination, teeth can be divided into completely impacted, when the tooth is fully surrounded by bone tissue, and partially impacted, when a fragment of the tooth is located outside the bone but has not reached the occlusal plane [2].

Third molars (M3s) are the most frequently impacted teeth in the permanent dentition of humans [3]. M3s make up 98% of all types of impacted teeth [4]. According to data, the prevalence of M3 impaction ranged from 16.7% to 66.86% [5]. A recent meta-analysis indicated worldwide M3 impaction prevalence at 24.40% [6]. The odds of M3 impaction in the mandible were 57.58% higher than in the maxilla ($p < 0.0001$). Neither sex nor population were found to significantly affect the frequency of M3 impaction. Mesioangular impaction was the most common variety (41.17%), followed by vertical (25.55%), distoangular (12.17%), and horizontal (11.06%). However, the prevalence of distoangular and bucco-lingual inclination was significantly higher in the upper I-M3 [7].

The primary reason for the retention of M3s is a deficit of space in the dental arch, resulting from evolutionary changes in the reduction in the bone base of the maxilla and mandible [8]. Less common causes of third molar impaction (I-M3) are incorrect positioning of the tooth bud, intraosseous pathologies, such as cysts or odontogenic tumors, or genetic diseases, such as cleidocranial dysplasia and ectodermal dysplasia [9,10]. The high incidence of third molar impaction makes the management of third molars an important role in public health. The retention of M3s may be asymptomatic or symptoms may occur due to troubles with eruption. Pain, swelling, trismus, and general symptoms such as fever and malaise are common reasons for patients to visit a dental office and may significantly affect their quality of life [11,12]. The literature also mentions long-term complications related to the presence of impacted third molars, which may affect not only the M3 but also surrounding tissues and teeth. Partially impacted M3s were associated with odontogenic infections, such as caries and periodontal diseases [13]. On the other hand, completely impacted M3s were predominantly related to non-inflammatory conditions, such as dentigerous cysts, odontogenic keratocysts, and ameloblastomas [14]. The aforementioned intraosseous pathologies, as well as an incorrect position of the third molar bud, may also contribute to second molar impaction. This rare phenomenon occurs in 0.03% to 0.65% of adolescents [15].

M3s may also be a factor impeding oral hygiene in the posterior areas. A high impaction rate, together with misalignment in all three spatial axes, especially in the mesial direction, causes extremely favorable conditions for the growth of oral cavity bacteria, which ultimately leads to the development of caries in adjacent second molar teeth (M2), and localized alveolar bone loss (ABL). Further development of those diseases may lead to either pulpitis or severe defects of periodontal tissues and increased mobility of M2s, thus carrying the risk of M2 loss. [16] Moreover, due to pressure exerted by eruption forces, there is a risk of external root resorption (ERR) in M2s adjacent to I-M3s, which may reach the root canal and lead to pulp inflammation and, consequently, pulp necrosis [17]. The cervical or apical location of contact points between the teeth, as well as mesioangular, horizontal, and inverted tooth inclination, were all associated with the highest risk of ERR [18,19]. A number of studies examined the relationship between the status of M3s and dental, as well as periodontal, lesions in adjacent M2s; however, to date, no systematic guidelines are available to allow for adequate predictions regarding the development of M3 pathologies, with respect to impaction status, angulation, and the comprehensive clinical picture [20]. To the best of our knowledge, the exact circumstances under which M3s should be extracted remain unclear [21].

On the basis of the available literature, we suspect that the presence of M3s increases the likelihood of caries, external root resorption, and alveolar bone loss occurring on the distal aspect of adjacent second molars. Therefore, the aim of this study was to evaluate this hypothesis based on panoramic radiographs taken among adult Poles. The null hypothesis (H_0) is that the presence and position of M3s do not raise the chances of any mentioned pathologies in M2s.

2. Materials and Methods

2.1. Patient Selection

This retrospective observational study was conducted in accordance with the Declaration of Helsinki and approved by the Ethics Committee of the Medical University of Warsaw (MUW, protocol code AKBE/291/2019). Panoramic radiographs of 2488 patients, referred to the Department of Periodontal and Oral Mucosa Diseases at MUW between January 2020 and December 2022, were evaluated retrospectively. The assessment was performed by a single examiner, who is a dental specialist in periodontology (D.P.). The minimum age for inclusion was 19 years since this is when M3s usually begin to erupt and are thus in the vicinity of M2s and might potentially affect them [22]. The upper age was not set.

Panoramic radiographs were taken in the Department of Dental and Maxillofacial Radiology at MUW. All projections were obtained using a Vatech Pax-I device (Vatech, Prague, Czech Republic, 70–85 kVp; 4–10 mA; exposure time of 9–19 s; 100.7 mGy $\times$ cm^2). The photographs were analyzed using a digital viewer (MicroDicom-DICOM viewer, MicroDicom Ltd., Sofia, Bulgaria, microdicom.com (accessed on 18 December 2023). The exclusion criteria applied to the panoramic radiographs are included in Table 1.

Table 1. Exclusion criteria for panoramic radiographs and dental quadrants.

Exclusion Criteria for Radiograph/Quadrant	Justification
Age < 18 years old	Eruption process of M3s usually starts later
Intraosseous and craniofacial disorders	Risk of misdiagnosing pathologies
Craniofacial trauma (e.g., fractures)	Risk of misdiagnosing pathologies
Patient undergoing orthodontic treatment	Risk of misdiagnosing pathologies
Artifacts or insufficient quality of a radiograph	Risk of misdiagnosing pathologies
M3 root formation below two-thirds of the expected length	Large potential of M3s to erupt in a proper position
Quadrant without an M2	No possibility to assess pathologies in M2s
Quadrant with an M2 being restored with a prosthetic crown	No possibility to assess which aspect of an M2 was damaged by caries
Quadrant with an M2 or M3 significantly damaged by caries	No possibility to assess the pathologies in an M2 or the influence of an M3

A total of 2783 panoramic radiographs were retrieved; 295 subjects were excluded on the basis of the exclusion criteria, and 2488 panoramic radiographs were accepted. Ultimately, 7912 dental quadrants were qualified for further evaluation (Figure 1). The age and sex of the patients were recorded based on the data provided in the documentation.

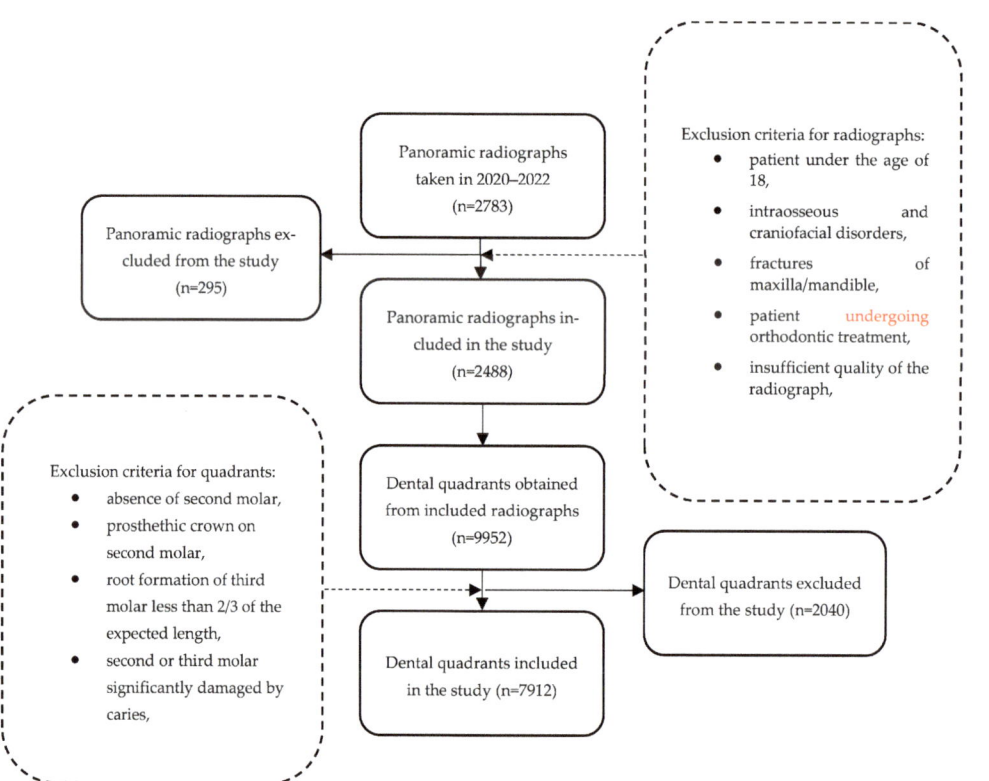

Figure 1. Flowchart of the qualification of dental quadrants.

2.2. Panoramic Radiograph Analysis

M3s were divided, according to the eruption status into (1) non-impacted (N-M3), when the tooth reached the occlusal plane, (2) completely impacted (I-M3), when the tooth was completely surrounded by bone, and (3) partially impacted M3, when the crown of a tooth was situated above the bone edge, but had not reached the occlusal plane (Figure 2) [2].

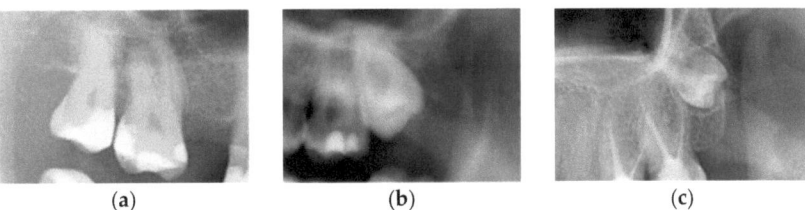

Figure 2. Third molars depending on the eruption status: (**a**) non-impacted (erupted) M3, (**b**) partially impacted M3, and (**c**) completely impacted M3.

Additionally, M3s were categorized based on Winter's classification in terms of their position in the dental arch relative to the long axis of M2s, according to the following criteria: (1) horizontal (angle between the long axes of an M2 and an M3 between 80° and 100°), (2) mesioangular (from 10° to 80°), (3) vertical (from −10° to 10°), and (4) distoangular (from −10° to −80°) (Figure 3) [23].

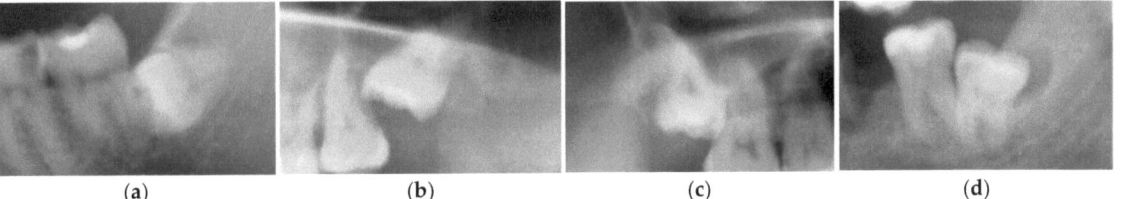

Figure 3. Third molar angulation: (**a**) horizontal, (**b**) mesioangular, (**c**) vertical, and (**d**) distoangular.

M2s and surrounding tissues were then analyzed for the presence of the following pathologies based on the guidelines by Al Khateeb et al. [24]: (1) caries on the distal surface of the tooth, described as a radiographically clear lesion with no direct contact with the crown of an M3, (2) external root resorption (ERR) on the distal surface of the root, defined as loss of tooth substance, caused by direct contact between M2s and the crown of an M3, (3) alveolar bone loss (ABL) of the alveolar process of the maxilla, or the alveolar part of the mandible distal to M2s, greater than 20% of the length of the distal root (Figure 4).

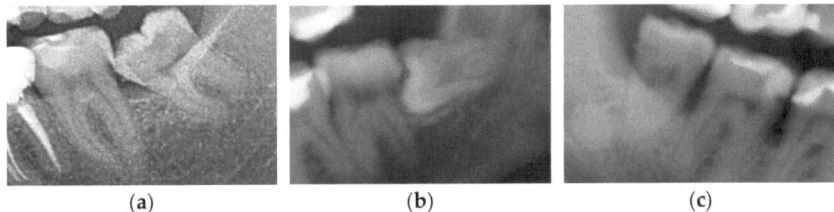

Figure 4. Radiologic view of pathologies in second molars and adjacent tissues: (**a**) caries on the distal surface of M2s, (**b**) external root resorption of the distal root of M2s, (**c**) bone loss on the distal aspect of M2s.

Only the occurrence of the above-mentioned diseases was assessed, not their advancement.

2.3. Statistical Analysis

Statistical analysis was conducted using Statistica 13.3 (Dell Technologies Inc., Round Rock, TX, USA (2016); Dell Statistica (data analysis software system), version 13.3; dell.com (accessed on 18 December 2023). Data are presented as frequencies and ratios. To evaluate the impact of M3 status on M2 pathologies, a multivariate logistic regression analysis was used. The odds ratio (OR) with 95% confidence intervals (CIs) was calculated separately for caries, ERR, and ABL. The presence of the analyzed pathologies was compared between M3s that were absent, partially impacted, and completely impacted. Moreover, the OR of the above-mentioned pathologies was assessed in relation to M3 angulation (horizontal, mesioangular, vertical, and distoangular), as well as patient age and sex. Quadrants with completely impacted M3s were used as reference groups for ORs. In the data set for logistic regression, the absence of multicollinearity was detected using the variance inflation factor method. The level of significance was set at 0.05.

3. Results

3.1. Demographic and Radiographic Findings

A total of 2488 X-rays were included in this study (1055 men and 1433 women; aged $\geq$ 19 years, mean age: 42.2 years). The exclusion criteria were applied to the quadrants, and 7912 quadrants qualified for this study. Among all 2488 subjects, 1842 participants (74.04%) had at least one N-M3, 631 participants (25.23%) had at least one partially impacted M3, and 303 participants (12.18%) had at least one completely impacted M3. With respect to the second molars, 1738 of which showed signs of distal caries, 141 had external resorption of the distal root and 1571 were diagnosed with bone loss on the distal aspect of the tooth (Tables 2–4).

Table 2. The presence of caries, root resorption, and bone loss in second molars depending on the presence or absence of a third molar.

		Caries		Root Resorption		Bone Loss	
		n	%	n	%	n	%
None		655	25.21	20	0.77	448	17.24
	Maxilla	419	28.22	16	1.08	335	22.56
	Mandible	236	21.20	4	0.36	113	10.15
Present		1083	20.38	121	2.28	1123	21.13
	Maxilla	542	20.70	74	2.83	632	24.14
	Mandible	541	20.07	47	1.74	491	18.21

Table 3. The presence of caries, root resorption, and bone loss in second molars depending on impaction or eruption of a third molar.

		Caries		Root Resorption		Bone Loss	
		n	%	n	%	n	%
Impacted		133	8.72	89	5.83	464	30.41
	Maxilla	54	7.84	51	7.40	199	28.89
	Mandible	79	9.44	38	4.54	265	31.66
Erupted		950	25.08	32	0.84	659	17.40
	Maxilla	488	25.30	23	1.19	433	22.45
	Mandible	462	24.85	9	0.48	226	12.16

Table 4. The presence of caries, root resorption, and bone loss in second molars depending on the degree of impaction of a third molar.

		Caries		Root Resorption		Bone Loss	
		n	%	n	%	n	%
Partially impacted		109	9.88	73	6.62	414	37.53
	Maxilla	43	9.70	44	9.93	184	41.53
	Mandible	66	10.00	29	4.39	230	34.85
Completely impacted		24	5.67	16	3.78	50	11.82
	Maxilla	11	4.47	7	2.85	15	6.10
	Mandible	13	7.34	9	5.08	35	19.77

The number of M3s, according to their angulation, is presented in Table 5. Vertically positioned M3s were the most prevalent in every category, followed by mesioangular M3s. Distoangular and horizontal M3s were observed in much smaller numbers.

Table 5. The number of third molars with respect to their position in the dental arch, relative to the long axis of a second molar.

	Erupted M3		Partially Impacted M3		Completely Impacted M3	
	n	%	n	%	n	%
Horizontal	6	0.16	114	10.33	48	11.35
Mesioangular	930	24.56	323	29.28	145	34.28
Vertical	2602	68.69	546	49.50	159	37.59
Distoangular	250	6.60	120	10.88	71	16.78

3.2. Multivariate Logistic Regression Analysis

The results of the analysis considering pathologies in M2s in comparison with erupted M3s are presented in Table 6. Completely impacted M3s were assigned as reference a group. All pathologies were more prevalent in the presence of both partially impacted and erupted M3s, although the ORs of carious lesions in M2s adjacent to erupted M3s in the mandible and in the maxilla and mandible altogether were not statistically significant.

Table 6. Odds ratios for caries, root resorption, and bone loss in second molars depending on the degree of impaction of a third molar.

M3 Status	Caries		Root Resorption		Bone Loss	
	OR (95% CI)	p-Value	OR (95% CI)	p-Value	OR (95% CI)	p-Value
Maxilla						
Completely impacted	Reference		Reference		Reference	
Partially impacted	1.44 (1.14–3.11)	<0.0001	9.43 (5.31–12.32)	<0.0001	5.32 (3.11–8.91)	<0.0001
Erupted	1.67 (1.09–2.11)	<0.0001	6.22 (2.18–9.07)	<0.0001	1.34 (1.11–2.20)	<0.0001
Mandible						
Completely impacted	Reference		Reference		Reference	
Partially impacted	1.32 (1.11–2.09)	<0.0001	4.36 (2.82–8.91)	<0.0001	4.94 (3.61–9.49)	<0.0001
Erupted	1.45 (1.09–1.65)	0.02	6.81 (3.92–10.61)	<0.0001	3.45 (1.90–8.93)	<0.0001
Maxilla + mandible						
Completely impacted	Reference		Reference		Reference	
Partially impacted	1.54 (1.11–2.82)	<0.0001	10.65 (7.81–20.19)	<0.0001	5.21 (3.38–10.81)	<0.0001
Erupted	1.39 (1.09–2.21)	0.02	6.51 (3.72–10.11)	<0.0001	2.42 (1.22–4.09)	<0.0001

Table 7 presents the ORs for caries, ERR, and ABL with respect to the angulation of M3s relative to the long axis of adjacent M2s. The risk of occurrence of every above-mentioned pathology was higher when M3s were placed either horizontally or mesioangularly. Moreover, vertically positioned M3s showed higher ORs for ERR in comparison with the ORs when an M3 was absent.

Table 7. Odds ratios for caries, root resorption, and bone loss in second molars depending on the angulation of a third molar.

M3 Status		M3 Angulation	Caries OR (95% CI)	p-Value	Root Resorption OR (95% CI)	p-Value	Bone Loss OR (95% CI)	p-Value
Maxilla								
	None		Reference		Reference		Reference	
	Present							
		Horizontal	1.23 (1.13–1.67)	0.0021	12.31 (7.32–23.90)	<0.0001	1.28 (1.13–3.31)	0.0031
		Mesioangular	1.34 (1.21 1.74)	0.0145	3.65 (2.59–4.04)	<0.0001	1.88 (1.50–2.08)	<0.0001
		Vertical	0.76 (0.43–1.12)	0.0892	1.82 (1.21–2.45)	<0.0001	0.83 (0.61–1.25)	0.6371
		Distoangular	0.26 (0.14–0.47)	<0.0001	0.59 (0.22–0.94)	<0.0001	0.89 (0.54–1.35)	0.7311
Mandible								
	None		Reference		Reference		Reference	
	Present							
		Horizontal	1.32 (0.62–1.78)	0.0036	17.02 (3.59–23.78)	<0.0001	1.30 (1.13–1.49)	<0.0001
		Mesioangular	1.49 (1.14–1.97)	0.0097	4.16 (2.04–7.56)	<0.0001	1.26 (1.04–1.53)	<0.0001
		Vertical	0.71 (0.51–0.96)	0.0309	1.67 (1.16–2.69)	<0.0001	1.05 (0.79–2.22)	0.2441
		Distoangular	0.57 (0.12–0.84)	<0.0001	0.48 (0.23–0.71)	<0.0001	0.37 (0.12–1.86)	0.7727
Maxilla + mandible								
	None		Reference		Reference		Reference	
	Present							
		Horizontal	1.68 (1.43–2.13)	<0.0001	10.09 (5.58–19.12)	<0.0001	1.67 (1.31–2.17)	<0.0001
		Mesioangular	1.18 (1.05–1.76)	<0.0001	5.17 (2.86–9.15)	<0.0001	1.73 (1.16–2.56)	<0.0001
		Vertical	0.77 (0.67–0.89)	<0.0001	1.55 (1.44–1.42)	0.0029	0.81 (0.24–1.16)	0.3317
		Distoangular	0.34 (0.19–0.56)	<0.0001	0.40 (0.08–1.08)	0.6721	0.91 (0.68–1.84)	0.3711

The ORs for the pathologies, taking into consideration patient age and sex, are presented in Table 8. The ORs for caries and ABL on the distal aspect of M2s increased with patient age, although the ORs for ERR were not statistically significant. Moreover, it was assessed that the likelihood of ABL was higher in male patients, whereas the risk of caries was greater in female patients.

Table 8. Odds ratios for caries, external root resorption, and bone loss in relation to patient age and sex.

		Caries OR (95% CI)	p-Value	Root Resorption OR (95% CI)	p-Value	Bone Loss OR (95% CI)	p-Value
Age							
	Maxilla	1.12 (1.04–1.45)	<0.0001	1.03 (0.99–1.11)	0.04353	1.11 (1.08–1.56)	<0.0001
	Mandible	1.03 (0.99–1.13)	0.04882	0.78 (0.45–1.31)	0.328829	1.03 (1.01–1.12)	<0.0001
	Maxilla + mandible	1.05 (1.02–1.13)	<0.0001	0.98 (0.94–1.11)	0.0872	1.04 (1.02–1.07)	<0.0001
Female		Reference		Reference		Reference	
Male		0.79 (0.69–0.89)	<0.0001	0.89 (0.61–1.28)	0.5140	1.16 (1.02–1.35)	<0.0001

4. Discussion

The aim of this study was to evaluate whether the presence of M3s poses a risk of caries, external root resorption, and alveolar bone loss on the distal aspect of adjacent M2s. Based on the data obtained from panoramic radiographs, it was found that the presence of N-M3s was associated with a higher incidence of caries, while the presence of I-M3s increased the incidence of ERR and ABL on the distal surface of M2s. The ORs of dental and periodontal lesions were significantly higher for horizontal and mesioangular I-M3s. The results of our study may assist in predicting which M3s are especially likely to cause the development of the aforementioned pathologies in M2s. This, in turn, may raise awareness among dental professionals and encourage the enrollment of patients in periodic clinical and radiological prophylactic protocols.

Our findings are consistent with prior research on caries in M2s associated with retained M3s. It was implied that plaque may be undisturbed in the approximal area, which is often inaccessible to cleaning devices. Subsequently, the presence of M3s may lead to the appearance of caries on the distal surface of M2s [25]. The prevalence of caries on the distal surface of mandibular M2s, associated with a semi-erupted M3, ranged from 7% to 32% [26–32]. A large longitudinal study with a 25-year follow-up reported a relative risk ratio (RR) of 2.53, which meant that patients with erupted M3s were at 153% greater risk of caries on the distal surface of M2s in comparison with subjects missing M3s [33]. Soft tissue I-M3s had a caries RR of 0.83, whereas bony I-M3s had a RR of 1.44 in comparison with patients with absent M3s. However, the sample of the above-mentioned study was composed exclusively of male patients. European studies suggested that M2 caries may be present in approximately one in four referrals for the assessment of M3s [34]. A recent meta-analysis confirmed that the presence of mandibular M3s increased the incidence of caries on the distal surface of M2s [35]. Moreover, the risk was higher when M3s were completely erupted (class A—Pell and Gregory), rather than non-erupted (class C—Pell and Gregory) (OR 3.45) when the horizontal position was compared with the vertical (OR 9.12) and distoangular (OR 9.75) positions and when the mesioangular position was compared with the vertical (OR 7.25) and distoangular (OR 9.54) positions. The overall pooled frequency of caries was 23% among patients [34]. A subgroup analysis yielded a prevalence of 36% for mesioangular I-M3s and 22% for horizontal I-M3s. As horizontal and mesioangular M3s exhibited a greater cement–enamel distance from M2s, food retention in the region also increased, leading to cleaning issues and a higher incidence of caries on the distal surface of M2s. It was also implied that the longer the M3s were exposed in the mouth, the greater the chance of caries occurring on the distal surface of M2s [36]. Similar to earlier studies, the present study found that horizontal and mesioangular M3s were most often correlated with the presence of caries on M2s. Given the above, caries on the distal surface of M2s is an associated long-term consequence of M3 retention. Thus, numerous authors recommended the prophylactic removal of semi-erupted, horizontal, and mesioangular M3s in order to prevent the appearance of caries on the distal surface of M2s [37,38].

ERR was associated with mechanical or inflammatory factors such as dental trauma, chronic periodontitis, pressure resulting from orthodontic appliances, cysts, benign or malignant tumors, and close proximity to an unerupted tooth [39]. Previous studies analyzing the ERR of M2s due to M3s, which used panoramic imaging or apical radiographs, reported prevalence varying between 0.3% and 24.2% [24,28,40–43]. In the present study, the prevalence of ERR was 2.28% when M3s were present and increased to 6.62% in case of partially impacted M3s. However, a prevalence rate as high as 49.43% was reported in previous studies that used CBCT [27,44]. Interestingly, a Chinese study carried out with the use of CBCT reported a lower incidence of ERR (20.17%), including only M3s that were mesially and horizontally impacted [45]. It must be highlighted that image acquisition parameters, such as the voxel size, influenced the detection of ERR, which may help explain some of the discrepancies [46]. In a study by Suter et al. [18], ERR was identified in 31.9% of M2s and was slight in 30.2%, moderate in 1.4%, and severe in 0.3% of the cases. The presence of ERR was significantly associated with direct contact between M2s and M3s, the angle between M2s and M3s with a mean angle measurement of 57.10°, the inclination of M3s, and the location of contact. Mesioangular, horizontal, and inverted impaction of M3s were correlated with increased ERR on the adjacent M2s. The risk percentage for the incidence of ERR was 62.5% for inverted inclination, 54.2% for horizontal inclination, and 47.2% for mesioangular inclination. Moreover, a male predilection was found with a risk percentage of 41.4%. In contrast, no significant sex predilection was found in other studies, as well as in our study. In a recent systematic review and meta-analysis, ERR in M2s was significantly associated with contact with I-M3s and the inclination of M3s [39]. The presence of ERR in mandibular M2s was higher (38.3%) than in the upper arch (33.8%). Taking into account the inclination of I-M3s, the incidence of ERR was higher with transverse, horizontal, and mesio-angular impacted M3s, with 54.5%, 47.5%, and 44.5% occurrence, respectively. M2s in close proximity to mesio-angular I-M3s showed a 50% higher risk of ERR than with vertical I-M3s (RR 0.50). Similar to our study, the majority of the research studies did not find an association between the incidence of ERR and age.

Increased levels of periodontal microbiota in M3 regions were observed, even with very limited clinical symptoms of periodontal issues [47]. The M3 pericoronal region may provide a favored niche for periodontal pathogens in otherwise healthy oral cavities. Another study reported an increased plaque index and bleeding on probing (BOP) around adjacent M2s [48]. The presence of N-M3s was indicated as a potential risk factor for the development of periodontitis in adjacent M2s [27,28,32,49]. N-M3s were correlated with a probing pocket depth (PPD) of at least 5 mm (OR 6.7) and BOP (OR 4.0). What is more, the periodontal status of adjacent M2s was affected by age [50]. Our study indicated that periodontal risk is associated with the presence of lower I-M3s, with higher odds for horizontal and mesioangular positions. The OR was higher in males and increased with age. A recent systematic review and meta-analysis by Yang et al. [51] found that the presence of M3s, especially mandibular N-M3s, negatively affected the periodontal status of adjacent M2s. The prevalence of ABL was 32% in the mandible when compared to 19% of M3s in general. It was higher with N-M3s (25%) than with I-M3s (19%). The higher prevalence of N-M3s might be associated with significant differences in periodontal pathologies between different impaction types. All in all, 19% of M2s showed distal early periodontal defects with the presence of M3s. Moreover, the pooled prevalence for deep periodontal pockets around M2s was 52%. Subgroup analyses showed the prevalence was higher in the mandible (62%) than in the maxilla (43%). In the case of N-M3s, the prevalence of deep periodontal pockets reached 50%. A wide range of studies observed that the removal of M3s, irrespective of being N-M3s or I-M3s, contributed to improvements in the periodontal status of adjacent M2s [48,52–54]. Baseline deep PPD, as well as advanced age, led to an unfavorable prognosis. A recent systematic review and meta-analysis reported that lower M3 surgery resulted in a moderate reduction in PPD, clinical attachment level (CAL), and alveolar bone defect (ABD) [55]. At 6 months, the PPD reduction was 1.06 mm, and the remaining PPD was 3.81 mm. Based on only four studies, PPD at 12 months was 4.79 mm, meaning that the periodontal pocket did not resolve completely after surgery. Baseline PPD was strongly associated with the remaining PPD at 6 months.

It is well-known that even asymptomatic M3s frequently become diseased with increased patient age and retention time. Caries and periodontal pathologies were most frequently reported, especially in partially erupted M3s and mesially inclined mandibular M3s [19,27]. Therefore, a number of authors recommend prophylactic removal of M3s since they are often nonfunctional and strategically non-important teeth. The advantages of such management are numerous. First of all, the earlier an M3 is extracted, the lower the odds for the development of caries, ERR, and ABL, as well as pericoronitis, odontogenic cysts, and tumors in that anatomical area. Interestingly, a recent study suggested that radiographic appearance may not be a reliable indicator of the absence of disease within the M3 dental follicle; hence, attention should be paid to peri-coronal radiolucency of follicles less than 2.5 mm in size [56]. Furthermore, there is a decreased likelihood of the occurrence of complications associated with M3 eruption, such as pain, swelling, purulent discharge, or trismus, which may increase the difficulty of extraction, as well as jeopardize postoperative healing. Moreover, as M3 roots may be underdeveloped, root separation may not be required, which makes the extraction easier and less time-consuming, and carries less risk of lingual nerve damage. On the other hand, some believe that there is little evidence for the benefits of M3 removal and there is a higher chance of postoperative complications than the risk of pathologies related to I-M3s. The occurrence of those complications might depend on a patient's general health and lifestyle, the dental surgeon's experience, and the anatomy of M3s and surrounding tissues. Apart from complications typical for tooth extraction, such as alveolitis, either sicca or purulent [57], facial swelling [58], or bleeding [59], there are those highly specific for third molar surgery. Postoperative trismus results from inflammatory infiltration of the masticatory muscles, especially the medial pterygoid muscle. It may significantly limit mouth opening and food intake. [60] Inferior alveolar nerve complications are specific to lower M3 surgery and may result either from edema pressing on the nerve or trauma caused by the tooth extraction instruments. In the first case, hypoesthesia lasts a few days as the swelling subsides, while in the second case, regaining the sensory function may take up to several months. Complete loss of sensation is very rare. As the innervation of the inferior alveolar nerve extends to the lower lip, eating and speaking may be problematic. Involuntary biting of the lip is also common, resulting in deep, long-healing traumatic ulcers [61]. Oroantral connection, on the other hand, might happen after upper M3 extraction due to a lack of or extremely thin alveolar bone proper in the apical part of the alveolus. Although radiographs, especially CBCT, might be useful to predict oroantral connection, the Valsalva maneuver or assessment using alveolar curette are far more reliable methods of detecting oroantral communication. After the closure of the communication, the patients must not sneeze or cough with their mouths closed. Airplane flights and diving are also prohibited to ensure the primary healing of the wound [62]. The above-mentioned issues may have a minor or considerable influence on a patient's quality of life. It is, therefore, of vital importance to use a scientific evidence-based approach in order to establish which variables increase the prevalence of certain pathologies associated with M3s, hence justifying their prophylactic removal. Understanding the risk factors of M3 impaction will aid in determining which clinical policy is optimal for a given patient. It is also important to assess the difficulty of M3 extraction based on, among others, M3 anatomy, alignment, and surrounding structures. For example, the relation between the M3 bud and the mandibular canal must be taken into account, especially if germectomy is considered. Numerous tools are available for these situations, which may help clinicians balance out indications and risk factors [63]. Although a plethora of clinical studies on this topic have been carried out, conflicting results were often observed. This might explain, at least partially, the lack of consensus among dental practitioners. The results of our study suggest that the retention of M3s, especially when impacted in horizontal or mesioangular positions over a long period of time, may constitute a risk factor for caries and ABL and is likely to result in harm to M2s. In this aspect, our observations are in line with other reports and enforce the evidence already present in the literature [13,18,32,55]. As PPD is more likely to increase with age, M3 surgery ought to be carried out before severe periodontitis occurs in order to avoid compromising periodontal defects and significant ABL [32,55]. Moreover, the horizontal or mesioangular position of I-M3s, and the direct contact between M2s and M3s, represent a further risk for ERR [18,27].

To the best of the authors' knowledge, this is the largest study of this kind that was carried out in Central Europe and in Poland. A total of 2488 panoramic radiographs and 7912 quadrants were positively qualified and meticulously evaluated. Ratios, frequencies, and ORs of caries, ERR, and ABL on the distal surface of the adjacent M2s were depicted. On the other hand, the results of this study have some feasible limitations and should be interpreted with caution. First of all, the examination was performed only on the basis of panoramic radiographs without clinical evaluation. The disease outcomes should ideally have been assessed both clinically and radiographically. Visual characteristics of caries and periodontal disease, such as changes in the color and opacity of dental tissues, redness and swelling of surrounding soft tissues, as well as periodontal indices, such as probing pocket depth (PPD), clinical attachment level (CAL), and bleeding on probing (BOP), are necessary to ensure a correct diagnosis. Furthermore, additional factors influencing the incidence of caries, ERR, and ABL in M2s ought to be considered and analyzed. Oral hygiene, recorded in the form of a suitable index, such as plaque index or approximal plaque index, plaque retention factors, such as tooth malposition in the buccolingual direction, or soft tissue defects, as well as saliva deficiency, could all have significantly impacted the presence of the above-mentioned pathologies. Furthermore, all included patients were referred to the Department of Periodontal and Oral Mucosal Diseases at MUW, which may have introduced bias, as these patients could potentially exhibit characteristics different from the general population, such as greater prevalence of periodontal disease—this had the potential to jeopardize the diagnosis of periodontal defects in the M3 area, as they may have originated due to generalized periodontitis. All in all, the presented results may not be applicable to all populations. What is more, the use of panoramic radiographs carried the risk of not detecting all the examined pathologies correctly. A minimum 30% loss of mineral substance, such as tooth or bone, must occur to be visible on a conventional radiograph, such as a panoramic X-ray [64]. Additionally, due to the two-dimensional nature of the projection, there was a risk of overlapping the image with surrounding healthy tissues, resulting in a pathology being unnoticed. This underestimation of the prevalence of caries and ERR could constitute one of the most significant limitations of the present study. As previously mentioned, panoramic radiographs were considered a valid, although less precise method to accurately assess the pathologies in question. Numerous studies confirmed that the best method of diagnosing caries or ERR in posterior teeth is the use of periapical inter-proximal radiographs and CBCT [65]. The greatest advantage of CBCT is the possibility to evaluate the root surface of an M2 in all three planes. On the other hand, periapical radiographs are more reliable in assessing periodontal tissues, and bitewing projections help to assess carious lesions more accurately using a much lower radiation dose. Nevertheless, the decision to use panoramic radiographs was made due to their wide availability, widespread use in general dental practice, and relatively low cost. It is also important to note that the state of M3s was not taken into account in our study. Pathologies in M3s, especially carious lesions, might have had an impact on M2s and their surrounding tissues. While significantly damaged M3s were not included in our study, less developed carious lesions might have contributed to M2 status and hindered a proper diagnosis.

Further longitudinal studies are required in a variety of populations, with well-described clinical and socio-demographic characteristics of the population, to better determine the incidence and the factors that increase the risk of caries, ERR, and ABL on the distal surface of the adjacent M2 with respect to M3 eruption status and angulation. Further studies ought to be conducted to explore this topic in a thorough manner, including the examination of participants' medical history, such as general diseases, medicaments, diet, and access to dental care, as well as clinical examinations including visual assessment of caries, probing pocket depth, clinical attachment level and oral hygiene indices, supported by radiographic imaging, such as CBCT.

5. Conclusions

Within the limitations of this radiological study, it may be concluded that:

- The presence of M3s might increase the incidence of caries, ERR, and ABL on the distal surface of M2s, especially in the long term;
- Caries were more commonly associated with N-M3s, whereas the presence of I-M3s was most likely to increase the risk of ERR and ABL;
- Mesioangular and horizontal positions of I-M3s were significantly more likely to cause caries, ERR, and ABL on the distal surface of M2s.

As the current study is cross-sectional and retrospective in nature, the absence of clinical status evaluations may be considered a serious limitation. On the other hand, the careful selection of patients with detailed exclusion criteria may be regarded as an advantage.

Author Contributions: Conceptualization, D.P. and B.G.; methodology, D.P. and B.G.; software, D.P.; validation, D.P.; formal analysis, D.P.; investigation, D.P.; resources, D.P.; data curation, D.P.; writing—original draft preparation, D.P. and B.G.; writing—review and editing, B.G.; visualization, D.P.; supervision, B.G.; project administration, D.P.; funding acquisition, D.P. All authors have read and agreed to the published version of the manuscript.

Funding: This research received no external funding.

Institutional Review Board Statement: This study was conducted in accordance with the Declaration of Helsinki and approved by the Institutional Ethics Committee of the Medical University of Warsaw (AKBE/291/2019).

Informed Consent Statement: Not applicable.

Data Availability Statement: The data presented in this study are available upon request from the corresponding author.

Conflicts of Interest: The authors declare no conflict of interest.

Abbreviations

ABL	alveolar bone loss
BOP	bleeding on probing
CAL	clinical attachment level
CBCT	cone beam computed tomography
CI	confidence interval
ERR	external root resorption
I-M3	impacted third molar
M2	second molar
M3	third molar
N-M3	non-impacted third molar
OR	odds ratio
PPD	probing pocket depth
RR	risk ratio

References

1. Kaczor-Urbanowicz, K.; Zadurska, M.; Czochrowska, E. Impacted Teeth: An Interdisciplinary Perspective. *Adv. Clin. Exp. Med.* **2016**, *25*, 575–585. [CrossRef] [PubMed]
2. Shoshani-Dror, D.; Shilo, D.; Ginini, J.G.; Emodi, O.; Rachmiel, A. Controversy regarding the need for prophylatic removal of impacted third molars: An overview. *Quintessence Int.* **2018**, *49*, 653–662. [CrossRef] [PubMed]
3. Hashemipour, M.A.; Tahmasbi-Arashlow, M.; Fahimi-Hanzaei, F. Incidence of impacted mandibular and maxillary third molars: A radiographic study in a Southeast Iran population. *Med. Oral Patol. Oral Cir. Bucal* **2013**, *18*, 140–145. [CrossRef] [PubMed]
4. Hassan, A.H. Pattern of third molar impaction in a Saudi population. *Clin. Cosmet. Investig. Dent.* **2010**, *2*, 109–113. [CrossRef] [PubMed]
5. Hartman, B.; Adlesic, E.C. Evaluation and Management of Impacted Teeth in the Adolescent Patient. *Dent. Clin. N. Am.* **2021**, *65*, 805–814. [CrossRef] [PubMed]
6. Carter, K.; Worthington, S. Predictors of Third Molar Impaction: A Systematic Review and Meta-analysis. *J. Dent. Res.* **2016**, *95*, 267–276. [CrossRef] [PubMed]
7. Shaari, R.B.; Awang Nawi, M.A.; Khaleel, A.K.; Al Rifai, A.S. Prevalence and pattern of third molars impaction: A retrospective radiographic study. *J. Adv. Pharm. Technol. Res.* **2023**, *14*, 46–50. [CrossRef]
8. Krecioch, J. Examining the relationship between skull size and dental anomalies. *Bull. Int. Assoc. Paleodont.* **2014**, *8*, 224–232.
9. Mello, F.W.; Melo, G.; Kammer, P.V.; Speight, P.M.; Rivero, E.R.C. Prevalence of odontogenic cysts and tumors associated with impacted third molars: A systematic review and meta-analysis. *J. Cranio-Maxillofac. Surg.* **2019**, *47*, 996–1002. [CrossRef]
10. Lyros, I.; Vasoglou, G.; Lykogeorgos, T.; Tsolakis, I.A.; Maroulakos, M.P.; Fora, E.; Tsolakis, A.I. The Effect of Third Molars on the Mandibular Anterior Crowding Relapse—A Systematic Review. *Dent. J.* **2023**, *11*, 131. [CrossRef]
11. Bruce, D.; Dudding, T.; Gormley, M.; Richmond, R.C.; Haworth, S. An observational analysis of risk factors associated with symptomatic third molar teeth. *Wellcome Open Res.* **2023**, *7*, 71. [CrossRef] [PubMed]
12. Kiencało, A.; Jamka-Kasprzyk, M.; Panaś, M.; Wyszyńska-Pawelec, G. Analysis of complications after the removal of 339 third molars. *Dent. Med. Probl.* **2021**, *58*, 75–80. [CrossRef] [PubMed]
13. Galvão, E.L.; da Silveira, E.M.; de Oliveira, E.S.; da Cruz, T.M.M.; Flecha, O.D.; Falci, S.G.M.; Gonçalves, P.F. Association between mandibular third molar position and the occurrence of pericoronitis: A systematic review and meta-analysis. *Arch. Oral Biol.* **2019**, *107*, 104486. [CrossRef] [PubMed]
14. Rakprasitkul, S. Pathologic changes in the pericoronal tissues of unerupted third molars. *Quintessence Int.* **2001**, *32*, 633–638. [PubMed]
15. Barone, S.; Antonelli, A.; Bocchino, T.; Cevidanes, L.; Michelotti, A.; Giudice, A. Managing Mandibular Second Molar Impaction: A Systematic Review and Meta-Analysis. *J. Oral Maxillofac. Surg.* **2023**, *81*, 1403–1421. [CrossRef] [PubMed]
16. Ye, Z.X.; Qian, W.H.; Wu, Y.B.; Yang, C. Pathologies associated with the mandibular third molar impaction. *Sci. Prog.* **2021**, *104*, 368504211013247. [CrossRef] [PubMed]
17. Qu, T.; Lai, Y.; Luo, Y.; Pan, W.; Liu, C.; Cao, Y.; Hua, C. Prognosis of Second Molars with External Root Resorption Caused by Adjacent Embedded Third Molars. *J. Endod.* **2022**, *48*, 1113–1120. [CrossRef]

18. Suter, V.G.A.; Rivola, M.; Schriber, M.; Leung, Y.Y.; Bornstein, M.M. Risk factors for root resorption of second molars associated with impacted mandibular third molars. *Int. J. Oral Maxillofac. Surg.* **2019**, *48*, 801–809. [CrossRef]
19. Skitioui, M.; Jaoui, D.; Haj Khalaf, L.; Touré, B. Mandibular Second Molars and Their Pathologies Related to the Position of the Mandibular Third Molar: A Radiographic Study. *Clin. Cosmet. Investig. Dent.* **2023**, *15*, 215–223. [CrossRef]
20. Vandeplas, C.; Vranckx, M.; Hekner, D.; Politis, C.; Jacobs, R. Does Retaining Third Molars Result in the Development of Pathology Over Time? A Systematic Review. *J. Oral Maxillofac. Surg.* **2020**, *78*, 1892–1908. [CrossRef]
21. Staderini, E.; Patini, R.; Guglielmi, F.; Camodeca, A.; Gallenzi, P. How to Manage Impacted Third Molars: Germectomy or Delayed Removal? A Systematic Literature Review. *Medicina* **2019**, *55*, 79. [CrossRef] [PubMed]
22. Jung, Y.H.; Cho, B.H. Radiohraphic evaluation of third molar development in 6- to 24-year-olds. *Imaging Sci. Dent.* **2014**, *44*, 185–191. [CrossRef] [PubMed]
23. Kalai Selvan, S.; Ganesh, S.K.N.; Natesh, P.; Moorthy, M.S.; Niazi, T.M.; Babu, S.S. Prevalence and Pattern of Impacted Mandibular Third Molar: An Institution-based Retrospective Study. *J. Pharm. Bioallied Sci.* **2020**, *12*, S462–S467. [CrossRef] [PubMed]
24. Al-Khateeb, T.H.; Bataineh, A.B. Pathology Associated with Impacted Mandibular Third Molars in a Group of Jordanians. *J. Oral Maxillofac. Surg.* **2006**, *64*, 1598–1602. [CrossRef] [PubMed]
25. Kang, F.; Huang, C.; Sah, M.K.; Jiang, B. Effect of eruption status of the mandibular third molar on distal caries in the adjacent second molar. *J. Oral Maxillofac. Surg.* **2016**, *74*, 684–692. [CrossRef] [PubMed]
26. Alsaegh, M.A.; Abushweme, D.A.; Ahmed, K.O.; Ahmed, S.O. The pattern of mandibular third molar impaction and its relationship with the development of distal caries in adjacent second molars among Emiratis: A retrospective study. *BMC Oral Health* **2022**, *22*, 306. [CrossRef] [PubMed]
27. Akkitap, M.P.; Gumru, B. Can the Position of the Impacted Third Molars Be an Early Risk Indicator of Pathological Conditions? A Retrospective Cone-Beam Computed Tomography Study. *J. Oral Maxillofac. Res.* **2023**, *14*, e3. [CrossRef]
28. Belam, A.; Rairam, S.G.; Patil, V.; Ratnakar, P.; Patil, S.; Kulkarni, S. Evaluation of detrimental effects of impacted Mandibular third molars on adjacent second molars—A retrospective observational study. *J. Conserv. Dent.* **2023**, *26*, 104–107. [CrossRef]
29. Chang, S.W.; Shin, S.Y.; Kum, K.Y.; Hong, J. Correlation study between distal caries in the mandibular second molar and the eruption status of the mandibular third molar in the Korean population. *Oral Surg. Oral Med. Oral Pathol. Oral Radiol. Endodontol.* **2009**, *108*, 838–843. [CrossRef]
30. Chu, F.C.; Li, T.K.; Lui, V.K.; Newsome, P.R.; Chow, R.L.; Cheung, L.K. Prevalence of impacted teeth and associated pathologies-a radiographic study of the Hong Kong Chinese population. *Hong Kong Med. J.* **2003**, *9*, 158–163.
31. Ozec, I.; Herguner Siso, S.; Tasdemir, U.; Ezirganli, S.; Goktolga, G. Prevalence and factors affecting the formation of second molar distal caries in a Turkish population. *Int. J. Oral Maxillofac. Surg.* **2009**, *38*, 1279–1282. [CrossRef] [PubMed]
32. Ates Yildirim, E.; Turker, N.; Goller Bulut, D.; Ustaoglu, G. The relationship of the position of mandibular third molar impaction with the development of dental and periodontal lesions in adjacent second molars. *J. Stomatol. Oral Maxillofac. Surg.* **2023**, *125*, 101610. [CrossRef] [PubMed]
33. Nunn, M.E.; Fish, M.D.; Garcia, R.I. Retained asymptomatic third molars and risk for second molar pathology. *J. Dent. Res.* **2013**, *92*, 1095–1099. [CrossRef] [PubMed]
34. Toedtling, V.; Devlin, H.; Tickle, M.; O'Malley, L. Prevalence of distal surface caries in the second molar among referrals for assessment of third molars: A systematic review and meta-analysis. *Br. J. Oral Maxillofac. Surg.* **2019**, *57*, 505–514. [CrossRef] [PubMed]
35. Glória, J.C.R.; Martins, C.C.; Armond, A.C.V.; Galvão, E.L.; Dos Santos, C.R.R.; Falci, S.G.M. Third Molar and Their Relationship with Caries on the Distal Surface of Second Molar: A Meta-analysis. *J. Maxillofac. Oral Surg.* **2018**, *17*, 129–141. [CrossRef] [PubMed]
36. Toedtling, V.; Devlin, H.; O'Malley, L.; Tickle, M. A systematic review of second molar distal surface caries incidence in the context of third molar absence and emergence. *Br. Dent. J.* **2020**, *228*, 261–266. [CrossRef] [PubMed]
37. Falci, S.G.; de Castro, C.R.; Santos, R.C.; de Souza Lima, L.D.; Ramos Jorge, M.L.; Botelho, A.M. Association between the presence of partially erupted mandibular third molar and the existence of caries in the distal of the second molars. *Int. J. Oral Maxillofac. Surg.* **2012**, *41*, 1270–1274. [CrossRef]
38. McArdle, L.W.; Renton, T.F. Distal cervical caries in the mandibular second molar: An indication for the prophylactic removal of the third molar? *Br. J. Oral Maxillofac. Surg.* **2006**, *44*, 42–45. [CrossRef]
39. Ma, Y.; Mu, D.; Li, X. Risk factors for root resorption of second molars with impacted third molars: A meta-analysis of CBCT studies. *Acta Odontol. Scand.* **2023**, *81*, 18–28. [CrossRef]
40. Akarslan, Z.Z.; Kocabay, C. Assessment of the associated symptoms, pathologies, positions and angulations of bilateral occurring mandibular third molars: Is there any similarity? *Oral Surg. Oral Med. Oral Pathol. Oral Radiol. Endodontol.* **2009**, *108*, 26–32. [CrossRef]
41. Nemcovsky, C.E.; Libfeld, H.; Zubery, Y. Effect of non-erupted 3rd molars on distal roots and supporting structures of approximal teeth. A radiographic survey of 202 cases. *J. Clin. Periodontol.* **1996**, *23*, 810–815. [CrossRef] [PubMed]
42. Nitzan, D.; Keren, T.; Marmary, Y. Does an impacted tooth cause root resorption of the adjacent one. *Oral Surg. Oral Med. Oral Pathol. Oral Radiol.* **1981**, *51*, 221–224. [CrossRef] [PubMed]
43. Van Der Linden, W.; Cleaton Jones, P.; Lownie, M. Diseases and lesions associated with third molars: Review of 1001 cases. *Oral Surg. Oral Med. Oral Pathol. Oral Radiol. Endodontol.* **1995**, *79*, 142–145. [CrossRef] [PubMed]

44. Oenning, A.C.; Melo, S.L.; Groppo, F.C.; Haiter Neto, F. Mesial inclination of impacted third molars and its propensity to stimulate external root resorption in second molars—A cone-beam computed tomographic evaluation. *J. Oral Maxillofac. Surg.* **2015**, *73*, 379–386. [CrossRef] [PubMed]
45. Wang, D.; He, X.; Wang, Y.; Li, Z.; Zhu, Y.; Sun, C.; Ye, J.; Jiang, H.; Cheng, J. External root resorption of the second molar associated with mesially and horizontally impacted mandibular third molar: Evidence from cone beam computed tomography. *Clin. Oral Investig.* **2017**, *21*, 1335–1342. [CrossRef]
46. Dalili, Z.; Taramsari, M.; Mousavi Mehr, S.Z.; Salamat, F. Diagnostic value of two modes of cone-beam computed tomography in evaluation of simulated external root resorption: An in vitro study. *Imaging Sci. Dent.* **2012**, *42*, 19–24. [CrossRef]
47. Mansfield, J.M.; Campbell, J.H.; Bhandari, A.R.; Jesionowski, A.M.; Vickerman, M.M. Molecular analysis of 16S rRNA genes identifies potentially periodontal pathogenic bacteria and archaea in the plaque of partially erupted third molars. *J. Oral Maxillofac. Surg.* **2012**, *70*, 1507–1514. [CrossRef]
48. Sun, L.J.; Qu, H.L.; Tian, Y.; Bi, C.S.; Zhang, S.Y.; Chen, F.M. Impacts of non-impacted third molar removal on the periodontal condition of adjacent second molars. *Oral Dis.* **2020**, *26*, 1010–1019. [CrossRef]
49. Li, Z.B.; Qu, H.L.; Zhou, L.N.; Tian, B.M.; Gao, L.N.; Chen, F.M. Nonimpacted Third Molars Affect the Periodontal Status of Adjacent Teeth: A Cross-Sectional Study. *J. Oral Maxillofac. Surg.* **2017**, *75*, 1344–1350. [CrossRef]
50. Blakey, G.H.; Golden, B.A.; White, R.P., Jr.; Offenbacher, S.; Phillips, C.; Haug, R.H. Changes over time in the periodontal status of young adults with no third molar periodontal pathology at enrollment. *J. Oral Maxillofac. Surg.* **2009**, *67*, 2425–2430. [CrossRef]
51. Yang, Y.; Tian, Y.; Sun, L.J.; Qu, H.L.; Chen, F.M. Relationship between Presence of Third Molars and Prevalence of Periodontal Pathology of Adjacent Second Molars: A Systematic Review and Meta-analysis. *Chin. J. Dent. Res.* **2022**, *25*, 45–55. [CrossRef] [PubMed]
52. Passarelli, P.C.; Lajolo, C.; Pasquantonio, G.; D'Amato, G.; Docimo, R.; Verdugo, F.; D'Addona, A. Influence of mandibular third molar surgical extraction on the periodontal status of adjacent second molars. *J. Periodontol.* **2019**, *90*, 847–855. [CrossRef] [PubMed]
53. Tian, Y.; Sun, L.; Qu, H.; Yang, Y.; Chen, F. Removal of nonimpacted third molars alters the periodontal condition of their neighbors clinically, immunologically, and microbiologically. *Int. J. Oral Sci.* **2021**, *13*, 5. [CrossRef] [PubMed]
54. Barbato, L.; Kalemaj, Z.; Buti, J.; Baccini, M.; La Marca, M.; Duvina, M.; Tonelli, P. Effect of Surgical Intervention for Removal of Mandibular Third Molar on Periodontal Healing of Adjacent Mandibular Second Molar: A Systematic Review and Bayesian Network Meta-Analysis. *J. Periodontol.* **2016**, *87*, 291–302. [CrossRef] [PubMed]
55. Pang, S.L.; Leung, K.P.Y.; Li, K.Y.; Pelekos, G.; Tonetti, M.; Leung, Y.Y. Factors affecting periodontal healing of the adjacent second molar after lower third molar surgery: A systematic review and meta-analysis. *Clin. Oral Investig.* **2023**, *27*, 1547–1565. [CrossRef]
56. Menditti, D.; Mariani, P.; Russo, D.; Rinaldi, B.; Fiorillo, L.; Cicciù, M.; Laino, L. Early pathological changes of peri-coronal tissue in the distal area of erupted or partially impacted lower third molars. *BMC Oral Health* **2023**, *23*, 380. [CrossRef]
57. Albanese, M.; Zangani, A.; Manfrin, F.; Bertossi, D.; De Manzoni, R.; Tomizioli, N.; Faccioni, P.; Pardo, A. Influence of Surgical Technique on Post-Operative Complications in the Extraction of the Lower Third Molar: A Retrospective Study. *Dent. J.* **2023**, *11*, 238. [CrossRef]
58. Antonelli, A.; Barone, S.; Bennardo, F.; Giudice, A. Three-dimensional facial swelling evaluation of pre-operative single-dose of prednisone in third molar surgery: A split-mouth randomized controlled trial. *BMC Oral Health* **2023**, *23*, 614. [CrossRef]
59. Cheng, Y.; Al-Aroomi, M.A.; Al-Worafi, N.A.; Al-Moraissi, E.A.; Sun, C. Influence of inflammation on bleeding and wound healing following surgical extraction of impacted lower third molars. *BMC Oral Health* **2023**, *23*, 83. [CrossRef]
60. Han, J.; Zhu, J.; Hu, S.; Li, C.; Zhang, X. Nd:YAG laser therapy on postoperative pain, swelling, and trismus after mandibular third molar surgery: A randomized double-blinded clinical study. *Lasers Med. Sci.* **2023**, *38*, 176. [CrossRef]
61. Li, Y.; Ling, Z.; Zhang, H.; Xie, H.; Zhang, P.; Jiang, H.; Fu, Y. Association of the Inferior Alveolar Nerve Position and Nerve Injury: A Systematic Review and Meta-Analysis. *Healthcare* **2022**, *10*, 1782. [CrossRef] [PubMed]
62. Lewusz-Butkiewicz, K.; Kaczor, K.; Nowicka, A. Risk factors in oroantral communication while extracting the upper third molar: Systematic review. *Dent. Med. Probl.* **2018**, *55*, 69–74. [CrossRef] [PubMed]
63. Gay-Escoda, C.; Sánchez-Torres, A.; Borrás-Ferreres, J.; Valmaseda-Castellón, E. Third molar surgical difficulty scales: Systematic review and preoperative assessment form. *Med. Oral Patol. Oral Cir. Bucal* **2022**, *27*, e68–e76. [CrossRef] [PubMed]
64. Wenzel, A. Radiographic display of carious lesions and cavitation in approximalsurfaces: Advantages and drawbacks of conventional and advanced modalities. *Acta Odontol. Scand.* **2014**, *72*, 251–264. [CrossRef]
65. Tarım Ertas, E.; Kucukyılmaz, E.; Ertas, H.; Savas, S.; Yırcalı Atıcı, M. A comparative study of different radiographic methods for detecting occlusal caries lesions. *Caries Res.* **2014**, *48*, 566–574. [CrossRef]

Disclaimer/Publisher's Note: The statements, opinions and data contained in all publications are solely those of the individual author(s) and contributor(s) and not of MDPI and/or the editor(s). MDPI and/or the editor(s) disclaim responsibility for any injury to people or property resulting from any ideas, methods, instructions or products referred to in the content.

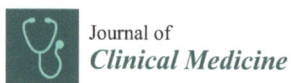 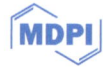

Article

Bismuth Shielding in Head Computed Tomography—Still Necessary?

Jana Di Rosso [1,†], Andreas Krasser [2,†], Sebastian Tschauner [1,*], Helmuth Guss [2] and Erich Sorantin [1]

[1] Division of Paediatric Radiology, Department of Radiology, Medical University of Graz, 8036 Graz, Austria; erich.sorantin@medunigraz.at (E.S.)

[2] Competence Centre for Medical Physics and Radiation Protection, University Hospital Graz, 8036 Graz, Austria

* Correspondence: sebastian.tschauner@medunigraz.at

† These authors contributed equally to this work.

Abstract: Introduction: Cranial CT scans are associated with radiation exposure to the eye lens, which is a particularly radiosensitive organ. Children are more vulnerable to radiation than adults. Therefore, it is essential to use the available dose reduction techniques to minimize radiation exposure. According to the European Consensus on patient contact shielding by the IRCP from 2021, shielding is not recommended in most body areas anymore. This study aims to evaluate whether bismuth shielding as well as its combination with other dose-saving technologies could still be useful. **Methods:** Cranial CT scans of a pediatric anthropomorphic phantom were performed on two up-to-date MDCT scanners. Eye lens dose measurements were performed using thermoluminescent dosimeters. Furthermore, the impact of BS and of the additional placement of standoff foam between the patient and BS on image quality was also assessed. **Results:** Bismuth shielding showed a significant lens dose reduction in both CT scanners (GE: 41.50 ± 4.04%, $p < 0.001$; Siemens: 29.75 ± 6.55%, $p = 0.00$). When combined with AEC, the dose was lowered even more (GE: 60.75 ± 3.30%, $p < 0.001$; Siemens: 41.25 ± 8.02%, $p = 0.00$). The highest eye dose reduction was achieved using BS + AEC + OBTCM (GE: 71.25 ± 2.98%, $p < 0.001$; Siemens: 58.75 ± 5.85%, $p < 0.001$). BS caused increased image noise in the orbital region, which could be mitigated by foam placement. Eye shielding had no effect on the image noise in the cranium. **Conclusions:** The use of BS in cranial CT can lead to a significant dose reduction, which can be further enhanced by its combination with other modern dose reduction methods. BS causes increase in image noise in the orbital region but not in the cranium. The additional use of standoff foam reduces image noise in the orbital region.

Keywords: bismuth; radiation; ionizing; radiation protection; lens; crystalline; multidetector computed tomography

Citation: Di Rosso, J.; Krasser, A.; Tschauner, S.; Guss, H.; Sorantin, E. Bismuth Shielding in Head Computed Tomography—Still Necessary? *J. Clin. Med.* **2024**, *13*, 25. https://doi.org/10.3390/jcm13010025

Academic Editor: Arutselvan Natarajan

Received: 20 November 2023
Revised: 11 December 2023
Accepted: 14 December 2023
Published: 20 December 2023

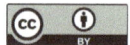

Copyright: © 2024 by the authors. Licensee MDPI, Basel, Switzerland. This article is an open access article distributed under the terms and conditions of the Creative Commons Attribution (CC BY) license (https://creativecommons.org/licenses/by/4.0/).

1. Introduction

Medical imaging plays an important role in patient management, including pediatric care. Growth is accomplished through elevated cell turnover, which means that a greater number of cells are in a vulnerable state. Therefore, children exhibit increased radiation sensitivity compared to adults. Due to this increased susceptibility and a long life expectancy post-exposure, children are at a higher risk of radiation-induced damage [1].

In pediatric radiology, the ultrasound and MRI are important methods used in order to avoid the risk of radiation. However, there are circumstances where CT is necessary to provide accurate diagnostic results.

Computed tomography (CT) is a powerful imaging modality widely used in medical diagnostics, especially for examining the brain and other structures within the skull. CT scans are still the main source of medical radiation exposure [2]. CT scans in pediatric radiology account for about 10% of the radiation-based imaging modalities. However, they are responsible for about 40–60% of the radiation exposure in children [1]. The radiation exposure associated with CT scans can cause harmful effects to the patient, especially to the lens of the eye. The lens is particularly sensitive to ionizing radiation, and exposure to even low levels can increase the risk of cataract formation. This risk is particularly concerning for patients who require repeated or frequent CT scans, such as those with head trauma, tumors, or neurological disorders.

To mitigate the risk of radiation-induced cataracts, various strategies have been proposed. Bismuth shielding (BS) has been described as an effective measure in reducing the dose to the eye lenses [3].

Structural shielding (e.g., blanket, rubber mat...) has been used in radiology for the last 70 years [4]. Bismuth shielding was first described by Hopper et al. in 1997 as the use of an in-plane overlying bismuth radioprotective material manufactured into form-fitting garments, which reduces radiation exposure to superficial organs [5]. Since then, shielding has been mainly used in CT to protect eyes, the thyroid gland, and breasts. By placing the shield over radiosensitive organs, the radiation exposition can be reduced by 30–50% [3].

However, in 2021 the International Commission on Radiological Protection (IRCP) released the European Consensus on patient contact shielding, in which it is recommended to discontinue shielding in most body areas including the eye lenses [4]. The main concerns related to shielding are a reduction in image quality and interference with other dose reduction systems, as well as factors related to the operator (inappropriate placement of the shield, infection control) and the patient (patient discomfort, movement during the examination). According to the IRCP, there are other, more effective dose-saving methods that reduce the dose while improving the image consistency, e.g., automatic exposure control systems [4].

This study assesses the eye lens dose and image quality when using BS and its combination with other currently used dose-saving technologies in paediatric cranial CT on two up-to-date multidetector computed tomography (MDCT) scanners. Moreover, it discusses practical considerations for implementing BS in clinical paediatric care and aims to inform its appropriate use in cranial MDCT with modern MDCT scanners.

2. Materials and Methods

This phantom study evaluates if there is an additional value of BS used on two modern MDCT scanners equipped with currently used dose reduction technologies, as well as the influence of BS on the image quality in head CT. Since the used CT machines differ considerably in their features and different scanning parameters were used, the radiation exposure differences were compared only for the individual CT machine and not between the scanners.

Ethical committee review and approval were not required because phantom studies were performed.

2.1. Phantoms, Bismuth Shield

An anthropomorphic pediatric phantom (CIRS ATOM® phantom, pediatric 5 years, 110 cm, 19 kg, Computerized Imaging Reference Systems, Inc. Norfolk, VA, USA) was used. After the localizer CT radiograph was acquired, a 1.27 mm thick bismuth shield (14 × 3.5 cm, Somatex, Berlin, Germany) was placed over both phantom lens areas (Figure 1).

2.2. MDCT Scanners, Scanning Protocols

The following two up-to-date CT scanners were used for the study: General Electric (GE) Revolution™ (GE, Milwaukee, WI, USA) and Siemens Somatom Definition AS™ (Siemens Healthineers, Erlangen, Germany). Scans on the GE scanner were performed in the helix and volume modes. Furthermore, in the GE scanner, scans in the volume mode with a fixed tube current were acquired. The Siemens scanner provides only the helix mode for the required ranges of this study.

On both scanners, age-adjusted scanning protocols were chosen (Table 1), as used in clinical practice, together with iterative reconstructions.

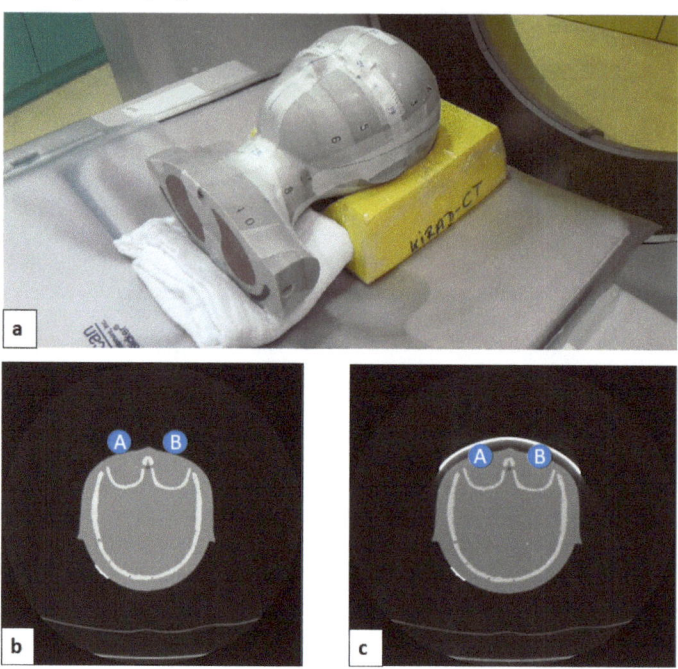

Figure 1. Positioning of the pediatric head phantom within the scanner (**a**) CT axial scans without bismuth shield (**b**) and with bismuth shield (**c**) (measurement points: A, right lens; B, left lens).

Table 1. Scanning protocols.

CT Scanner	GE Revolution™				Siemens Somatom Definition AS™		
Scan mode	Volume	Helix	Helix	Helix	Helix	Helix	Helix
Tube voltage (kV)	100	100	100	100	100	100	100
kV modulation	-	-	-	-	-	-	-
Average tube current (mA)	300	230	223	184	253	192	189
AEC (z-direction)	-	-	yes	yes	-	yes	yes
OBTCM (x,y-direction)	-	-	-	yes	-	-	yes
Slice thickness (mm), collimation (rows)	0.625	0.625 × 40	0.625 × 80	0.625 × 80	0.6 × 40	0.6 × 40	0.6 × 128
Scan length (mm)	157.5	160	160	160	160	160	160
Pitch	0	0.516	0.507	0.507	0.55	0.55	0.55
Rotation time (s)	0.5	0.5	0.5	0.5	0.5	1	1
Adaptive dose shield	-	-	-	-	yes	yes	yes
FOV	250 mm	250 mm	250 mm	250 mm	250 mm	250 mm	250 mm
Focus	0.6 mm	0.6 mm	0.6 mm	0.6 mm	0.7 mm	0.7 mm	0.7 mm
CTDIvol (mGy)	12.04	19.15	16.34	13.64	24.08	19.96	16.81
DLPvol (mGy × cm)	192.6	384.6	261.5	223.6	401.0	332.6	291.2
Filtering	4.2 mm Al				6.8 mm Al		

2.3. Dose-Saving Techniques

Automated exposure control (AEC) and organ-based tube current modulation (OBTCM) are modern dose-saving techniques available on the used MDCT scanners. These techniques have vendor-specific characteristics. The GE scanner offers smart mA™ (AEC) and ODM™ (OBTCM). Care Dose 4D™ (AEC) and X-care™ (OBTCM) are provided by the Siemens scanner.

The scans for surface dose and image quality assessment were conducted under different conditions, as shown in Table 2: (a) reference scan without any dose reduction method, (b) AEC, (c) AEC + OBTCM, (d) BS, (e) BS + AEC, (f) BS + AEC + OBTCM.

Table 2. Different scanning conditions used for eye lens dose and image quality evaluation.

CT Machine	Scan Mode	Dose Modulation
GE Revolution™	Volume	—
	Helix	—
	Helix	+ smart mA
	Helix	+ smart mA + ODM
Siemens Somatom Definition AS™	Helix	—
	Helix	+ Care Dose 4D
	Helix	+ Care Dose 4D + X-care

Automated exposure control (AEC) is a dose reduction technique used to provide automatic adaptation of mA based on the user-specified image quality and X-ray attenuation characteristics of the scanned body region. The goal of the AEC is to apply radiation to the patient more efficiently and keep the image quality constant. Smart mA™ is GE's technology for automated exposure control. The technology offered by Siemens is called Care Dose 4D™.

Organ-based tube current modulation (OBTCM) is used to reduce the dose delivered to superficial radiosensitive organs in CT by reducing the tube current when the X-ray tube passes over the organs. GE and Siemens have developed different OBTCM techniques called Organ Dose Modulation (ODM™) and X-care™, respectively.

Organ Dose Modulation (ODM™) is offered by GE and it is used to reduce the tube current in a 180° radial arc in body protocols and in a 90° radial arc in head protocols. ODM™ does not increase tube current in other projections, which leads to a reduction in the radiation dose.

X-care™ is Siemens's technology for organ-based tube current modulation. This dose-saving technique is used to allocate the tube current more to the lateral and posterior tube positions than to the anterior tube positions while keeping the total scanner output the same. It reduces the tube current in a 120° radial arc above the anterior organs and increases the tube current posteriorly in the remaining 240° of the scanning range, so that the radiation dose and image quality remain constant. Superficially located organs have a reduced exposure within the 120° radial arc and increased exposure over the 240°.

2.4. Dosimetry

The eye lens dose was estimated using thermoluminescent dosimeters (TLD-100™, Rods 1 × 6 mm, LiF:Mg,Ti , Thermo Scientific™ Waltham, MA, USA) placed over the eye areas of the anthropomorphic pediatric head phantom.

To obtain reasonable dose values, all scans were conducted 15 times, and afterwards measured values were divided by 15 to obtain the dose of an individual scan. The factor 15 was empirically determined in a pre-study. The whole procedure was repeated three times and dose values of dosimeters were averaged.

2.5. Image Quality Assessment, ROI Measurements

Image noise represents a marker of image quality. In many studies, increases in image noise and artifacts has been reported as the biggest disadvantage of BS [6].

In order to overcome this disadvantage, the following approach proved to be successful at the authors' institution: a 2.0 cm standoff foam is placed between the patient and BS to reduce artifacts in superficial areas. To assess the influence of BS as well as the influence of foam on image quality, CT scans were acquired in the following way: phantom alone, phantom + foam, phantom + BS, and phantom + foam + BS, as depicted in Figure 2. These scans were conducted only for the assessment of image quality; therefore, no dosimetric values were acquired.

Image noise was estimated using the standard deviation of density values (Hounsfield units, HU) within a circular region of interest (ROI—Figure 3) and served as a quantitative parameter of image quality.

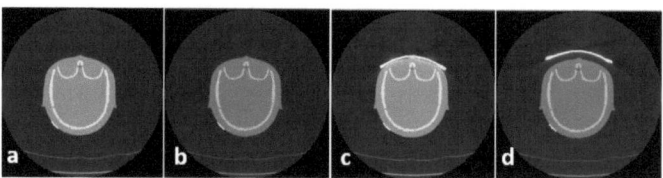

Figure 2. Protocol for quality assessment included 4 scans pro series: phantom (**a**), phantom + foam (**b**), phantom + bismuth shield (**c**), phantom + foam + bismuth shield (**d**).

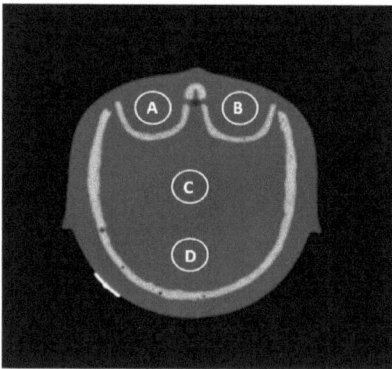

Figure 3. Different points of ROI measurement: orbital right (A), orbital left (B), central in the cranium (C), and occiput (D).

2.6. Statistical Analysis

Dose savings were calculated in % based on a scanner reference scan.

t-tests, one-way analysis of variance, and post hoc tests were performed. Dose savings under different scanning conditions were compared (reference scan without any dose reduction method, AEC, AEC + OBTCM, BS, BS + AEC, and BS + AEC + OBTCM). Furthermore, the influence of the foam on the image quality was evaluated comparing different imaging conditions (phantom alone, phantom + foam, phantom + BS, phantom + foam + BS).

$p < 0.05$ was considered to indicate a statistically significant difference. The tests were performed in statistical software IBM SPSS Statistics for Windows, Version 21.0 (Armonk, NY, USA: IBM Corp. Released 2012).

3. Results

3.1. Eye Lens Dose Evaluation

All scan modes showed symmetrical doses between the two eye areas.

AEC led to a statistically significant dose reduction in the GE scanner (21.50 ± 10.28%, $p = 0.025$) but not in the Siemens scanner (−0.75 ± 11.87%, $p = 0.907$).

A dose reduction of over 40% was also achieved without BS, using only the combination of AEC and OBTCM (GE: 50.5. ± 5.07%, $p < 0.001$; Siemens: 43.50 ± 4.36%, $p < 0.001$).

Bismuth shielding alone showed a significant dose reduction (GE: 41.50 ± 4.04%, $p < 0.001$; Siemens: 29.75 ± 6.55%, $p = 0.003$). A further reduction in dose was observed in combinations of BS with other dose-saving methods, such as BS with AEC

(GE: 60.75 ± 3.30%, $p < 0.001$; Siemens: 41.25 ± 8.02%, $p = 0.002$). The highest eye dose reduction was achieved using BS + AEC + OBTCM (GE: 71.25 ± 2.98%, $p < 0.001$; Siemens: 58.75 ± 5.85%, $p < 0.001$).

The impact of different dose-saving methods and their combination on the dose is shown in Figure 4.

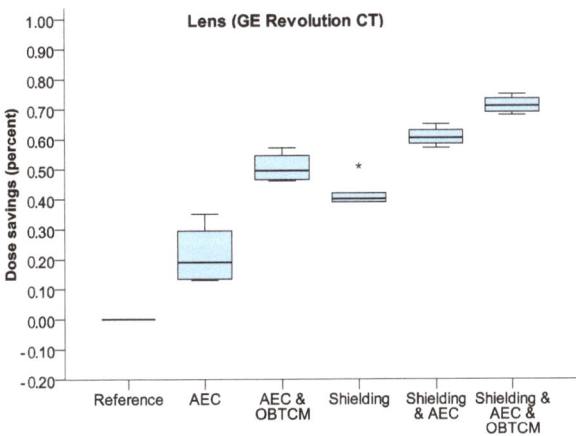

(a) Lens (GE)

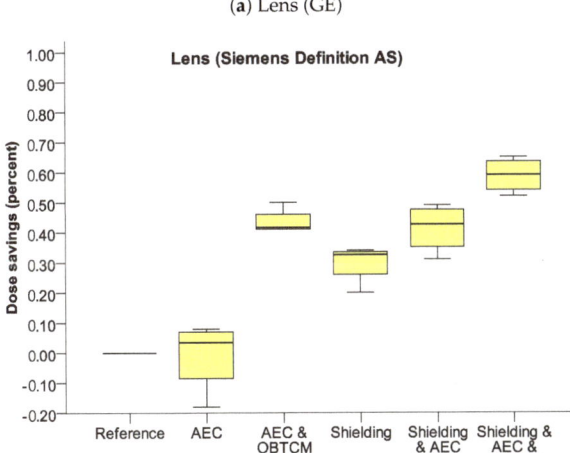

(b) Lens (Siemens)

Figure 4. Average relative dose savings of both CT scanners for lens. 1.00 = 100%. Note particularly the difference between AEC and OBTCM without/with shielding. Asterisks (*) represent outliers in the box plot.

A direct comparison between different dose-saving methods provided by the two different scanners is not possible, since there different scanning parameters were used, as shown previously in Table 2.

3.2. Image Quality Assessment

There was no significant difference in image noise between ROI A and ROI B (orbit right and left). As shown in Figure 5, relative to the reference scan, bismuth shielding caused a significant increase in the image noise in the orbit in both CT scanners. However, the placement of plastic foam between the eye areas and BS lowered the image noise on both CT scanners.

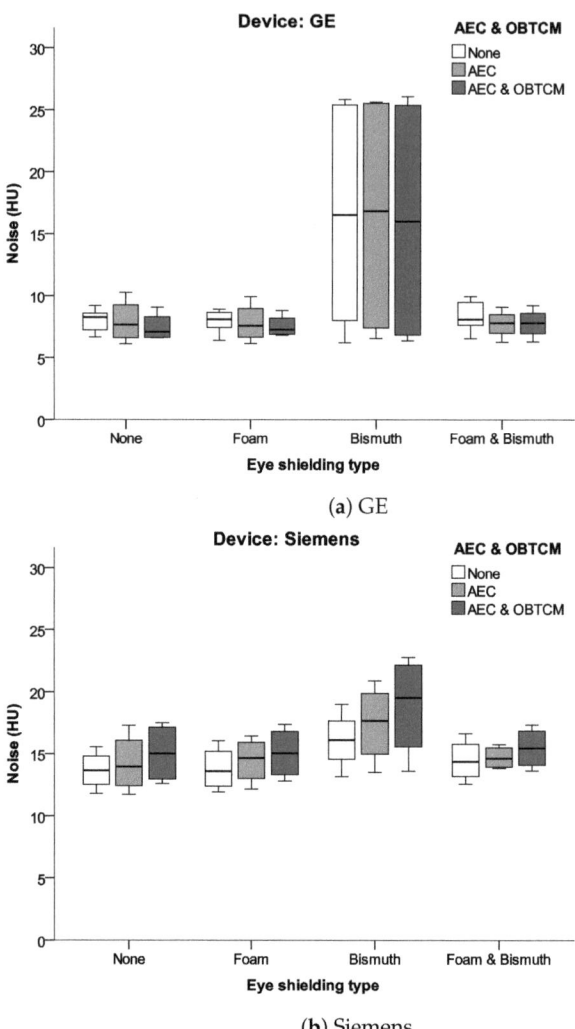

Figure 5. Box plots of mean noise values in the orbital region for different shielding types and different dose reduction methods (AEC and OBTCM). Note the positive effects of placing plastic foam between the bismuth shielding and the eyes.

Spacing foam is composed of homogeneous materials with low X-ray attenuation properties; therefore, it should not affect the image quality. Plastic foam placed on the eye areas without the use of bismuth shielding did not influence image quality.

As shown in Figure 6, eye shielding had no effect on image noise centrally in the cranium and in the occiput, which is crucial for the purpose of brain diagnostics. The additional use of foam in these regions did not lead to a significant decrease in the image noise.

Different scan modes (volume, helix) and dose-saving techniques (AEC, AEC + OBTCM) did not influence the image quality related to shielding.

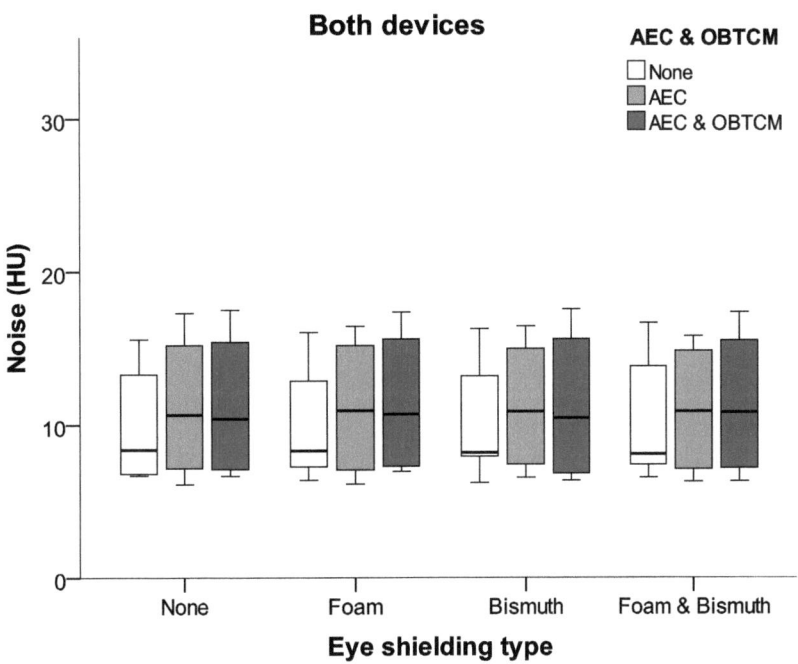

Figure 6. Image noise in the cranium centrally and occipitally for different eye shielding types. Note that shielding apparently had no effect on image noise intracranially.

4. Discussion

4.1. Results of This Study vs. Current Literature

Bismuth shielding is a practical and effective method for reducing radiation exposure to the eye lens during cranial CT imaging. In the presented study, BS showed a significant lens dose reduction in both CT scanners, which could be enhanced by its combination with other dose reduction techniques. The highest eye dose reduction of up to 70% was achieved using BS + AEC + OBTCM.

Relative to the reference scan, BS led to a significant increase in the image noise in the orbital region. However, the combination of BS with foam lowered the image noise in the orbit significantly. Shielding, as well as its combination with foam, had no effect on image noise intracranially. These results are compatible with the results published in the currently available literature.

A meta-analysis of the effects of BS for the protection of superficial radiosensitive organs from 2019 included pediatric and adult anthropomorphic phantoms, as well as patients undergoing CT. The fixed-effects pooled estimate of eye lens dose reduction was 34%. Shielding was recommended in 88.89% of the studies [6].

There is a study from 2012 that combined BS with OBTCM (XCare™, Siemens) for dose reduction to the eye in head CT. The dose to the eye was reduced by 26.4% with bismuth shielding. A combination of OBTCM with one bismuth shield reduced the dose by 47.0%, but the CT number accuracy and image quality (noise and artifacts) were affected. The image noise in the brain region was slightly increased for all dose reduction methods [3].

In a study from 2020, the effect of barium sulfate and bismuth-antimony shields on the dose reduction to the eye lens and image quality in cranial CT on a MDCT scanner (Somatom Definition Flash; Siemens Healthcare) was investigated. It showed a significant lens dose reduction (by 28.60–31.92% and 43.87–47.00%, respectively) while causing substantial image artifacts. Shielding combined with AEC did not exhibit a significant difference compared to the dose measured under the fixed tube current (FTC). In comparison to a fixed tube current, employing AEC yielded improved signal-to-noise and contrast-to-noise ratios within the intracranial structures when using the bismuth-antimony and barium sulfate shields, respectively [7].

In the available literature, the use of eye shielding has been associated with a moderate increase in image noise of about 1–2 HU. The additional use of foam has led to a decrease in the image noise near the orbit but not in the brain region [3].

To the best of the authors' knowledge, no current study has been performed evaluating the use of BS and its combination with other currently available dose reduction techniques and its effects on the dose reduction and image quality on up-to-date MDCT scanners.

4.2. IRCP Statement

According to the European Consensus on patient contact shielding released in 2021, shielding is not recommended anymore to protect eye lens in cranial CT [4]. However, it might still be used to protect the breast and thyroid if the potential benefit of its use could outweigh the risks, e.g., in numerous examinations and interventional procedures, where the cumulative dose is high. Anxious and radiosensitive patients could also benefit from the use of shielding [6].

4.3. Limitations of BS and Potential Solutions

When it comes to eye lens shielding with bismuth in cranial CT, there are several problematic points and limitations that need to be considered, especially in children:

- Dose reduction: While bismuth shields are effective in reducing the radiation dose to the eye lens, they do not eliminate it entirely. Moreover, the shielding effect is highly dependent on the design and placement of the shield. In children, who are more susceptible to radiation-induced damage than adults, it is important to balance the benefits of dose reduction with the potential risks associated with additional imaging.
- Image artifacts: BS effects the image quality due to increased image noise and streak artifacts. Artifacts may interfere with the interpretation of CT images and can be especially problematic in the context of pediatric CT, where image quality is critical for accurate diagnosis and treatment planning. Foams have been used to increase the distance between the bismuth shield and the superficial structures, reducing the image noise and artifacts under shielding [6], which also proved to be useful in the presented study.
- Interference with the automatic exposure control systems: This can lead to increased radiation. Therefore, the shield should be placed after acquiring the scout view, as conducted in the presented study [6].
- Practical considerations: Bismuth shields can be difficult to apply in pediatric patients, who may be more prone to movement and require specialized techniques to maintain a stable head position during imaging. In addition, the use of bismuth shields may require additional time and effort on the part of the technologist (placement of the shield, infection control), which can increase the overall imaging time.
- Patient comfort: Children may be uncomfortable with the use of bismuth shields, which can be heavy and difficult to position. Moreover, the use of shields may increase anxiety or fear, leading to more difficulties in imaging or even sedation.

4.4. Alternative Techniques

There are alternative techniques that can be used to reduce radiation the dose to the eye lens in cranial CT, such as automatic exposure control systems, low-dose protocols, globally lowering the tube current (GLTC), reducing the tube voltage (RTV), or gantry tilting [8].

Gantry tilting is one of the most effective ways to protect the eye lens in head CT but it is not always possible in pediatric radiology, due, e.g., to patient positioning limitations or contraindications of head tilting.

However, the effectiveness of these techniques may vary depending on the patient and the clinical indication, and bismuth shielding may still be necessary in some cases.

4.5. Optimization of Bismuth Shielding Utilization

Overall, the use of bismuth shields for eye lens protection in pediatric CT requires careful consideration of the potential risks and benefits, as well as the practical limitations and patient comfort. The decision to implement shielding at individual institutions should involve a collaborative effort by a multidisciplinary team, including medical physics experts. Furthermore, it should be documented in the examination protocols.

Comprehensive training for staff should encompass proper shielding usage, effective communication with patients, shield selection, and precise positioning, as well as procedures for the cleaning, disinfection, and storage of BS.

Clinical decisions should be made based on the individual patient's clinical indication, age, size, and imaging characteristics. The use of BS should be optimized to balance the benefits of radiation dose reduction with the potential risks associated with image quality deterioration and additional imaging.

4.6. Limitations of This Study

The phantom used in this study represented only the head of a 5-year-old child. At this age, skull calcification is already complete; therefore, the results of this study should also be applicable to older children. X-ray beam attenuation in a less calcified skull of younger children is more similar to that of a toddler torso, which has been evaluated in previous studies and showed similar results [9].

The presented phantom study had a small sample size. Extensive research with patients is necessary, especially regarding image quality under BS and its influence on specific diagnostic tasks.

Dose assessment was limited to the eye lens area because it is a particularly radiosensitive organ and its repeated exposure to radiation is associated with cataract formation.

5. Conclusions

The results of this study suggest that bismuth shielding can be beneficial in clinical practice using up-to-date MDCT scanners. Bismuth shielding has proven useful, especially in combination with other dose reduction methods, such as AEC and OBTCM. BS leads to an increase in the image noise in the orbital region, which can be significantly decreased by the placement of plastic foam between the shield and the eyes. Shielding had no effect on image noise intracranially, which is crucial for brain diagnostics.

Author Contributions: J.D.R., A.K., H.G. and E.S. contributed to the conceptualization and design of this study. A.K. and H.G. conducted experiments and collected data. J.D.R., S.T. and E.S. contributed to the drafting of this manuscript. S.T. and E.S. conducted statistical analyses and contributed to data interpretation. J.D.R., S.T. and E.S. critically reviewed and revised this manuscript. All authors have read and agreed to the published version of this manuscript.

Funding: This research received no external funding.

Institutional Review Board Statement: Not applicable.

Informed Consent Statement: Not applicable.

Data Availability Statement: Data can be obtained from the corresponding author (ST) on request.

Conflicts of Interest: The authors declare no conflicts of interest.

References

1. Sorantin, E.; Weissensteiner, S.; Hasenburger, G.; Riccabona, M. CT in children–dose protection and general considerations when planning a CT in a child. *Eur. J. Radiol.* **2013**, *82*, 1043–1049. [CrossRef] [PubMed]
2. Kubo, T. Vendor free basics of radiation dose reduction techniques for CT. *Eur. J. Radiol.* **2019**, *110*, 14–21. [CrossRef] [PubMed]

3. Wang, J.; Duan, X.; Christner, J.A.; Leng, S.; Grant, K.L.; McCollough, C.H. Bismuth shielding, organ-based tube current modulation, and global reduction of tube current for dose reduction to the eye at head CT. *Radiology* **2012**, *262*, 191–198. [CrossRef] [PubMed]
4. Hiles, P.; Gilligan, P.; Damilakis, J.; Briers, E.; Candela-Juan, C.; Faj, D.; Foley, S.; Frija, G.; Granata, C.; de las Heras Gala, H.; et al. European consensus on patient contact shielding. *Insights Imaging* **2021**, *12*, 194. [CrossRef] [PubMed]
5. Hopper, K.D.; King, S.H.; Lobell, M.; TenHave, T.; Weaver, J. The breast: In-plane x-ray protection during diagnostic thoracic CT–shielding with bismuth radioprotective garments. *Radiology* **1997**, *205*, 853–858. [CrossRef] [PubMed]
6. Mehnati, P.; Malekzadeh, R.; Sooteh, M.Y. Use of bismuth shield for protection of superficial radiosensitive organs in patients undergoing computed tomography: A literature review and meta-analysis. *Radiol. Phys. Technol.* **2019**, *12*, 6–25. [CrossRef] [PubMed]
7. Lee, Y.H.; Yang, S.H.; Lin, Y.K.; Glickman, R.D.; Chen, C.Y.; Chan, W.P. Eye shielding during head CT scans: Dose reduction and image quality evaluation. *Acad. Radiol.* **2020**, *27*, 1523–1530. [CrossRef] [PubMed]
8. Karami, V.; Albosof, M.; Gholami, M.; Adeli, M.; Hekmatnia, A.; Sheidaei, M.F.B.; Behbahani, A.T.; Sharif, H.S.; Jafrasteh, S. Tradeoffs between radiation exposure to the lens of the eyes and diagnostic image quality in pediatric brain computed tomography. *J. Med. Signals Sens.* **2023**, *13*, 208–216. [PubMed]
9. Geleijns, J.; Salvado Artells, M.; Veldkamp, W.; Lopez Tortosa, M.; Calzado Cantera, A. Quantitative assessment of selective in-plane shielding of tissues in computed tomography through evaluation of absorbed dose and image quality. *Eur. Radiol.* **2006**, *16*, 2334–2340. [CrossRef] [PubMed]

Disclaimer/Publisher's Note: The statements, opinions and data contained in all publications are solely those of the individual author(s) and contributor(s) and not of MDPI and/or the editor(s). MDPI and/or the editor(s) disclaim responsibility for any injury to people or property resulting from any ideas, methods, instructions or products referred to in the content.

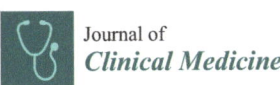

Article

Evaluating a Periapical Lesion Detection CNN on a Clinically Representative CBCT Dataset—A Validation Study

Arnela Hadzic [1], Martin Urschler [1,*], Jan-Niclas Aaron Press [2], Regina Riedl [1], Petra Rugani [2], Darko Štern [3] and Barbara Kirnbauer [2]

1. Institute for Medical Informatics, Statistics and Documentation, Medical University of Graz, 8036 Graz, Austria; arnela.hadzic@medunigraz.at (A.H.); regina.riedl@medunigraz.at (R.R.)
2. Division of Oral Surgery and Orthodontics, Medical University of Graz, 8010 Graz, Austria; petra.rugani@medunigraz.at (P.R.); barbara.kirnbauer@medunigraz.at (B.K.)
3. Institute of Computer Graphics and Vision, Graz University of Technology, 8010 Graz, Austria
* Correspondence: martin.urschler@medunigraz.at

Abstract: The aim of this validation study was to comprehensively evaluate the performance and generalization capability of a deep learning-based periapical lesion detection algorithm on a clinically representative cone-beam computed tomography (CBCT) dataset and test for non-inferiority. The evaluation involved 195 CBCT images of adult upper and lower jaws, where sensitivity and specificity metrics were calculated for all teeth, stratified by jaw, and stratified by tooth type. Furthermore, each lesion was assigned a periapical index score based on its size to enable a score-based evaluation. Non-inferiority tests were conducted with proportions of 90% for sensitivity and 82% for specificity. The algorithm achieved an overall sensitivity of 86.7% and a specificity of 84.3%. The non-inferiority test indicated the rejection of the null hypothesis for specificity but not for sensitivity. However, when excluding lesions with a periapical index score of one (i.e., very small lesions), the sensitivity improved to 90.4%. Despite the challenges posed by the dataset, the algorithm demonstrated promising results. Nevertheless, further improvements are needed to enhance the algorithm's robustness, particularly in detecting very small lesions and the handling of artifacts and outliers commonly encountered in real-world clinical scenarios.

Keywords: artificial intelligence; deep learning; digital imaging/radiology; inflammation; oral diagnosis; periapical lesions; image segmentation; convolutional neural network

1. Introduction

Artificial intelligence (AI) models have made remarkable advancements in various fields, with deep convolutional neural networks (CNNs) [1] emerging as a powerful subset of AI, especially for processing and analyzing images. These networks, inspired by the structure of the visual cortex in the human brain, show superior performance in tasks such as image classification, object detection, and image segmentation [2]. In the field of medical imaging, these networks have demonstrated promising capabilities in detecting and diagnosing various diseases such as breast cancer, heart disease, and brain tumors [3,4]. Their performance is often reported to be comparable to that of experienced professionals, significantly reducing the time required for diagnosis [5–7].

Recently, dental medicine has also started to benefit from such deep learning techniques [8]. Specifically, these techniques have been applied to panoramic radiographs and cone-beam computed tomography (CBCT) images with the aim of assisting clinicians in detecting and analyzing dental conditions and diseases in the maxillofacial region [9–11]. Examples include the detection of maxillary sinus mucosa [12], pharyngeal airway space [13], calcifications of the cervical carotid artery [14], jaw cysts [15,16], supernumerary mesiobuccal root canals on maxillary molars [17], vertical root fractures [18], and periapical lesions (PALs).

PALs are one of the most frequent pathological occurrences in dental images. They resemble usually bacteria-induced osteolytic areas around the tip of the roots within a few millimeters in diameter [19,20]. PALs are conventionally analyzed in radiographs, whereas CBCT images often reveal these lesions as incidental findings [20,21]. While widely used conventional intra- and extra-oral radiographs [22] lead to lower radiation doses but suffer from superimposition issues due to their projective nature, CBCT allows fully three-dimensional (3D) imaging of the maxillofacial region at the cost of higher dose requirements. However, due to its volumetric nature, CBCT has been shown to improve the detection of PALs when compared with radiographs [23–25]. Manually identifying PALs with high sensitivity (recall) in both imaging modalities requires a certain amount of experience to prevent overlooked findings. As a result, automated deep learning-based methods for PAL detection in radiographs or CBCT imaging data have been proposed [16,26–34]. Serving as the foundation of this study, the promising CNN-based approach for periapical lesion detection in CBCT images proposed in [32] achieved a sensitivity of 97.1% and a specificity of 88.0% when evaluated on 144 CBCT volumes with 206 lesions.

The great success of any deep CNN-based approach is based upon the assumption that training and testing data come from the same data distribution. However, when the test data deviates from the training data distribution, the ability of deep neural networks to generalize and perform well on the new data degrades [35]. This phenomenon is often observed in clinical datasets due to factors such as anatomical anomalies, image artifacts, or occlusions, which shift the data distribution. In light of this, our validation study aims to provide a thorough statistical evaluation regarding the effectiveness and generalization capability of the CNN-based PAL-detection model proposed in [32] on an entirely new, previously unseen clinical CBCT dataset with a shifted data distribution compared to the data used to train the model. The null hypothesis of this validation study is that the method proposed in [32] delivers an inferior result when applied to our new, challenging evaluation dataset from clinical practice.

2. Materials and Methods

2.1. Study Design

The research protocol for this retrospective study was performed following the guidelines of the Declaration of Helsinki. Ethical approval for retrospective collection of the evaluation dataset used in this study was provided by the local Ethics Committee of the Medical University of Graz, Austria (review board number "34-519 ex 21/22").

2.2. Sample Size Calculation

The sample size for this study is based on assumptions for the lesion detection sensitivity. We assumed observation of a sensitivity of 95%, corresponding to the lower limit of the 95% confidence interval for the sensitivity observed in the prior study of Kirnbauer et al. [32]. To show that the sensitivity is non-inferior to 90% (using a margin of 5%), a sample size of 243 lesions is necessary to achieve a power of >80%, using a one-sided non-inferiority binomial test with an alpha of 2.5%. Assuming that about 10% of the teeth have lesions, a sample size of 2430 teeth is required. For an assumed specificity of 87% and to show that the specificity is non-inferior to 82% (margin of 5%), the sample size of 2187 teeth yields a power of >99%.

2.3. Dataset

Dataset collection was performed similarly to Kirnbauer et al. [32], but in a less selective manner, so that clinical practice was better reflected (see the comparison of inclusion and exclusion criteria between studies in Table 1). CBCT volumes from routine clinical operations performed for different diagnostic indications (i.e., implant planning, radiological assessment of impacted teeth, assessment of odontogenic tumors or other lesions, and orthodontic reasons) from the year 2018 were retrospectively screened and selected according to the criteria listed in Table 1. All scans were performed on a Planmeca ProMax® 3D Max (Planmeca, Helsinki, Finland) device.

Table 1. Comparison of inclusion and exclusion criteria for dataset collection in this study and the study conducted by Kirnbauer et al. [32].

Criterion	Kirnbauer et al. [32]	This Study
Field of view with a representation of the entire dental arch (upper jaw, lower jaw, or both)	Included	Included
Device and assessment parameters: Field of view of 10.0 × 5.9 cm or 10.0 × 9.3 cm, covering at least one completely visible dental arch, with a 200-µm voxel size (96 kV, 5.6–9.0 mA, 12 s), which is labeled as "normal" mode by the manufacturer	Included	Included
An acceptable degree of scatter and/or artifacts (exclusion of clinically insufficient interpretable datasets, i.e., severe metal artifacts inhibiting individual crown visualization, and ghost effects/double images due to long-motion artifacts)	Included	Included
Completed root development	Included	Included
No edentulism	Included Additional: as few missing teeth as possible	Included Additional: up to 11 missing teeth per jaw
Tooth gaps	Excluded	Included
Partially and totally impacted teeth	Excluded	Included
Dental implants	Excluded	Included
Augmentations	Excluded	Included

The collected dataset was pseudonymized, so that patient names were replaced with a sequential code and no conclusions could be drawn about patient data when they were used during the investigation. All investigators who received access to encrypted and non-encrypted data were subject to the General Data Protection Regulation (GDPR) and the Austrian Data Protection Regulation in the currently valid version (http://www.dsb.gv.at, accessed on 14 December 2023). An initial dataset screening was performed by one dentist on an MDNC-2221 monitor (resolution 1600 × 1200; size 432 mm × 324 mm; 59.9 Hz; Barco Control Rooms GmbH, Karlsruhe, Germany) using the Planmeca Romexis® software version 6.0 (Planmeca, Helsinki, Finland).

The ground-truth detection of PALs was performed by three investigators (two senior oral surgeons with >15 years of experience and one junior dentist), who did an initial round of lesion detection separately from each other on the whole dataset. Within a second round, lesion results were consensually determined including PAL classification, according to the periapical index scoring scheme of Estrela et al. [20], thus establishing the expert ground truth. The collected dataset consisted of a total of 196 CBCT images from unique patients. One patient image had to be excluded due to the software failing to read the file, leaving 195 patient images (99.5%) for the comparison of software-based PAL detections with expert ground truth within this study. Out of these 195 images, 164 showed only one jaw, and 31 images displayed both jaws. In total, there were 2947 present teeth across the 226 jaws (101 lower jaws, 125 upper jaws) in the dataset. In the images of these jaws, there were 669 teeth missing due to various possible reasons, such as caries, periodontitis, dental trauma, periapical disease, or orthodontic reasons [36].

During the investigation, a total of 300 periapical lesions were identified by the expert consensus, and the remaining 2647 present teeth were determined to be lesion-free. Table 2 provides a summary of the dataset characteristics, including lesion classification according to the lesion diameter-based periapical index scoring scheme proposed by Estrela et al. [20], while Table 3 gives a detailed distribution of tooth groups per lesion class.

Table 2. Overview of dataset characteristics used for the evaluation in this study.

	Number	Additional Information
Images	195	One jaw: 164 Both jaws: 31
Jaws	226	Upper: 125 Lower: 101
Teeth present	2947	With lesion: 300 (10.2%) Without lesion: 2647 (89.8%)
Lesion classification [1]	Score 1: 28 (9.3%) Score 2: 59 (19.7%) Score 3: 67 (22.3%) Score 4: 85 (28.3%) Score 5: 61 (20.3%)	Diameter > 0.5–1 mm Diameter > 1–2 mm Diameter > 2–4 mm Diameter > 4–8 mm Diameter > 8 mm

[1] Lesion classification performed according to Estrela et al. [20].

Table 3. Distribution of lesions over periapical index scores for each tooth group.

Periapical Index Score	1	2	3	4	5	Total
Third molars	3 (27.3%)	4	0	2	2	11
Second molars	4 (6.0%)	12	9	20	22	67
First molars	3 (3.5%)	17	19	25	21	85
Second premolars	6 (14.0%)	9	10	14	4	43
First premolars	2 (5.7%)	9	11	8	5	35
Canines	1 (7.7%)	3	4	2	3	13
Lateral incisors	3 (21.4%)	1	4	4	2	14
Central incisors	6 (18.8%)	4	10	10	2	32
Total	28 (9.3%)	59	67	85	61	300

2.4. Automatic PAL Detection

To facilitate the evaluation of the CNNs' performances on the newly collected dataset, we have developed a user-friendly Windows software program. The program incorporates the PAL-detection method proposed in [32] and includes a graphical user interface built using the tkinter library in Python. This interface eliminates the need for any programming operations, thus simplifying the evaluation process and hiding the details of the software for the purpose of this independent evaluation. The user can select the CBCT image to be processed and choose the specific jaw they want to investigate. The software then creates a segmentation map of the detected lesions in the CBCT input image and saves it automatically. The time required to generate a segmentation map depends on the GPU used. Here, we utilized the Asus GeForce® GTX 1660 Ti 6GB TUF Gaming EVO OC graphics card, and the generation of a segmentation map took at most 3 min.

The PAL-detection method [32] integrated into the software consists of three main steps, as illustrated in Figure 1. First, the SpatialConfiguration-Net (SCN) [37] is trained to predict the 3D coordinates of teeth in the original images at a lower resolution. The original image is resized to a fixed aspect ratio of [64, 64, 32] before being input into the SCN. The resulting teeth locations are then utilized to crop the input image for each present tooth, where the center coordinates of the cropped images correspond to the predicted coordinates of teeth. Each cropped image is resampled using trilinear interpolation and an isotropic voxel size of 0.4 mm and has a size of [64, 64, 64]. Finally, these cropped images are fed into a modified U-Net, trained to generate binary segmentation maps that visualize the detected periapical lesions for individual teeth. The SCN and the U-Net were trained and tested on a dataset consisting of 144 CBCT images, with 2128 present teeth and 206 manually annotated periapical lesions. Within that dataset, there were 54 images of the lower jaw, 74 images of the upper jaw, and 16 images of both jaws. The method underwent a four-fold cross-validation, where the dataset was divided into four subsets of equal sizes, and the teeth with lesions were uniformly distributed over the folds. Each fold involved training on the three subsets and testing on the single remaining subset. As a result, four different trained models were obtained, with each model being trained on 108 images and tested on 36 different images. The models were trained in such a manner that the imbalance between positive and negative samples, i.e., cases with and without lesions, did not affect their performances. The training and testing procedures were performed using an Intel(R) CPU 920 with an NVIDIA GeForce GTX TITAN X on the Ubuntu 20.04 operating system with Python 3.7 and TensorFlow 1.15.0. The SCN required approximately 20 h for training per cross-validation fold, while the modified U-Net took approximately 17 h. For additional details on the network's architecture, training/testing procedure, and prediction performance, we refer to [32,38].

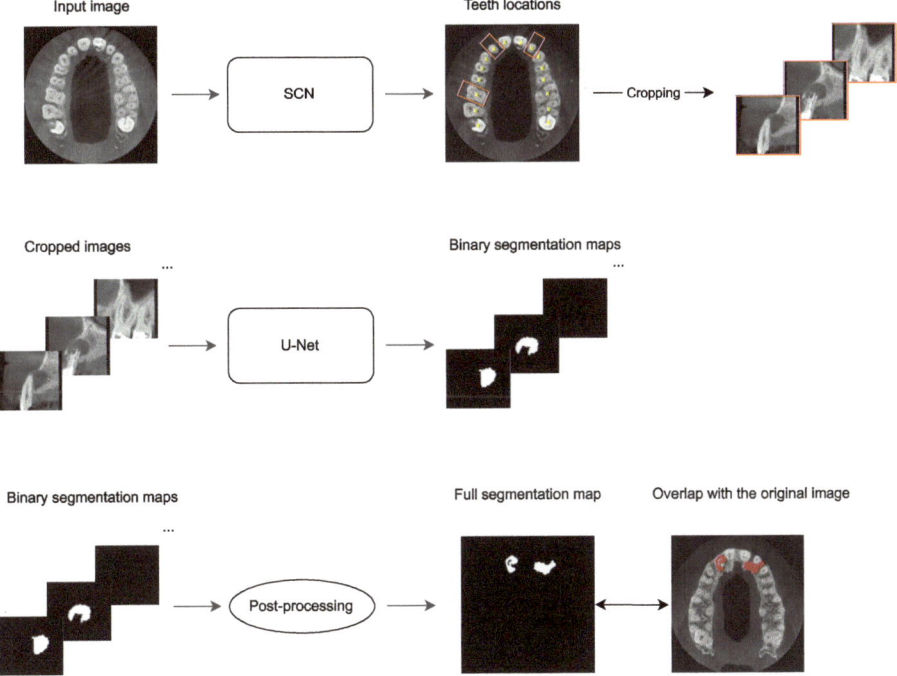

Figure 1. Method overview: First, the SpatialConfiguration-Net (SCN) is utilized to generate the locations of teeth in a given CBCT image. These locations are then used to crop the input image for each tooth, ensuring that the center coordinate of each cropped image matches the predicted coordinate of the corresponding tooth. In the second stage, the cropped images are fed into a modified U-Net, which generates binary segmentation maps that visualize detected lesions in these cropped images. Lastly, the binary segmentation maps are resampled and merged to create a full segmentation map that visualizes all detected lesions in the input CBCT image.

The software used in this study utilizes one of the four pre-trained models from [32] to evaluate the lesion detection performance of the model on a new, independent dataset consisting of 195 CBCT images. The dataset used in this study is a pure test dataset that the model has not seen before, i.e., its images have not been used during training of the PAL-detection method or to tune its hyperparameters. Before generating the final output image, the software applies an additional post-processing step, as illustrated in the bottom row of Figure 1. After the PAL-detection method generates binary segmentation maps for the cropped teeth images, we implement a resampling and merging procedure to create a full segmentation map that includes detected lesions for all teeth within the original image. To achieve this, first, a blank segmentation map of the identical size and spacing as the original image is generated. Subsequently, the original input image and the blank segmentation map are resampled to match the spacing of the cropped images. The predicted teeth coordinates obtained from the SCN, which were used for cropping the images, are also transformed using the spacing of the cropped images. These transformed coordinates determine the regions where the predicted binary segmentation maps are copied. Finally, the full segmentation map containing the detected lesions is resampled back to match the size and spacing of the original image.

2.5. Expert Assessment of Software PAL Detections

After applying the automatic PAL-detection software (based on the pre-trained model from [32]) to the new dataset, lesion segmentation results were assessed in consensus by two of the three dental investigators (one senior, one junior), who first did the expert ground-truth annotation. For assessment, they used the ITK-SNAP software [39] and loaded the CBCT volume as well as the corresponding resampled lesion segmentation for visualization. Investigators marked the segmentation results, which were defined as regions of at least one voxel in size, as true or false positives on the level of individual teeth. As soon as the segmentation affected two or more neighboring teeth, all of those teeth were noted to have a CNN-detected PAL. Furthermore, segmentations that were lying in areas far away from the periapical regions, within nerve channels, pulp chambers of impacted teeth, or even outside the alveolar crest were also documented and detected as false positives.

2.6. Statistical Analysis

To evaluate the algorithm's performance in identifying PALs, sensitivity and specificity metrics are used, comparing positive and negative detections with the expert ground truth. Sensitivity (recall) measures the method's accuracy in identifying the presence of lesions, while specificity measures its ability to correctly identify the absence of lesions. Sensitivity and specificity with their corresponding exact 95% confidence intervals (CIs) are presented for all teeth and stratified by upper/lower jaw and tooth type. Non-inferiority tests were performed using one-sided binomial tests with an alpha of 2.5%. Differences in sensitivity and specificity between lower and upper jaws were assessed by Fisher's exact tests. For statistical analysis, SAS version 9.4 was used.

3. Results

From Table 4, it can be seen that the overall sensitivity of the deep learning-based lesion detection approach evaluated on all present teeth was 86.7% (95% CI: 82.3–90.3%) when compared with the expert-derived ground truth. The specificity of the software was 84.3% (95% CI: 82.8–85.6%). The null hypothesis of inferiority of the software with respect to sensitivity could not be rejected ($p = 0.975$), while the null hypothesis of inferiority with respect to specificity could be rejected ($p = 0.001$). In our dataset consisting of images, where either one or both jaws were available, any of the jaws could have missing teeth. Out of a total of 669 missing teeth, the software found 42 false positive (6.3%) lesion predictions, while 627 missing teeth were correctly identified as negatives (93.7%). The confusion matrices of the overall results for present teeth, as well as for present and missing teeth combined, are given in Tables 5 and 6.

Table 4. Lesion detection results. We show sensitivities and specificities including confidence intervals (CIs) for all present teeth in three result categories: overall for all teeth, stratified by jaws, and stratified by tooth type (combining jaws).

Category	Lesion count	Sensitivity (%)	95% CI Exact	Specificity (%)	95% CI Exact
Overall	300	86.67	82.29–90.30%	84.25	82.80–85.61%
Upper jaw	196	87.76	82.33–91.99%	82.31	80.21–84.27%
Lower jaw	104	84.62	76.22–90.94%	86.43	84.40–88.28%
Third molars	11	63.64	30.79–89.07%	81.61	75.04–87.07%
Second molars	67	91.04	81.52–96.64%	70.59	64.97–75.78%
First molars	85	91.76	83.77–96.62%	70.51	64.22–76.28%
Second premolars	43	88.37	74.92–96.11%	81.63	77.03–85.64%
First premolars	35	82.86	66.35–93.44%	87.37	83.60–90.54%
Canines	13	69.23	38.57–90.91%	89.70	86.41–92.41%
Lateral incisors	14	64.29	35.14–87.24%	92.68	89.72–95.01%
Central incisors	32	90.63	74.98–98.02%	88.03	84.44–91.04%

Table 5. Confusion matrix of lesion detection for present teeth.

		Predicted condition		
		Lesion	Non-lesion	Total
Actual condition	Lesion	260	40	300
	Non-lesion	417	2230	2647
	Total	677	2270	2947

Table 6. Confusion matrix of lesion detection for present and missing teeth combined.

		Predicted condition		
		Lesion	Non-lesion	Total
Actual condition	Lesion	260	40	300
	Non-lesion	459	2857	3316
	Total	719	2897	3616

Table 4 also illustrates individual lesion detection results stratified per jaw. For the upper jaw ($N = 125$ patients with a total of 1598 present teeth), the sensitivity is 87.8% (95% CI: 82.3–92.0%), and the specificity is 82.3% (95% CI: 80.2–84.3%). For the lower jaw ($N = 101$ patients with a total of 1349 present teeth), the sensitivity is 84.6% (95% CI: 76.2–90.9%), and the specificity is 86.4% (95% CI: 84.4–88.3%). The difference in sensitivity between the upper jaw and lower jaw is 3.2% (95% CI: −5.2–11.5%). This difference is not significant according to Fisher's exact test when comparing the two jaws ($p = 0.478$). The difference in specificity between the upper jaw and lower jaw is −4.1% (95% CI: −6.9–1.4%), which is significant ($p = 0.004$) according to Fisher's exact test.

Moreover, we illustrate lesion detection results stratified per tooth type (combined for both jaws) in Table 4. Sensitivities are below 70% for the three categories where also the total number of lesions was comparatively lower (third molars, canines, lateral incisors). On the other hand, for the remaining five tooth categories, the average sensitivity is 88.9%.

Finally, we analyze the lesion detection results with respect to lesion classifications (periapical index scores according to Estrela et al. [20]). In Figure 2, we plot a histogram of true positives and false negatives per lesion type, illustrating that for the smallest lesion type (class 1, with a diameter of periapical radiolucency between 0.5 and 1 mm), the sensitivity is low, while for classes 2 through 5 (diameters of periapical radiolucency larger than 1 mm, see also Table 2), the sensitivities are much higher.

Exemplary qualitative results of the software are shown in Figure 3.

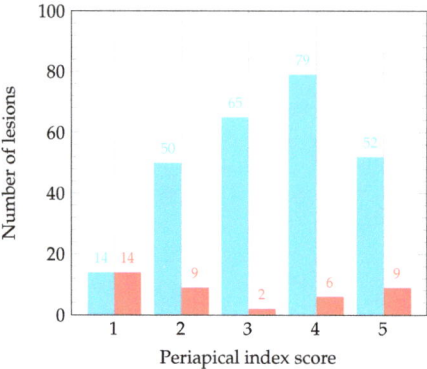

Figure 2. Distribution of predicted lesions across different periapical index scores according to Estrela et al. [20]. Blue bins represent true positive (TP) predictions, while red bins represent false negative (FN) predictions for a specific periapical index score.

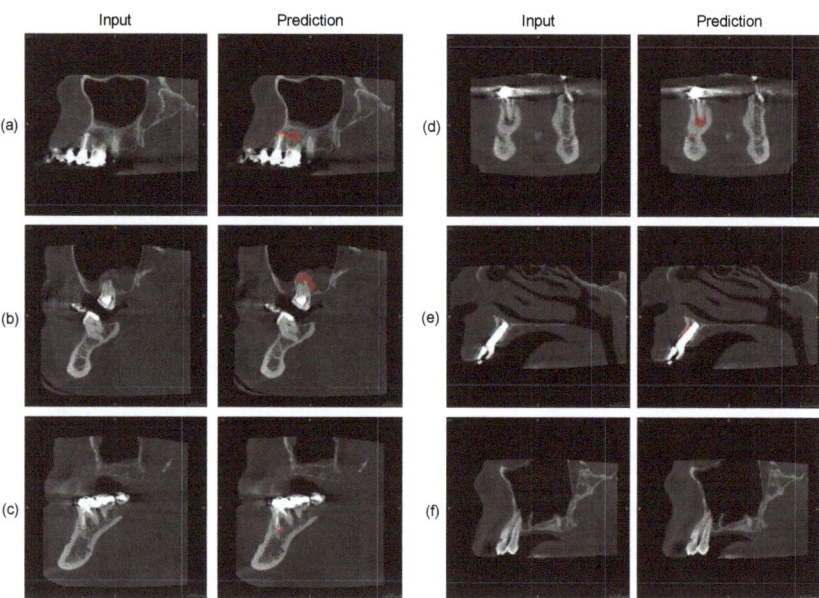

Figure 3. Qualitative results: (**a**) Two true positive (TP) lesions are detected at the second premolar and the first molar, and one false positive (FP) lesion is identified at the second molar in the upper jaw. (**b**) One TP lesion is found at the second molar in the upper jaw at a challenging location close to the sinus. (**c**) One TP lesion is detected at the first molar in the lower jaw. (**d**) One TP lesion is identified at the second premolar, along with one FP lesion at the mental nerve in the lower jaw. (**e**) One FP lesion is observed at the anterior tooth position in the upper jaw due to artifacts at an implant site. (**f**) One FP lesion is detected at the first premolar in the upper jaw (close to the sinus). The qualitative results are best visualized in PDF format.

4. Discussion

Recent machine learning methods, especially deep neural networks for assisting experts in the detection and segmentation of lesions in medical imaging data, have shown tremendous success, but they struggle with issues due to a lack of generalization to datasets from clinical practice [35]. We have performed a thorough evaluation and non-inferiority testing of a recently published algorithm for automated periapical lesion segmentation from dental CBCT images [32]. This algorithm was hidden behind a graphical user interface that solely produced a lesion segmentation given an input image from the new, single-use testing dataset used in this study. The dataset comprises 196 subjects with images of adult upper and lower jaws, including tooth gaps, dental restorations, implants, and impacted third molars (see Table 1). Additionally, the new dataset was obtained with a specific criterion that allowed the inclusion of up to 11 missing teeth per jaw. This led to a significantly higher number of missing teeth compared to the dataset in [32], where the aim was to include jaws with a minimal number of missing teeth. Thus, our new evaluation dataset reflects the presence of challenging circumstances in clinical practice. Moreover, our evaluation protocol was very strict in defining false positive findings, since one false positive (FP) voxel in the segmentation had already led to an FP prediction (see Figure 3a), thus imposing a hard but realistic scenario for the algorithm.

The algorithm could be successfully applied to present and missing teeth from 195 subjects, i.e., 99.5% of subjects in the total dataset. Our main result is a sensitivity of 86.7% and a specificity of 84.3% in detecting PALs at present teeth. The non-inferiority tests, which were designed upon sensitivity and specificity estimates derived from the proof of concept evaluation in [32], provided enough evidence to reject the null hypothesis for specificity but did not do so for sensitivity. Despite this drop in sensitivity, we still consider our absolute performance on this challenging dataset as very promising (see also our qualitative results in Figure 3a–c), since both the sensitivity and specificity are better than the threshold of 80%, which, according to the systematic review in [24], can be interpreted as the threshold indicating excellent results. One of the reasons for false positives occurring might be that some lesions are located close to the incisive, the inferior alveolar, and the mental nerve, as illustrated in Figure 3d. Furthermore, artifacts in general, caused by root canal fillings or dental implants potentially pose problems for the deep CNN (see Figure 3e). We also studied the algorithm's performance at missing teeth and found that the overall specificity for present and missing teeth combined increases from 84.3% to 86.2% (see confusion matrix in Table 6).

Regarding the related work for automated detection of PALs in CBCT images, only a limited number of studies have been published. Zheng et al. [28] proposed an anatomically constrained Dense U-Net model, which they evaluated on 20 CBCT images, obtaining a sensitivity of 84.0% and a precision of 90.0% in a root-based evaluation. In addition, Orhan et al. [29] used a U-Net-based model to evaluate PAL detection in CBCT images and achieved a sensitivity of 92.8%. Setzer et al. [27] evaluated a U-Net-based model on 2D slices from 20 CBCT images and achieved a sensitivity of 93.0% and a specificity of 88.0% in PAL detection. Recently, Calazans et al. [34] proposed a classification model based on a 2D Siamese Network combined with a DenseNet-121 CNN [40]. Their model was evaluated on 1000 coronal and sagittal slices extracted from CBCT images and achieved a sensitivity of 64.5% and a specificity of 75.8% in classifying PALs.

Comparing our study with those conducted by Zheng et al. [28] and Orhan et al. [29] is difficult due to the lack of reported specificities and details regarding negative class examples in their research. Relying on the precision metric for comparison may be misleading since our dataset is highly imbalanced, whereas their datasets have a well-balanced distribution that does not reflect real-world clinical scenarios. The precision metric is sensitive to class distribution, making it less suitable in this context. In terms of sensitivity and specificity, our study outperforms the results of Calazans et al. [34], as they report a higher number of false negatives and false positives. While our sensitivity and specificity results are lower than those of the closely related and best-performing work by Setzer et al. [27], it is important to note that their evaluation solely consisted of 20 CBCT test images with 61 roots. Therefore, we claim that our evaluation protocol is more strict than theirs, due to our extensive single-use testing dataset collected from clinical practice. Furthermore, many of these works use models trained on 2D slices, thus neglecting valuable 3D information.

In CBCT imaging, PALs are often not the primary clinical question, however, secondary PAL findings occur frequently, and, furthermore, they have to be documented by dentists who are often not radiological experts or may not have sufficient time to assess the CBCT images in great detail. In such cases, the help of an algorithm is invaluable to prevent findings from being overlooked, even at the cost of a larger number of false positives, which, however, can be ruled out comparatively straightforwardly, either visually or via additional clinical assessment of the respective tooth.

To study our evaluation results in more detail, we also analyze different stratifications of the testing dataset. While collecting the expert ground truth of the lesions, a lesion classification of lesion diameters into five different periapical index score categories [20] was used. We see from Figure 2 that for lesion classes 2 through 5 (lesions with diameters larger than 1 mm), the algorithm leads to few false negatives, i.e., high recall, while for lesion class 1 (lesions between 0.5 and 1 mm of diameter), 50% of the lesions in our dataset were missed. From a radiological point of view, such small lesions are generally challenging to detect, which was previously reported by Tsai et al. [41] when studying simulated lesions in vitro on radiographs and CBCTs. If we use the lesion class stratification to compute the sensitivity solely for lesion classes 2 through 5, it reaches 90.4% (95% CI: 86.3–93.7%), which we consider to be a meaningful recall in clinical practice, such that the use of the algorithm can be suggested for lesions of sizes larger than 1 mm.

Another stratification that we investigated was from the anatomical point of view. Our results indicate that the algorithm provides a significantly higher specificity for teeth in the lower jaw, while the sensitivity difference between the lower and upper jaw was not statistically significant. We assume that this decrease in false positive findings for the lower jaw is due to its better radiological assessability compared with the upper jaw since the contrast between radiolucent lesions and alveolar bone or teeth is higher in the lower jaw (see Figure 3a (at the second molar), c and d). Moreover, teeth in the upper jaw are located close to the maxillary sinus, such that the thin bony maxillary sinus floor or potential sinus membrane alterations might lead to confusion for the algorithm (see Figure 3b,f).

When looking at different tooth categories in Table 4, where teeth are assessed for both jaws combined, we notice that there are three tooth groups for which sensitivity is lower (below 70%), i.e., wisdom teeth (3rd molars), canines, and lateral incisors. Wisdom teeth are rarer in the population in general since many of them are removed when reaching adulthood or never show up. This is also reflected in our dataset, thus leading to a low number of lesions as well (see Table 4). Moreover, different from lateral incisors and canines, molars are the teeth most affected by PALs, according to [42]. Due to the lower number of lesions in the abovementioned three tooth groups (see Table 4 for numbers of lesions), false negatives have a larger relative influence. Additionally, class 1 lesions of a smaller diameter are more strongly represented in two out of these three tooth categories in our dataset (third molars, lateral incisors, see Table 3). We assume that the combination of these aspects leads to the lower sensitivity, while the average sensitivity of the remaining five tooth categories, where a larger number of lesions is present in each category, is 88.9%.

One limitation of our study is that the dataset collection for this evaluation was performed at the same hospital as in [32]. While the focus was on the evaluation of generalizability via the inclusion of challenging data representative for clinical practice, we can therefore not draw any conclusions regarding generalizing to data from different sites. Moreover, the impact of anatomic variability due to differences in ethnicities, as, e.g., demonstrated in [43], regarding the occurrence of radix entomolaris in an Asian population, has not been taken into account. Another limitation was that our testing dataset only contained a low number of lesions of periapical lesion index score 1. We conclude that in order to improve the algorithm and to draw stronger conclusions for small lesions as well, a re-training of the machine learning method on more data with the class 1 lesion diameter is required, which we see as potential future work.

In summary, we see our results as a very promising indication that machine learning can play an important role in assisting experts in dental practice, where high recall is needed to prevent overlooked findings.

5. Conclusions

In this validation study, we performed a thorough evaluation and non-inferiority test of the periapical lesion (PAL)-detection algorithm proposed in [32] using a new, real-world clinical CBCT dataset. Despite the presence of challenging scenarios in the dataset, such as dental restorations, implants, and impacted third molars, the algorithm demonstrated promising results in accurately detecting PALs. Our evaluation covered all present teeth in the dataset and yielded a sensitivity of 86.7% and a specificity of 84.3% when compared with expert ground truth. The non-inferiority test rejected the null hypothesis for specificity for the non-inferiority threshold of 82%, but it did not reject the null hypothesis for sensitivity for the non-inferiority threshold of 90%. We also found that for lesions smaller than 1 mm, the sensitivity was low. However, when evaluating solely on lesions with periapical index scores 2 through 5, the sensitivity increased to 90.4%, thus indicating that the algorithm has the potential to assist clinicians to prevent overlooked lesions with a diameter above 1 mm. Overall, we conclude that the algorithm is promising but not yet fully robust to all the artifacts and outliers that were present in this clinically representative dataset.

Author Contributions: A.H.: Conceptualization, Methodology, Software, Visualization, Writing—original draft. M.U.: Conceptualization, Methodology, Writing—original draft, Writing—review and editing. J.-N.A.P.: Data curation, Investigation, Methodology. R.R.: Formal analysis, Validation, Visualization. P.R.: Data curation, Investigation. D.Š.: Methodology, Supervision. B.K.: Conceptualization, Data curation, Funding acquisition, Investigation, Project Administration, Supervision, Writing—review and editing. All authors have read and agreed to the published version of the manuscript.

Funding: This research received no external funding.

Institutional Review Board Statement: This study was conducted according to the guidelines of the Declaration of Helsinki and approved by the Ethics Committee of the Medical University of Graz (Review Board number: 34-519 ex 21/22; date of approval: 5 December 2022).

Informed Consent Statement: Not applicable.

Data Availability Statement: The data presented in this study are available on request from the corresponding author. The data are not publicly available due to ethical restrictions.

Acknowledgments: The authors would like to thank Norbert Jakse for supporting this study.

Conflicts of Interest: The authors declare no conflict of interest.

Abbreviations

The following abbreviations are used in this manuscript:

CBCT	Cone-beam computed tomography
AI	Artificial intelligence
CNN	Convolutional neural network
3D	Three-dimensional
PAL	Periapical lesion
GDPR	General Data Protection Regulation
SCN	SpatialConfiguration-Net
CI	Confidence interval
TP	True positive
FN	False negative
FP	False positive

References

1. Goodfellow, I.; Bengio, Y.; Courville, A. *Deep Learning*; MIT Press: Cambridge, MA, USA, 2016.
2. Li, Z.; Liu, F.; Yang, W.; Peng, S.; Zhou, J. A Survey of convolutional neural networks: Analysis, applications, and prospects. *IEEE Trans. Neural Netw. Learn. Syst.* **2022**, *33*, 6999–7019. [CrossRef] [PubMed]
3. Litjens, G.; Kooi, T.; Bejnordi, B.E.; Setio, A.A.A.; Ciompi, F.; Ghafoorian, M.; van der Laak, J.A.W.M.; van Ginneken, B.; Sánchez, C.I. A survey on deep learning in medical image analysis. *Med. Image Anal.* **2017**, *42*, 60–88. [CrossRef] [PubMed]
4. Yu, H.; Yang, L.T.; Zhang, Q.; Armstrong, D.; Deen, M.J. Convolutional neural networks for medical image analysis: State-of-the-art, comparisons, improvement and perspectives. *Neurocomputing* **2021**, *444*, 92–110. [CrossRef]
5. Esteva, A.; Kuprel, B.; Novoa, R.A.; Ko, J.; Swetter, S.M.; Blau, H.M.; Thrun, S. Dermatologist-level classification of skin cancer with deep neural networks. *Nature* **2017**, *542*, 115–118. [CrossRef] [PubMed]
6. De Fauw, J.; Ledsam, J.R.; Romera-Paredes, B.; Nikolov, S.; Tomasev, N.; Blackwell, S.; Askham, H.; Glorot, X.; O'Donoghue, B.; Visentin, D.; et al. Clinically applicable deep learning for diagnosis and referral in retinal disease. *Nat. Med.* **2018**, *24*, 1342–1350. [CrossRef] [PubMed]
7. McKinney, S.M.; Sieniek, M.; Godbole, V.; Godwin, J.; Antropova, N.; Ashrafian, H.; Back, T.; Chesus, M.; Corrado, G.S.; Darzi, A.; et al. International evaluation of an AI system for breast cancer screening. *Nature* **2020**, *577*, 89–94. [CrossRef] [PubMed]
8. Schwendicke, F.; Samek, W.; Krois, J. Artificial intelligence in dentistry: Chances and challenges. *J. Dent. Res.* **2020**, *99*, 769–774. [CrossRef] [PubMed]
9. Shukla, S.; Chug, A.; Afrashtehfar, K.I. Role of cone beam computed tomography in diagnosis and treatment planning in dentistry: An update. *J. Int. Soc. Prev. Community Dent.* **2017**, *7*, S125. [CrossRef]
10. Khanagar, S.B.; Alfadley, A.; Alfouzan, K.; Awawdeh, M.; Alaqla, A.; Jamleh, A. Developments and performance of artificial intelligence models designed for application in endodontics: A systematic review. *Diagnostics* **2023**, *13*, 414. [CrossRef]
11. Issa, J.; Jaber, M.; Rifai, I.; Mozdziak, P.; Kempisty, B.; Dyszkiewicz-Konwińska, M. Diagnostic Test Accuracy of Artificial Intelligence in Detecting Periapical Periodontitis on Two-Dimensional Radiographs: A Retrospective Study and Literature Review. *Medicina* **2023**, *59*, 768. [CrossRef]
12. Hung, K.F.; Ai, Q.Y.H.; Wong, L.M.; Yeung, A.W.K.; Li, D.T.S.; Leung, Y.Y. Current applications of deep learning and radiomics on CT and CBCT for maxillofacial diseases. *Diagnostics* **2022**, *13*, 110. [CrossRef] [PubMed]
13. Sin, Ç.; Akkaya, N.; Aksoy, S.; Orhan, K.; Öz, U. A deep learning algorithm proposal to automatic pharyngeal airway detection and segmentation on CBCT images. *Orthod. Craniofacial Res.* **2021**, *24* (Suppl. S2), 117–123. [CrossRef] [PubMed]
14. Ajami, M.; Tripathi, P.; Ling, H.; Mahdian, M. Automated detection of cervical carotid artery calcifications in cone beam computed tomographic images using deep convolutional neural networks. *Diagnostics* **2022**, *12*, 2537. [CrossRef] [PubMed]
15. Chai, Z.K.; Mao, L.; Chen, H.; Sun, T.G.; Shen, X.M.; Liu, J.; Sun, Z.J. Improved diagnostic accuracy of ameloblastoma and odontogenic keratocyst on cone-beam CT by artificial intelligence. *Front. Oncol.* **2022**, *11*, 793417. [CrossRef] [PubMed]
16. Lee, J.H.; Kim, D.H.; Jeong, S.N. Diagnosis of cystic lesions using panoramic and cone beam computed tomographic images based on deep learning neural network. *Oral Dis.* **2020**, *26*, 152–158. [CrossRef] [PubMed]
17. Albitar, L.; Zhao, T.; Huang, C.; Mahdian, M. Artificial intelligence (AI) for detection and localization of unobturated second mesial buccal (MB2) canals in cone-beam computed tomography (CBCT). *Diagnostics* **2022**, *12*, 3214. [CrossRef] [PubMed]
18. Yang, P.; Guo, X.; Mu, C.; Qi, S.; Li, G. Detection of vertical root fractures by cone-beam computed tomography based on deep learning. *Dentomaxillofacial Radiol.* **2023**, *52*, 20220345. [CrossRef]
19. Mosier, K.M. Lesions of the Jaw. *Semin. Ultrasound CT MR* **2015**, *36*, 444–450. [CrossRef]
20. Estrela, C.; Bueno, M.R.; Azevedo, B.C.; Azevedo, J.R.; Pécora, J.D. A new periapical index based on cone beam computed tomography. *J. Endod.* **2008**, *34*, 1325–1331. [CrossRef]
21. Becconsall-Ryan, K.; Tong, D.; Love, R.M. Radiolucent inflammatory jaw lesions: A twenty-year analysis. *Int. Endod. J.* **2010**, *43*, 859–865. [CrossRef]
22. Keerthana, G.; Singh, N.; Yadav, R.; Duhan, J.; Tewari, S.; Gupta, A.; Sangwan, P.; Mittal, S. Comparative analysis of the accuracy of periapical radiography and cone-beam computed tomography for diagnosing complex endodontic pathoses using a gold standard reference—A prospective clinical study. *Int. Endod. J.* **2021**, *54*, 1448–1461. [CrossRef]
23. Estrela, C.; Bueno, M.R.; Leles, C.R.; Azevedo, B.; Azevedo, J.R. Accuracy of cone beam computed tomography and panoramic and periapical radiography for detection of apical periodontitis. *J. Endod.* **2008**, *34*, 273–279. [CrossRef] [PubMed]
24. Leonardi Dutra, K.; Haas, L.; Porporatti, A.L.; Flores-Mir, C.; Nascimento Santos, J.; Mezzomo, L.A.; Corrêa, M.; De Luca Canto, G. Diagnostic Accuracy of Cone-beam Computed Tomography and Conventional Radiography on Apical Periodontitis: A Systematic Review and Meta-analysis. *J. Endod.* **2016**, *42*, 356–364. [CrossRef] [PubMed]
25. Antony, D.P.; Thomas, T.; Nivedhitha, M.S. Two-dimensional Periapical, Panoramic Radiography Versus Three-dimensional Cone-beam Computed Tomography in the Detection of Periapical Lesion After Endodontic Treatment: A Systematic Review. *Cureus* **2020**, *12*, e7736. [CrossRef] [PubMed]
26. Ekert, T.; Krois, J.; Meinhold, L.; Elhennawy, K.; Emara, R.; Golla, T.; Schwendicke, F. Deep Learning for the Radiographic Detection of Apical Lesions. *J. Endod.* **2019**, *45*, 917–922.e5. [CrossRef] [PubMed]
27. Setzer, F.C.; Shi, K.J.; Zhang, Z.; Yan, H.; Yoon, H.; Mupparapu, M.; Li, J. Artificial intelligence for the computer-aided detection of periapical lesions in cone-beam computed tomographic images. *J. Endod.* **2020**, *46*, 987–993. [CrossRef]

28. Zheng, Z.; Yan, H.; Setzer, F.C.; Shi, K.J.; Mupparapu, M.; Li, J. Anatomically constrained deep learning for automating dental CBCT segmentation and lesion detection. *IEEE Trans. Autom. Sci. Eng.* **2020**, *18*, 603–614. [CrossRef]
29. Orhan, K.; Bayrakdar, I.; Ezhov, M.; Kravtsov, A.; Özyürek, T. Evaluation of artificial intelligence for detecting periapical pathosis on cone-beam computed tomography scans. *Int. Endod. J.* **2020**, *53*, 680–689. [CrossRef]
30. Ezhov, M.; Gusarev, M.; Golitsyna, M.; Yates, J.M.; Kushnerev, E.; Tamimi, D.; Aksoy, S.; Shumilov, E.; Sanders, A.; Orhan, K. Clinically applicable artificial intelligence system for dental diagnosis with CBCT. *Sci. Rep.* **2021**, *11*, 15006. [CrossRef]
31. Yüksel, A.E.; Gültekin, S.; Simsar, E.; Özdemir, Ş.D.; Gündoğar, M.; Tokgöz, S.B.; Hamamcı, İ.E. Dental enumeration and multiple treatment detection on panoramic X-rays using deep learning. *Sci. Rep.* **2021**, *11*, 12342. [CrossRef]
32. Kirnbauer, B.; Hadzic, A.; Jakse, N.; Bischof, H.; Štern, D. Automatic detection of periapical osteolytic lesions on cone-beam computed tomography using deep convolutional neuronal networks. *J. Endod.* **2022**, *48*, 1434–1440. [CrossRef] [PubMed]
33. Hamdan, M.H.; Tuzova, L.; Mol, A.; Tawil, P.Z.; Tuzoff, D.; Tyndall, D.A. The effect of a deep-learning tool on dentists' performances in detecting apical radiolucencies on periapical radiographs. *Dentomaxillofac. Radiol.* **2022**, *51*, 20220122. [CrossRef] [PubMed]
34. Calazans, M.A.A.; Ferreira, F.A.B.S.; Alcoforado, M.d.L.M.G.; Santos, A.d.; Pontual, A.d.A.; Madeiro, F. Automatic classification system for periapical lesions in cone-beam computed tomography. *Sensors* **2022**, *22*, 6481. [CrossRef] [PubMed]
35. Varoquaux, G.; Cheplygina, V. Machine learning for medical imaging: Methodological failures and recommendations for the future. *npj Digit. Med.* **2022**, *5*, 48. [CrossRef] [PubMed]
36. Broers, D.L.; Dubois, L.; de Lange, J.; Su, N.; de Jongh, A. Reasons for tooth removal in adults: A systematic review. *Int. Dent. J.* **2022**, *72*, 52–57. [CrossRef] [PubMed]
37. Payer, C.; Štern, D.; Bischof, H.; Urschler, M. Integrating spatial configuration into heatmap regression based CNNs for landmark localization. *Med. Image Anal.* **2019**, *54*, 207–219. [CrossRef]
38. Hadzic, A.; Kirnbauer, B.; Štern, D.; Urschler, M. Teeth Localization and Lesion Segmentation in CBCT Images using SpatialConfiguration-Net and U-Net. *arXiv* **2023**, arXiv:2312.12189. [CrossRef]
39. Yushkevich, P.A.; Piven, J.; Hazlett, H.C.; Smith, R.G.; Ho, S.; Gee, J.C.; Gerig, G. User-guided 3D active contour segmentation of anatomical structures: Significantly improved efficiency and reliability. *Neuroimage* **2006**, *31*, 1116–1128. [CrossRef]
40. Huang, G.; Liu, Z.; Van Der Maaten, L.; Weinberger, K.Q. Densely connected convolutional networks. In Proceedings of the 2017 IEEE Conference on Computer Vision and Pattern Recognition (CVPR), Honolulu, HI, USA, 21–26 July 2017; pp. 4700–4708. [CrossRef]
41. Tsai, P.; Torabinejad, M.; Rice, D.; Azevedo, B. Accuracy of cone-beam computed tomography and periapical radiography in detecting small periapical lesions. *J. Endod.* **2012**, *38*, 965–970. [CrossRef]
42. Jakovljevic, A.; Nikolic, N.; Jacimovic, J.; Pavlovic, O.; Milicic, B.; Beljic-Ivanovic, K.; Miletic, M.; Andric, M.; Milasin, J. Prevalence of apical periodontitis and conventional nonsurgical root canal treatment in general adult population: An updated systematic review and meta-analysis of cross-sectional studies published between 2012 and 2020. *J. Endod.* **2020**, *46*, 1371–1386.e8. [CrossRef]
43. Javed, M.Q.; Srivastava, S.; Alotaibi, B.B.R.; Bhatti, U.A.; Abulhamael, A.M.; Habib, S.R. A Cone Beam Computed Tomography-Based Investigation of the Frequency and Pattern of Radix Entomolaris in the Saudi Arabian Population. *Medicina* **2023**, *59*, 2025. [CrossRef] [PubMed]

Disclaimer/Publisher's Note: The statements, opinions and data contained in all publications are solely those of the individual author(s) and contributor(s) and not of MDPI and/or the editor(s). MDPI and/or the editor(s) disclaim responsibility for any injury to people or property resulting from any ideas, methods, instructions or products referred to in the content.

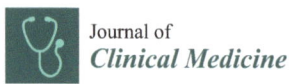 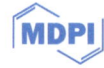

Review

AI in Orthodontics: Revolutionizing Diagnostics and Treatment Planning—A Comprehensive Review

Natalia Kazimierczak [1,†], Wojciech Kazimierczak [1,2,*,†], Zbigniew Serafin [2], Paweł Nowicki [1], Jakub Nożewski [3] and Joanna Janiszewska-Olszowska [4]

1. Kazimierczak Private Medical Practice, Dworcowa 13/u6a, 85-009 Bydgoszcz, Poland
2. Department of Radiology and Diagnostic Imaging, Collegium Medicum, Nicolaus Copernicus University in Torun, Jagiellońska 13-15, 85-067 Bydgoszcz, Poland
3. Department of Emeregncy Medicine, University Hospital No 2 in Bydgoszcz, Ujejskiego 75, 85-168 Bydgoszcz, Poland
4. Department of Interdisciplinary Dentistry, Pomeranian Medical University in Szczecin, 70-111 Szczecin, Poland
* Correspondence: wojtek.kazimierczak@gmail.com; Tel.: +48-606670881
† These authors contributed equally to this work.

Abstract: The advent of artificial intelligence (AI) in medicine has transformed various medical specialties, including orthodontics. AI has shown promising results in enhancing the accuracy of diagnoses, treatment planning, and predicting treatment outcomes. Its usage in orthodontic practices worldwide has increased with the availability of various AI applications and tools. This review explores the principles of AI, its applications in orthodontics, and its implementation in clinical practice. A comprehensive literature review was conducted, focusing on AI applications in dental diagnostics, cephalometric evaluation, skeletal age determination, temporomandibular joint (TMJ) evaluation, decision making, and patient telemonitoring. Due to study heterogeneity, no meta-analysis was possible. AI has demonstrated high efficacy in all these areas, but variations in performance and the need for manual supervision suggest caution in clinical settings. The complexity and unpredictability of AI algorithms call for cautious implementation and regular manual validation. Continuous AI learning, proper governance, and addressing privacy and ethical concerns are crucial for successful integration into orthodontic practice.

Keywords: orthodontics; artificial intelligence; deep learning; cephalometric analysis; radiology; CBCT; skeletal age; treatment planning

1. Introduction

Artificial intelligence (AI), a term first introduced in 1955 by John McCarthy, describes the ability of machines to perform tasks that are classified as intelligent [1]. During these 70 years, there have been cycles of significant optimism associated with the development of AI, alternating with periods of failure, reductions in research funding, and pessimism [2]. The 2015 victory of AlphaGo, a Google-developed AI application, over the "GO" world champion represented a breakthrough [2]. This AI success over a human player sparked further development and interest, which was raised by the introduction of the Chat-GPT in 2022. These events served as precursors to the remarkable growth of AI applications in various fields, including everyday life and medicine [2].

AI algorithms have already proven effective in various medical specialties, surpassing the capabilities of experienced clinicians [3–7]. These algorithms enable the analysis, organization, visualization, and classification of healthcare data. The development of AI algorithms in medicine has gained momentum in recent years, particularly in radiology, where medical imaging accounts for approximately 85% of FDA-approved AI programs (data for 2023) [8].

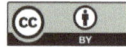

In the field of diagnostic imaging, AI can be categorized into three main domains: operational AI, which enhances healthcare delivery; diagnostic AI, which aids in the interpretation of clinical images; and predictive AI, which forecasts future outcomes [9]. Currently, the primary goals of AI in diagnostic imaging are to detect and segment structures and classify pathologies [10]. AI tools can analyze images obtained from various imaging modalities, ranging from X-ray to MRI [11–15].

Orthodontics, with its emphasis on cephalometric analysis and pretreatment imaging, is particularly well suited for the implementation of AI. However, AI is also being utilized in orthodontics for applications beyond cephalometric analysis. The literature on the use of AI in orthodontics can be divided into five main areas: diagnosis and treatment planning, automated landmark detection and cephalometric analysis, assessment of growth and development, treatment outcome evaluation, and miscellaneous applications [16].

The number of AI companies in the healthcare industry has experienced a remarkable increase, indicating significant growth in commercial prospects for AI [9]. AI tools are no longer limited to researchers and scientists involved in research and development projects. They are now accessible through commercially available web-based products as well. In orthodontics, the adoption of AI has led to the creation of various AI-based programs, such as WeDoCeph (Audax, Ljubljana, Slovenia), WebCeph (Assemble Circle, Seoul, Republic of Korea), and CephX (ORCA Dental AI, Las Vegas, NV, USA). These systems can automatically identify cephalometric landmarks, compute angles and distances, and generate cephalometric reports with significant findings. AI programs are now easily accessible on mobile devices, making AI tools widely available and promoting equal access for all interested users. As a result, orthodontic practices and scientific researchers utilizing AI applications have notably increased. However, this accessibility has also sparked concerns about patient safety, especially when AI is used for diagnosis and treatment.

The main objectives of this article are as follows: elucidate the principles of AI, outline its applications in the diagnostic process of modern orthodontic practices, and discuss the concerns associated with the implementation of AI algorithms in clinical practice.

2. Materials and Methods

2.1. Search Strategy

To conduct this review, literature searches for free text and MeSH terms were performed using several search engines: Medline (PubMed), Web of Science, Scopus, and Google Scholar. The search engines were used to find studies that focused on the application of AI in orthodontics. The last search date was 20 December 2023. For Google Scholar, the search was restricted to the first 100 most relevant articles published over the last 10 years. The search was preceded by a presearch to find the best search terms. The keywords used in the search strategy were as follows: "artificial intelligence", "orthodontics", "deep learning", "neural networks", "automatic detection", "automated", "caries", "periapical lesion", "periapical lucency", "CBCT", "vertebral maturation", "skeletal age assessment", "temporomandibular joint", "temporomandibular joint disorders", "osteoarthritis", "extraction decision making", and "cephalometric landmarks identification". The cited articles explored the subject of AI applications in orthodontics and dentistry: dental diagnostics, cephalometric analysis, TMJ evaluation, determination of skeletal age, and treatment planning.

2.2. Eligibility Criteria

The following inclusion criteria were employed for this review: (1) a randomized clinical trial (RCT), (2) a cohort study, (3) a case–control study, (4) articles published in the last 10 years, and (5) articles published in English.

The following exclusion criteria were applied: (1) case reports; (2) abstracts and author debates or editorials; and (3) papers not related to practical implementations of AI programs in dentistry, particularly in orthodontics.

2.3. Data Extraction

Titles and abstracts were independently selected by two authors (NK and WK) following the inclusion criteria. The full text of each identified article was then analyzed to verify whether the article was suitable for inclusion. Whenever disagreement occurred, it was resolved by discussion with the third author (JJO). The authorship, year of publication, type of each eligible study, and relevance of the study for the application of AI in orthodontics were extracted by one author (NK) and examined by another author (WK).

3. Results and Discussion

There were 509 potential articles identified. After the removal of 183 duplicates, 226 titles and abstracts were assessed. Then, 89 papers were excluded because they did not meet the inclusion criteria and were not related to the topic of this review. All the remaining 139 papers were retrieved and analyzed to conduct this review.

3.1. AI Categories

AI can be classified into two main categories: symbolic AI and machine learning (ML) [17]. Symbolic AI involves structuring an algorithm in a way that is easily understandable to humans. This approach, known as Good Old-Fashioned AI (GOFAI), was dominant in AI research until the late 1980s. Symbolic AI is still useful when problems have limited outcomes, computational power is limited, or human interpretability is important. However, in healthcare, the efficiency of the GOFAI is low due to the complexity of the problems, multiple variables, and limited sets of rules [18]. Therefore, advancements in technology and computer sciences have led to the emergence of more powerful iterations of AI that are replacing the GOFAI in medical applications. Figure 1 provides a schematic representation of AI.

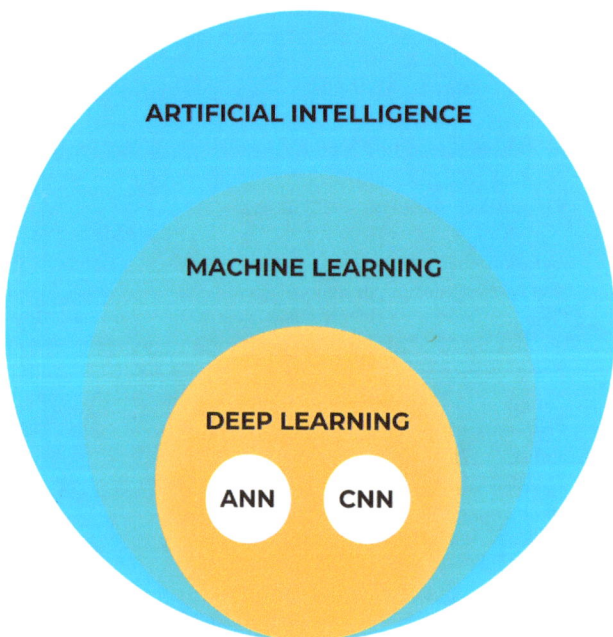

Figure 1. Simplified AI diagram.

3.1.1. Machine Learning

Machine learning (ML) is the predominant paradigm in the field of AI. Coined by Arthur Samuel in 1952, ML differs from symbolic AI because it relies on models learned from examples rather than predefined rules set by humans [19]. By utilizing statistical and probabilistic techniques, machines can enhance their performance by learning from previous models and adapting their actions when new data are introduced. This can involve making predictions, identifying new patterns, or classifying new data.

ML methods can be categorized into three types based on the learning approach and desired outcome. The first type is supervised learning, which is used for classification or prediction tasks where the outcome is already known. In this case, the algorithm learns from a labeled dataset and generalizes its knowledge to make accurate predictions with respect to unseen data. The second type is unsupervised learning, which aims to discover hidden patterns and structures in data without any prior knowledge of the outcome. This type of learning is useful for tasks such as clustering and anomaly detection. Finally, reinforcement learning involves a machine in the development of an algorithm that maximizes a predefined reward based on previous versions of the machine. This type of learning is often used in scenarios where an agent interacts with an environment and learns through trial and error [20].

3.1.2. Deep Learning

Deep learning (DL) is a subset of ML that involves machines independently computing specific characteristics of an input. DL builds upon artificial neural networks (ANNs) developed in the 1990s. Recent advancements in computational technology have allowed researchers to construct more complex neural networks, referred to as "deeper" networks, to handle increasingly challenging tasks. In the field of medical imaging, DL algorithms predominantly utilize convolutional neural networks (CNNs) with high diagnostic accuracy [21–23].

DL differs from traditional ML methods because it enables machines to automatically extract relevant features from input data. Unlike traditional ML, DL models do not rely on human engineers to manually point these features. DL algorithms can learn and identify patterns directly from raw data, eliminating the need for time-consuming feature identification and extraction [23]. This capability has proven particularly valuable in imaging, where DL tools have shown superior diagnostic accuracy compared to experienced readers [21,24,25]. However, DL is not limited to image analysis tasks. It has shown promise in various other applications, such as medical disease diagnosis and personalized treatment recommendation [26–29].

3.2. AI Applications in Orthodontics

3.2.1. Dental Diagnostics

The use of medical imaging methods is essential in dental patient care because they aid in the clinical diagnosis of pathologies related to teeth and their surrounding structures [30–32]. Radiological methods, such as orthopantomograms (OPGs) and cone-beam computed tomography (CBCT), play crucial roles in orthodontic diagnosis, treatment planning, and monitoring [33–35]. However, with the increasing number of radiological examinations being performed [36], there is a need for a comprehensive tool to support the process of radiological diagnosis. In response to this demand, multimodular diagnostic systems based on AI have emerged.

One such AI-based system, developed by Diagnocat Ltd. (San Francisco, CA, USA), utilizes CNNs and provides precise and comprehensive dental diagnostics. The system enables tooth segmentation and enumeration, oral pathology diagnosis (including periapical lesions and caries), and volumetric assessment. Several scientific papers have validated the diagnostic performance of this program, demonstrating its high efficacy and accuracy [37–41]. A study by Orhan et al. [37] reported that the AI system achieved 92.8% accuracy in the detection of periapical lesions in CBCT images and showed no statistically significant difference in volumetric measurements compared to manual methods. Similarly, a study evaluating the diagnostic accuracy of the program for periapical lesion detection on periapical radiographs (PRs) yielded comparable results [38]. However, conflicting results have also been reported, particularly regarding the accuracy of AI in the assessment of periapical lesions in OPGs [42].

In a recent study by Ezhov (2021) [43], the overall diagnostic performance of two groups, one aided by AI and the other unaided, was compared in oral CBCT evaluation. The AI system used in this study included modules for tooth and jaw segmentation, tooth localization and enumeration, periodontitis, caries, and periapical lesion detection. The results showed that the AI system significantly improved the diagnostic capabilities of dentists, with higher sensitivity and specificity values observed in the AI-aided group than in the unaided group (sensitivity: 0.8537 vs. 0.7672; specificity: 0.9672 vs. 0.9616).

Several systematic reviews and meta-analyses have been conducted on the utilization of AI for identifying caries and periapical lucencies [44–55]. In a recent comprehensive study by Rahimi [54], the accuracy of classification models for caries detection was evaluated across 48 studies. The reported diagnostic accuracy varied significantly based on the imaging modality, ranging from 68% to 99.2%. The diagnostic odds ratio, which indicates the effectiveness of the test, also varied greatly from 2.27 to 32,767 across studies. The study concluded that deep learning models show promise for caries detection and may aid clinical workflows. One of the earliest meta-analyses conducted in 2019 on the computer-aided detection of radiolucent lesions in the maxillofacial region [46] yielded a pooled accuracy estimate of 88.75% (95% CI = 85.19–92.30); however, only four studies were included. A more recent meta-analysis by Sadr [52] included 18 studies and revealed that the pooled sensitivity and specificity were 0.925 (95% CI, 0.862–0.960) and 0.852 (95% CI, 0.810–0.885), respectively. The authors concluded that deep learning showed highly accurate results in detecting periapical radiolucent lesions in dental radiographs. These findings suggest that multimodal AI programs may serve as first-line diagnostic aids and decision support systems, improving patient care at multiple levels. Figure 2 shows a sample of the Diagnocat report.

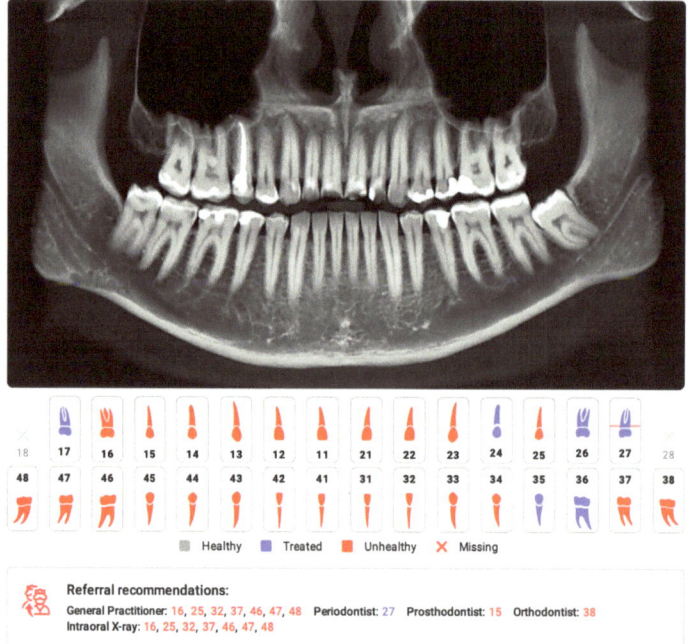

Figure 2. Part of the automatic diagnostic report from a CBCT scan was obtained prior to orthodontic treatment on a 24-year-old male. The software automatically identified the absence of teeth 18 and 28, as well as changes in the remaining teeth, primarily consisting of attrition and the presence of dental fillings. The program has recommended further consultations as necessary.

3.2.2. Cephalometric Analysis

Cephalometric analysis (CA) is an important diagnostic tool in orthodontics that has been in use since 1931 [56]. Over the years, advancements in technology have revolutionized CA by replacing manual assessments with digital software. This approach simplifies the measurement process and provides an automatic display of the analysis results. Automated CA has been shown to be more stable and repeatable than manual analyses, which rely heavily on operator-dependent landmark identification and often exhibit significant variability [57–60]. Accurate and repeatable landmark identification is crucial for reliable CA outcomes. Several studies have demonstrated the effectiveness of AI in identifying cephalometric landmarks. Although lateral radiography remains the most commonly used method in CA, recent AI advancements have sparked renewed interest in the use of cone-beam computed tomography (CBCT) [61].

The effectiveness of AI in identifying cephalometric landmarks has been studied since 1998 [62]. Numerous studies have used various automated methods and have consistently achieved high accuracy in landmark identification [59,60,63–72]. A recent study by Hwang et al. (2020) [60] concluded that automated cephalometric landmark identification can be as reliable as an experienced human reader. Similarly, Kim et al. [65], Lee et al. [71], and Dobratulin et al. [63] achieved landmark definition accuracies between 88% and 92% using AI. These authors also found that, compared with manual methods, AI methods demonstrated greater accuracy in landmark identification and reduced the time and human labor required. In other studies conducted by Hwang et al. [59] and Yu et al. [70], the authors found no statistically significant differences between the results of automated cephalometric analysis and those calculated via manually identified landmarks. Additionally, AI has been shown to significantly improve the workflow of practices, reducing analysis time by up to 80 times compared to manual analysis [72]. Figure 3 shows the definitions of the sampled cephalometric landmarks.

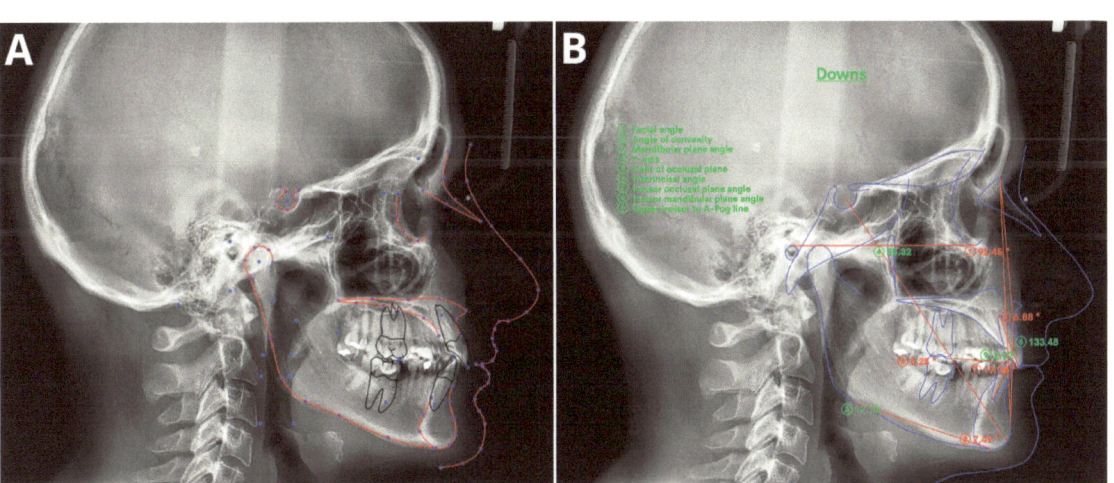

Figure 3. Sample of automatic cephalometric landmark tracings performed using CephX (**A**) and WebCeph (**B**) on an 18-year-old male. The results of Downs cephalometric analysis superimposed on tracings (**B**). Measurements outside the standard range marked in red and with asterix *.

The utilization of CBCT in CA was first reported in the 2000s [73], but its use has remained limited due to inefficiency and time constraints. However, recent advancements in AI have revived interest in CBCT-based CA. Several studies [74–81] have shown that AI techniques are accurate and efficient for automatically identifying and analyzing landmarks, surpassing manual approaches. Kim et al. [80] found that the repeatability of artificial neural networks was higher than achieved by human reades, while Muraev et al. [81]

reported that artificial neural networks (ANNs) performed as well as or better than inexperienced readers in identifying landmarks. However, Bao et al. (2023) [82] recently revealed that manual tracing is still necessary to increase the accuracy of automated AI analysis, indicating the importance of manual supervision.

Meta-analyses have generally shown high accuracy in identifying cephalometric landmarks [83–89]. However, the results are strongly dependent on predefined thresholds, with lower accuracies reported at a 2 mm threshold [83,85,88]. Serafin et al. [89] conducted a study in 2023 and reported a mean difference of 2.44 mm between three-dimensional (3D) automated and manual landmarking. A meta-regression analysis indicated a significant association between publication year and mean error, suggesting that recent advances in deep learning (DL) algorithms have significantly improved landmark annotation accuracy. Overall, AI tools have shown promising results in automated cephalometric analyses, but caution is advised due to potential biases in evaluated studies [83–85,87].

3.2.3. Determination of Skeletal Age

Growth and maturation play crucial roles in orthodontics because they directly impact the effectiveness of orthodontic treatments, which are often timed to coincide with periods of rapid growth and developmental changes in facial structure. Previous studies have demonstrated that tailoring treatments to align with the patient's growth phases can enhance treatment outcomes [90,91]. Additionally, some studies suggest that dental maturation is linked to the patient's skeletal class [92]. Accurately assessing the rate of growth and stage of facial development is crucial in orthodontic treatment to achieve long-term results and minimize post-treatment changes caused by ongoing facial growth [93]. However, growth dynamics during adolescence differ greatly among individuals, making it insufficient to rely solely on chronological age for estimating the amount of remaining growth [94,95].

Skeletal age, which can be assessed using cervical vertebral maturation (CVM) or wrist X-rays, is a more suitable parameter for evaluating individual growth [90,96–99]. While wrist X-rays are contraindicated in standard diagnostic orthodontic routines, the CVM can be assessed using lateral cephalometric X-rays [33]. In recent years, there has been a growing body of scientific evidence supporting the diagnostic accuracy and effectiveness of AI in assessing skeletal age based on both wrist X-rays and CVM [100–105]. Despite the proven diagnostic accuracy of AI in skeletal age assessment, particularly with wrist X-rays and even index finger X-rays, concerns remain regarding the accuracy of CVM-based models [106,107]. Studies on this topic have yielded varied results, with agreement rates with human observers ranging from 58% to more than 90% [107–112]. Seo et al. (2021) reported that CNN-based models achieved more than 90% accuracy in CVM assessments, suggesting that automatic diagnosis using lateral cephalometric radiographs can accurately determine skeletal maturity [109]. However, exercise caution is important when evaluating the results of AI in CVM assessments. Other studies have reported notable discrepancies, particularly during crucial orthodontic treatment stages around the growth peak, when accuracy tends to decrease [95,110].

Caution is advised when interpreting AI-assisted CVM assessment studies due to the limited number of expert readers used to establish the gold standard for evaluation. Errors made by these readers may have influenced the study results and subsequently impacted the performance of the AI algorithm [104]. The lack of scientific evidence in meta-analyses highlights the need for a broader examination of the role of AI in CMR. A recent systematic review by The Angle Orthodontist reported that the model accuracy for test data ranged from 50% to more than 90%. The authors emphasized the importance of conducting new studies to develop robust models and reference standards that can be applied to external datasets. While these findings are encouraging, we anticipate that future advancements in AI technology will enhance the diagnostic accuracy of CMR tools, potentially making them comparable to wrist X-ray assessments for skeletal maturity.

3.2.4. TMJ Evaluation

Osteoarthritis (OA) is a condition that affects joints and is characterized by the gradual deterioration of joint cartilage, bone remodeling, and the formation of osteoproliferative bodies [113]. Temporomandibular joint osteoarthritis (TMJOA) is a specific type of temporomandibular disorder that can cause significant joint pain, dysfunction, and dental malocclusion and a decrease in overall quality of life [113]. The examination of TMJ function and morphology is crucial in orthodontic and dental treatments [114]. TMJOA is one of the causes of malocclusion and facial asymmetry [115,116]. Radiographic examination, such as OPG/CBCT, confirms the presence of TMJOA by revealing bony changes [117], while MRI is the preferred modality for evaluating joint discs [114].

Recent studies have demonstrated the high diagnostic performance of AI in detecting and staging TMJOA [117–121]. These studies have shown the potential for automated, detailed assessment of joint morphology using various imaging techniques, including OPG, CBCT, and MRI. Therefore, the authors anticipate that the use of AI systems for TMJ diagnostic imaging will contribute to future research on early detection and personalized treatments for OA.

The few reviews and meta-analyses conducted on this topic showed the overall moderate-to-good accuracy of the tested models in TMJOA detection [122–126]. The 2023 study by Almasan [123] showed that the pooled sensitivity and specificity of AI in panoramic radiograph TMJOA detection accounted for 0.76 (95% CI 0.35–0.95) and 0.79 (95% CI 0.75–0.83), respectively. Similar results related to this topic were reported by Xu [126], who reported a pooled sensitivity, specificity, and area under the curve (AUC) of 80%, 90%, and 92%, respectively. A more comprehensive study carried out by Jha et al. [125] analyzed 17 articles for the automated diagnosis of masticatory muscle disorders, TMJ osteoarthrosis, internal derangement, and disc perforation. The results of the meta-analysis showed the high diagnostic accuracy of the tested AI models, with accuracy and specificity ranging from 84% to 99.9% and 73% to 100%, respectively.

3.2.5. Extraction Decision Making

One of the most challenging issues during orthodontic treatment is deciding whether extraction is mandatory in a particular case. A variety of factors associated with the identified orthodontic defect, patient preferences, expected outcomes, sociocultural factors, and the professional position of the orthodontist influence the patient's attitude toward the proposed orthodontic extraction therapy [127–129]. On the other hand, decisions related to extractions are influenced by the experience, training, and philosophy of the orthodontist [130–133]. All these factors render the extraction decision during orthodontic treatment very challenging, even for an experienced practitioner. Furthermore, conclusions regarding the treatment undertaken can greatly vary among experts, especially in borderline cases [134–137].

Several AI tools have been introduced in recent years to support therapeutic decision making in orthodontics [94,138,139]. Initial studies on extraction decision aids have shown promising results, with AI algorithms achieving over 80% agreement with expert decisions [140–144]. Xie's study (2010) [144] revealed an 80% concurrence in extraction decisions between AI and experts, although only 20 cases were analyzed. Jung and King evaluated an ANN system [142], which achieved a 93% success rate in diagnosing extraction versus nonextraction cases based on 12 cephalometric variables and an 84% success rate for the detailed diagnosis of specific extraction patterns.

Similar results were achieved by Li et al. (2019) [143], who reported a 94% accuracy for extraction versus nonextraction predictions, 84.2% for extraction patterns, and 92.8% for anchorage patterns. These studies identified several features that are important in predicting treatment efficacy, such as crowding of the upper arch, position of anterior teeth, lower incisor inclination, overjet, overbite, and capability for lip closure. However, it is important to note that these studies have significant limitations that may introduce bias. For instance, the AI systems were trained using examples provided by a limited number of experts, which may reflect the treatment philosophies of those experts without considering the validity of those approaches. Additionally, important dental findings, such as large dental fillings, periapical lesions, periodontal damage, previous endodontic treatment, and missing teeth, were not considered [129,141–144].

Given these limitations, it is important to acknowledge that making a definitive decision on whether to proceed with orthodontic extraction therapy is often challenging, especially in borderline cases. Clinicians need to carefully evaluate the advantages and disadvantages of each treatment approach and consider the overall clinical situation. Additionally, the use of extraction decision-making tools in clinical practice carries the risk of being influenced by a specific treatment philosophy, which could impact patient care. Practitioners should strive to develop individualized treatment plans for their patients and not be influenced by rigid treatment "philosophies" [128].

3.2.6. Orthognathic Surgery Decision Making and Planning

Despite significant developments in orthodontics and surgery, there is a lack of clearly established criteria for qualifying patients for surgical procedures. This issue becomes particularly problematic in borderline cases, where the orthodontist faces the decision of whether to refer the patient for surgical treatment or camouflage treatment [145,146]. The primary issue that determines the further fate of a patient is the identification of patients who benefit from orthognathic surgery. The diagnosis of a surgical case is usually confirmed via lateral cephalograms, which are the primary method for assessing sagittal skeletal deformities. The effectiveness of both the AI and ML algorithms has already been proven to identify orthognathic surgery diagnoses with over 90% accuracy [117,147–150]. One interesting study carried out by Jeong et al. [151] evaluated soft tissue profiles based on facial photographs. The evaluated CNN yielded 89% accuracy in correctly classifying surgical cases [151].

There is a limited yet promising body of literature that assesses the performance of AI in orthognathic surgery treatment planning [140,152,153]. Knoops et al. conducted a study in which they applied a 3D morphable model (3DMM) to automatically diagnose patients, categorize their risk levels, and generate simulations for orthognathic surgery treatment plans [153]. This approach achieved a sensitivity of 95.5% and a specificity of 95.2%, with an average accuracy of 1.1 ± 0.3 mm. Additionally, the positive and negative predictive values were 87.5% and 98.3%, respectively [153]. Chung et al. proposed a technique for the automatic alignment of CBCT images with optically scanned models using a DeepPose regression neural network [152]. This method surpassed the accuracy of previously top-performing techniques by 33.09% [152]. In a previously mentioned study by Choi et al., a model accurately predicted the need for surgery and provided an extraction plan for surgical patients, achieving an accuracy ranging from 88% to 97% [140].

However, it is important to mention that the research discussed above is subject to the same limitations mentioned in the chapter on extraction decision making. These limitations stem from the lack of strict guidelines, which results in a heavy reliance on expert decisions and opinions. A systematic review conducted by Smith et al. [154] further supports this notion by indicating that the results of current studies cannot be easily generalized due to their significant heterogeneity. The authors carefully concluded that AI might be a useful tool in planning orthognathic surgery. However, additional studies are needed.

It is worth noting that the abovementioned research shares the same limitations as those discussed in the extraction decision-making chapter, primarily due to the absence of clear guidelines. This leads to a heavy dependence on expert decisions and opinions. A systematic review by Smith et al. [154] further highlighted the significant heterogeneity among current studies and the difficulty in generalizing their results. The authors cautiously concluded that AI could be a valuable tool in orthognathic surgery planning, but further research is necessary.

3.2.7. Treatment Outcome Prediction

Orthodontists face the challenge of selecting the most appropriate treatment strategy for each patient based on their individual expectations, socioeconomic conditions, cultural background, and skills. However, procedures such as extractions and orthognathic surgeries are irreversible and can result in permanent patient dissatisfaction. Therefore, accurately predicting treatment outcomes is crucial for both practitioners and patients. Fortunately, a growing body of literature demonstrates the effectiveness of AI in predicting orthodontic and orthognathic treatment outcomes [155–163].

The model proposed by Park et al. [161] achieved high accuracy in predicting treatment outcomes for Class II patients, with a mean error of 1.79 ± 1.77 mm. In a recent study by Tanikawa et al. [163], a DL model was used to predict the 3D outcomes of orthodontic and orthognathic treatment in Japanese patients, resulting in mean errors of 0.69 ± 0.28 mm and 0.94 ± 0.43 mm for the orthodontic and surgical patient groups, respectively. Similarly, Park et al. [160] evaluated a DL algorithm that accurately predicted treatment outcomes in terms of 3D facial changes, with a mean prediction error of 1.2 ± 1.01 mm. Other studies have also achieved high accuracies in predicting facial symmetry in orthognathic patients [156,158] and 3D facial soft tissue changes in cleft patients after orthognathic surgery [164].

In addition to treatment outcomes, AI has also been used to predict patients' experiences during clear aligner treatment. Xu et al. [159] developed a system that achieved close to 90% prediction accuracy in predicting patients' pain, anxiety, and quality of life. This study highlights the importance of considering patient experience and shifting the focus from solely cosmetic or functional outcomes.

A recent scoping review [165] revealed that AI models are not only efficient but also outperform conventional methods in orthognathic treatment planning and outcome prediction. This review highlighted the reliability and reproducibility of these models, suggesting their potential to improve clinical outcomes, especially for less experienced practitioners. However, a recent meta-analysis [166] emphasized the need for caution and restraint when adopting AI advancements in orthodontics.

3.2.8. Patient Monitoring

The COVID-19 pandemic has brought attention to the importance of social distancing, remote work, and telemedicine [167]. Orthodontic treatment typically lasts approximately 20 months [168] and requires regular progress monitoring and potential complications. Traditional methods of monitoring can be time-consuming and repetitive. However, recent advancements in orthodontics, such as self-ligating systems and aligners, along with the implementation of telemedicine, have led to the development of dental monitoring (DM) [169].

The DM system consists of three integrated platforms: a mobile app for patients, a web-based Doctor Dashboard®, and a movement-tracking algorithm that analyzes pictures taken by the patient. The goal of DM is to reduce in-office visits, detect aligner incidents and misfitting, and personalize treatment for each patient [170]. Several studies have already demonstrated the value of DM in orthodontic treatment, including reducing chairside time, improving patient compliance [171,172], early detection of orthodontic emergencies [173], reducing orthodontic relapse [174], remote monitoring of aligner fit [169,174,175], and improving oral hygiene status [176]. Interestingly, Homsi et al. [177] reported that digitally reconstructed models obtained remotely were as accurate as those obtained through intraoral scans.

However, the implementation of AI in remote care for orthodontic patients is still an underexplored topic with limited evidence. A recent systematic review [178] showed that DM showed promise in improving aligner fit and reducing the number of in-office visits during ongoing orthodontic therapy. These findings emphasize the need for further research in this area.

3.3. Implementation Considerations

While the potential of AI to improve patient management in orthodontics is vast, its impact has been proven in only a limited number of cases. Most of the literature on this subject consists of retrospective studies without support from large randomized controlled trials. However, we might expect such studies in the coming years due to the exciting nature of this topic and the increasing supply of AI solutions. Financial investments and the number of introduced AI technologies are rapidly growing; in 2022, there were 69 new FDA-approved products associated with USD 4.8 billion in funding. By 2035, product-year funding is projected to reach USD 30.8 billion, resulting in 350 new AI products [8].

Despite many optimistic studies demonstrating the high performance of AI algorithms in a variety of tasks, the further incorporation of AI algorithms into everyday clinical practice remains a matter for the future. Most of the aforementioned programs were introduced within the past 2–3 years. On average, 17 years are required for medical innovations to be implemented in clinical practice [179,180]. The process of implementing AI in workflows and clinical practice requires meeting a number of requirements to ensure sufficient clinical quality and patient safety. As indicated by Pianykh [9], there are still important issues to overcome. The first issue is the lack of reproducibility. AI models are typically developed using limited and specific datasets, which makes it challenging for them to perform well on a wide range of data. The second issue is the lack of adaptivity. Existing AI models are not designed to constantly adjust to changes in their environment. The third issue is the absence of robust quality control mechanisms for AI, which increases susceptibility to data errors, outliers, and sudden shifts in trends. Finally, there is a lack of integration between AI algorithms and workflows, which prevents them from effectively adapting to changes in the data environment. To address these issues, continuous learning AI needs to be developed. This approach enables the AI tool to adapt continuously to changes in the data [9]. With continuous learning, AI algorithms can make live adjustments, preventing performance deterioration over time. Like in any technology used in medicine, there is a need for a sufficient AI governance process to maintain the quality of results and ensure patient safety [181,182]. The need for continuous evaluation of algorithm quality should be kept in mind to prevent degradation in performance and to allow appropriate early intervention. Moreover, privacy issues, safety concerns, and health inequities (such as AI algorithms that exacerbate racial or income disparities) are a few more general issues related to the application of AI in medicine, and they have recently been highlighted in The Lancet [183]. While a wide range of AI products are available, scientific evidence regarding their validation and effectiveness in general medicine and specific fields such as orthodontics remains limited [184].

Despite the availability of a wide range of products, there is still limited scientific evidence regarding the validation and effectiveness of AI products in general medicine and narrow fields such as orthodontics [184]. Despite the generally optimistic results of various AI tools, the issues highlighted above underscore the necessity of exercising considerable caution when introducing AI into daily practice.

4. Conclusions

Undoubtedly, AI has the potential to revolutionize medicine, particularly in the field of diagnostic imaging, including orthodontics. The continuous advancement of AI algorithms that support pretreatment diagnostic processes allows the visualization of outcomes and facilitates decision making during treatment, placing orthodontics among the disciplines benefiting the most from the introduction of AI technology. However, due to the high complexity and associated unpredictability of AI, these tools should be treated with caution, and their results should be regularly and manually validated.

Funding: This research received no external funding.

Institutional Review Board Statement: Not applicable.

Informed Consent Statement: Not applicable.

Data Availability Statement: Not applicable.

Conflicts of Interest: The authors declare no conflicts of interest.

References

1. McCarthy, J.; Minsky, M.L.; Rochester, N.; Shannon, C.E. A Proposal for the Dartmouth Summer Research Project on Artificial Intelligence. *AI Mag.* **2006**, *27*, 12.
2. Haenlein, M.; Kaplan, A. A Brief History of Artificial Intelligence: On the Past, Present, and Future of Artificial Intelligence. *Calif. Manag. Rev.* **2019**, *61*, 5–14. [CrossRef]
3. Schwendicke, F.; Golla, T.; Dreher, M.; Krois, J. Convolutional Neural Networks for Dental Image Diagnostics: A Scoping Review. *J. Dent.* **2019**, *91*, 103226. [CrossRef] [PubMed]
4. Esteva, A.; Kuprel, B.; Novoa, R.A.; Ko, J.; Swetter, S.M.; Blau, H.M.; Thrun, S. Dermatologist-Level Classification of Skin Cancer with Deep Neural Networks. *Nature* **2017**, *542*, 686. [CrossRef] [PubMed]
5. Gulshan, V.; Peng, L.; Coram, M.; Stumpe, M.C.; Wu, D.; Narayanaswamy, A.; Venugopalan, S.; Widner, K.; Madams, T.; Cuadros, J.; et al. Development and Validation of a Deep Learning Algorithm for Detection of Diabetic Retinopathy in Retinal Fundus Photographs. *JAMA* **2016**, *316*, 2402–2410. [CrossRef]
6. Mazurowski, M.A.; Buda, M.; Saha, A.; Bashir, M.R. Deep Learning in Radiology: An Overview of the Concepts and a Survey of the State of the Art with Focus on MRI. *J. Magn. Reson. Imaging* **2019**, *49*, 939–954. [CrossRef]
7. Saida, T.; Mori, K.; Hoshiai, S.; Sakai, M.; Urushibara, A.; Ishiguro, T.; Satoh, T.; Nakajima, T. Differentiation of Carcinosarcoma from Endometrial Carcinoma on Magnetic Resonance Imaging Using Deep Learning. *Pol. J. Radiol.* **2022**, *87*, 521–529. [CrossRef]
8. McNabb, N.K.; Christensen, E.W.; Rula, E.Y.; Coombs, L.; Dreyer, K.; Wald, C.; Treml, C. Projected Growth in FDA-Approved Artificial Intelligence Products Given Venture Capital Funding. *J. Am. Coll. Radiol.* **2023**. [CrossRef]
9. Pianykh, O.S.; Langs, G.; Dewey, M.; Enzmann, D.R.; Herold, C.J.; Schoenberg, S.O.; Brink, J.A. Continuous Learning AI in Radiology: Implementation Principles and Early Applications. *Radiology* **2020**, *297*, 6–14. [CrossRef]
10. Milam, M.E.; Koo, C.W. The Current Status and Future of FDA-Approved Artificial Intelligence Tools in Chest Radiology in the United States. *Clin. Radiol.* **2023**, *78*, 115–122. [CrossRef]
11. Giełczyk, A.; Marciniak, A.; Tarczewska, M.; Kloska, S.M.; Harmoza, A.; Serafin, Z.; Woźniak, M. A Novel Lightweight Approach to COVID-19 Diagnostics Based on Chest X-Ray Images. *J. Clin. Med.* **2022**, *11*, 5501. [CrossRef] [PubMed]
12. Kloska, A.; Tarczewska, M.; Giełczyk, A.; Kloska, S.M.; Michalski, A.; Serafin, Z.; Woźniak, M. Influence of Augmentation on the Performance of the Double ResNet-Based Model for Chest X-Ray Classification. *Pol. J. Radiol.* **2023**, *88*, 244–250. [CrossRef] [PubMed]
13. Fujima, N.; Kamagata, K.; Ueda, D.; Fujita, S.; Fushimi, Y.; Yanagawa, M.; Ito, R.; Tsuboyama, T.; Kawamura, M.; Nakaura, T.; et al. Current State of Artificial Intelligence in Clinical Applications for Head and Neck MR Imaging. *Magn. Reson. Med. Sci.* **2023**, *22*, 401–414. [CrossRef] [PubMed]
14. Matsubara, K.; Ibaraki, M.; Nemoto, M.; Watabe, H.; Kimura, Y. A Review on AI in PET Imaging. *Ann. Nucl. Med.* **2022**, *36*, 133–143. [CrossRef] [PubMed]
15. Wang, B.; Jin, S.; Yan, Q.; Xu, H.; Luo, C.; Wei, L.; Zhao, W.; Hou, X.; Ma, W.; Xu, Z.; et al. AI-Assisted CT Imaging Analysis for COVID-19 Screening: Building and Deploying a Medical AI System. *Appl. Soft Comput.* **2021**, *98*, 106897. [CrossRef] [PubMed]
16. Bichu, Y.M.; Hansa, I.; Bichu, A.Y.; Premjani, P.; Flores-Mir, C.; Vaid, N.R. Applications of Artificial Intelligence and Machine Learning in Orthodontics: A Scoping Review. *Prog. Orthod.* **2021**, *22*, 18. [CrossRef]
17. Williams, M.; Haugeland, J. Artificial Intelligence: The Very Idea. *Technol. Cult.* **1987**, *28*, 706. [CrossRef]
18. Schwartz, W.B.; Patil, R.S.; Szolovits, P. Artificial Intelligence in Medicine. Where Do We Stand? *N. Engl. J. Med.* **1987**, *316*, 685–688. [CrossRef]
19. Faber, J.; Faber, C.; Faber, P. Artificial Intelligence in Orthodontics. *APOS Trends Orthod.* **2019**, *9*, 201–205. [CrossRef]
20. Bishop, C. *Pattern Recognition and Machine Learning*; Springer: Berlin/Heidelberg, Germany, 2007; Volume 16.
21. Rajpurkar, P.; Irvin, J.; Ball, R.L.; Zhu, K.; Yang, H.; Mehta, H.; Duan, T.; Ding, D.; Bagul, A.; Langlotz, C.P.; et al. Deep Learning for Chest Radiograph Diagnosis: A Retrospective Comparison of the CheXNeXt Algorithm to Practicing Radiologists. *PLoS Med.* **2018**, *15*, e1002686. [CrossRef]
22. Chilamkurthy, S.; Ghosh, R.; Tanamala, S.; Biviji, M.; Campeau, N.G.; Venugopal, V.K.; Mahajan, V.; Rao, P.; Warier, P. Deep Learning Algorithms for Detection of Critical Findings in Head CT Scans: A Retrospective Study. *Lancet* **2018**, *392*, 2388–2396. [CrossRef] [PubMed]
23. Yu, A.C.; Mohajer, B.; Eng, J. External Validation of Deep Learning Algorithms for Radiologic Diagnosis: A Systematic Review. *Radiol. Artif. Intell.* **2022**, *4*, e210064. [CrossRef] [PubMed]
24. Wu, N.; Phang, J.; Park, J.; Shen, Y.; Huang, Z.; Zorin, M.; Jastrzebski, S.; Fevry, T.; Katsnelson, J.; Kim, E.; et al. Deep Neural Networks Improve Radiologists' Performance in Breast Cancer Screening. *IEEE Trans. Med. Imaging* **2020**, *39*, 1184–1194. [CrossRef] [PubMed]
25. Kuo, W.; Häne, C.; Mukherjee, P.; Malik, J.; Yuh, E.L. Expert-Level Detection of Acute Intracranial Hemorrhage on Head Computed Tomography Using Deep Learning. *Proc. Natl. Acad. Sci. USA* **2019**, *116*, 22737–22745. [CrossRef] [PubMed]

26. Bulten, W.; Pinckaers, H.; van Boven, H.; Vink, R.; de Bel, T.; van Ginneken, B.; van der Laak, J.; Hulsbergen-van de Kaa, C.; Litjens, G. Automated Deep-Learning System for Gleason Grading of Prostate Cancer Using Biopsies: A Diagnostic Study. *Lancet Oncol.* **2020**, *21*, 233–241. [CrossRef] [PubMed]
27. Hosny, A.; Aerts, H.J.; Mak, R.H. Handcrafted versus Deep Learning Radiomics for Prediction of Cancer Therapy Response. *Lancet Digit. Health* **2019**, *1*, e106–e107. [CrossRef]
28. Lou, B.; Doken, S.; Zhuang, T.; Wingerter, D.; Gidwani, M.; Mistry, N.; Ladic, L.; Kamen, A.; Abazeed, M.E. An Image-Based Deep Learning Framework for Individualising Radiotherapy Dose: A Retrospective Analysis of Outcome Prediction. *Lancet Digit. Health* **2019**, *1*, e136–e147. [CrossRef]
29. Haug, C.J.; Drazen, J.M. Artificial Intelligence and Machine Learning in Clinical Medicine, 2023. *New Engl. J. Med.* **2023**, *388*, 1201–1208. [CrossRef]
30. Vandenberghe, B.; Jacobs, R.; Bosmans, H. Modern Dental Imaging: A Review of the Current Technology and Clinical Applications in Dental Practice. *Eur. Radiol.* **2010**, *20*, 2637–2655. [CrossRef]
31. Drage, N. Cone Beam Computed Tomography (CBCT) in General Dental Practice. *Prim. Dent. J.* **2018**, *7*, 26–30. [CrossRef]
32. Gallichan, N.; Albadri, S.; Dixon, C.; Jorgenson, K. Trends in CBCT Current Practice within Three UK Paediatric Dental Departments. *Eur. Arch. Paediatr. Dent.* **2020**, *21*, 537–542. [CrossRef] [PubMed]
33. Kapetanović, A.; Oosterkamp, B.C.M.; Lamberts, A.A.; Schols, J.G.J.H. Orthodontic Radiology: Development of a Clinical Practice Guideline. *Radiol. Medica* **2021**, *126*, 72–82. [CrossRef] [PubMed]
34. de Grauwe, A.; Ayaz, I.; Shujaat, S.; Dimitrov, S.; Gbadegbegnon, L.; Vande Vannet, B.; Jacobs, R. CBCT in Orthodontics: A Systematic Review on Justification of CBCT in a Paediatric Population Prior to Orthodontic Treatment. *Eur. J. Orthod.* **2019**, *41*, 381–389. [CrossRef] [PubMed]
35. Garlapati, K.; Gandhi Babu, D.B.; Chaitanya, N.C.S.K.; Guduru, H.; Rembers, A.; Soni, P. Evaluation of Preference and Purpose of Utilisation of Cone Beam Computed Tomography (CBCT) Compared to Orthopantomogram (OPG) by Dental Practitioners—A Cross-Sectional Study. *Pol. J. Radiol.* **2017**, *82*, 248–251. [CrossRef] [PubMed]
36. Hajem, S.; Brogårdh-Roth, S.; Nilsson, M.; Hellén-Halme, K. CBCT of Swedish Children and Adolescents at an Oral and Maxillofacial Radiology Department. A Survey of Requests and Indications. *Acta Odontol. Scand.* **2020**, *78*, 38–44. [CrossRef] [PubMed]
37. Orhan, K.; Bayrakdar, I.S.; Ezhov, M.; Kravtsov, A.; Özyürek, T. Evaluation of Artificial Intelligence for Detecting Periapical Pathosis on Cone-Beam Computed Tomography Scans. *Int. Endod. J.* **2020**, *53*, 680–689. [CrossRef]
38. Issa, J.; Jaber, M.; Rifai, I.; Mozdziak, P.; Kempisty, B.; Dyszkiewicz-Konwińska, M. Diagnostic Test Accuracy of Artificial Intelligence in Detecting Periapical Periodontitis on Two-Dimensional Radiographs: A Retrospective Study and Literature Review. *Medicina* **2023**, *59*, 768. [CrossRef]
39. Orhan, K.; Shamshiev, M.; Ezhov, M.; Plaksin, A.; Kurbanova, A.; Ünsal, G.; Gusarev, M.; Golitsyna, M.; Aksoy, S.; Mısırlı, M.; et al. AI-Based Automatic Segmentation of Craniomaxillofacial Anatomy from CBCT Scans for Automatic Detection of Pharyngeal Airway Evaluations in OSA Patients. *Sci. Rep.* **2022**, *12*, 11863. [CrossRef]
40. Vujanovic, T.; Jagtap, R. Evaluation of Artificial Intelligence for Automatic Tooth and Periapical Pathosis Detection on Panoramic Radiography. *Oral. Surg. Oral. Med. Oral. Pathol. Oral. Radiol.* **2023**, *135*, e51. [CrossRef]
41. Brignardello-Petersen, R. Artificial Intelligence System Seems to Be Able to Detect a High Proportion of Periapical Lesions in Cone-Beam Computed Tomographic Images. *J. Am. Dent. Assoc.* **2020**, *151*, e83. [CrossRef]
42. Zadrożny, Ł.; Regulski, P.; Brus-Sawczuk, K.; Czajkowska, M.; Parkanyi, L.; Ganz, S.; Mijiritsky, E. Artificial Intelligence Application in Assessment of Panoramic Radiographs. *Diagnostics* **2022**, *12*, 224. [CrossRef] [PubMed]
43. Ezhov, M.; Gusarev, M.; Golitsyna, M.; Yates, J.M.; Kushnerev, E.; Tamimi, D.; Aksoy, S.; Shumilov, E.; Sanders, A.; Orhan, K. Clinically Applicable Artificial Intelligence System for Dental Diagnosis with CBCT. *Sci. Rep.* **2021**, *11*, 15006. [CrossRef] [PubMed]
44. Li, S.; Liu, J.; Zhou, Z.; Zhou, Z.; Wu, X.; Li, Y.; Wang, S.; Liao, W.; Ying, S.; Zhao, Z. Artificial Intelligence for Caries and Periapical Periodontitis Detection. *J. Dent.* **2022**, *122*, 104107. [CrossRef] [PubMed]
45. Ramezanzade, S.; Laurentiu, T.; Bakhshandah, A.; Ibragimov, B.; Kvist, T.; Bjørndal, L.; Bjørndal, L.; Dawson, V.S.; Fransson, H.; Frisk, F.; et al. The Efficiency of Artificial Intelligence Methods for Finding Radiographic Features in Different Endodontic Treatments—A Systematic Review. *Acta Odontol. Scand.* **2023**, *81*, 422–435. [PubMed]
46. Silva, V.K.S.; Vieira, W.A.; Bernardino, Í.M.; Travençolo, B.A.N.; Bittencourt, M.A.V.; Blumenberg, C.; Paranhos, L.R.; Galvão, H.C. Accuracy of Computer-Assisted Image Analysis in the Diagnosis of Maxillofacial Radiolucent Lesions: A Systematic Review and Meta-Analysis. *Dentomaxillofacial Radiol.* **2020**, *49*, 20190204. [CrossRef] [PubMed]
47. Setzer, F.C.; Shi, K.J.; Zhang, Z.; Yan, H.; Yoon, H.; Mupparapu, M.; Li, J. Artificial Intelligence for the Computer-Aided Detection of Periapical Lesions in Cone-Beam Computed Tomographic Images. *J. Endod.* **2020**, *46*, 987–993. [CrossRef] [PubMed]
48. Prados-Privado, M.; Villalón, J.G.; Martínez-Martínez, C.H.; Ivorra, C.; Prados-Frutos, J.C. Dental Caries Diagnosis and Detection Using Neural Networks: A Systematic Review. *J. Clin. Med.* **2020**, *9*, 3579. [CrossRef]
49. Reyes, L.T.; Knorst, J.K.; Ortiz, F.R.; Ardenghi, T.M.H. Machine Learning in the Diagnosis and Prognostic Prediction of Dental Caries: A Systematic Review. *Caries Res.* **2022**, *56*, 161–170. [CrossRef]
50. Badr, F.F.; Jadu, F.M. Performance of Artificial Intelligence Using Oral and Maxillofacial CBCT Images: A Systematic Review and Meta-Analysis. *Niger. J. Clin. Pract.* **2022**, *25*, 1918–1927. [CrossRef]

51. Khanagar, S.B.; Alfouzan, K.; Awawdeh, M.; Alkadi, L.; Albalawi, F.; Alfadley, A. Application and Performance of Artificial Intelligence Technology in Detection, Diagnosis and Prediction of Dental Caries (DC)—A Systematic Review. *Diagnostics* **2022**, *12*, 1083. [CrossRef]
52. Sadr, S.; Mohammad-Rahimi, H.; Motamedian, S.R.; Zahedrozegar, S.; Motie, P.; Vinayahalingam, S.; Dianat, O.; Nosrat, A. Deep Learning for Detection of Periapical Radiolucent Lesions: A Systematic Review and Meta-Analysis of Diagnostic Test Accuracy. *J. Endod.* **2023**, *49*, 248–261.e3. [CrossRef] [PubMed]
53. Abesi, F.; Maleki, M.; Zamani, M. Diagnostic Performance of Artificial Intelligence Using Cone-Beam Computed Tomography Imaging of the Oral and Maxillofacial Region: A Scoping Review and Meta-Analysis. *Imaging Sci. Dent.* **2023**, *53*, 101–108. [CrossRef] [PubMed]
54. Mohammad-Rahimi, H.; Motamedian, S.R.; Rohban, M.H.; Krois, J.; Uribe, S.E.; Mahmoudinia, E.; Rokhshad, R.; Nadimi, M.; Schwendicke, F. Deep Learning for Caries Detection: A Systematic Review. *J. Dent.* **2022**, *122*, 104115. [CrossRef] [PubMed]
55. Abesi, F.; Jamali, A.S.; Zamani, M. Accuracy of Artificial Intelligence in the Detection and Segmentation of Oral and Maxillofacial Structures Using Cone-Beam Computed Tomography Images: A Systematic Review and Meta-Analysis. *Pol. J. Radiol.* **2023**, *88*, 256–263. [CrossRef]
56. Leonardi, R.; Giordano, D.; Maiorana, F.; Spampinato, C. Automatic Cephalometric Analysis: A Systematic Review. *Angle Orthod.* **2008**, *78*, 145–151. [CrossRef]
57. Chen, Y.J.; Chen, S.K.; Yao, J.C.C.; Chang, H.F. The Effects of Differences in Landmark Identification on the Cephalometric Measurements in Traditional versus Digitized Cephalometry. *Angle Orthod.* **2004**, *74*, 155–161.
58. Dias Da Silveira, H.L.; Dias Silveira, H.E. Reproducibility of Cephalometric Measurements Made by Three Radiology Clinics. *Angle Orthod.* **2006**, *76*, 394–399.
59. Hwang, H.-W.; Moon, J.-H.; Kim, M.-G.; Donatelli, R.E.; Lee, S.-J. Evaluation of Automated Cephalometric Analysis Based on the Latest Deep Learning Method. *Angle Orthod.* **2021**, *91*, 329–335. [CrossRef]
60. Hwang, H.W.; Park, J.H.; Moon, J.H.; Yu, Y.; Kim, H.; Her, S.B.; Srinivasan, G.; Aljanabi, M.N.A.; Donatelli, R.E.; Lee, S.J. Automated Identification of Cephalometric Landmarks: Part 2-Might It Be Better than Human? *Angle Orthod.* **2020**, *90*, 69–76. [CrossRef]
61. Chung, E.J.; Yang, B.E.; Park, I.Y.; Yi, S.; On, S.W.; Kim, Y.H.; Kang, S.H.; Byun, S.H. Effectiveness of Cone-Beam Computed Tomography-Generated Cephalograms Using Artificial Intelligence Cephalometric Analysis. *Sci. Rep.* **2022**, *12*, 20585. [CrossRef]
62. Rudolph, D.J.; Sinclair, P.M.; Coggins, J.M. Automatic Computerized Radiographic Identification of Cephalometric Landmarks. *Am. J. Orthod. Dentofac. Orthop.* **1998**, *113*, 173–179. [CrossRef] [PubMed]
63. Dobratulin, K.; Gaidel, A.; Kapishnikov, A.; Ivleva, A.; Aupova, I.; Zelter, P. The Efficiency of Deep Learning Algorithms for Detecting Anatomical Reference Points on Radiological Images of the Head Profile. In Proceedings of the ITNT 2020–6th IEEE International Conference on Information Technology and Nanotechnology, Samara, Russia, 26–29 May 2020.
64. Park, J.H.; Hwang, H.W.; Moon, J.H.; Yu, Y.; Kim, H.; Her, S.B.; Srinivasan, G.; Aljanabi, M.N.A.; Donatelli, R.E.; Lee, S.J. Automated Identification of Cephalometric Landmarks: Part 1—Comparisons between the Latest Deep-Learning Methods YOLOV3 and SSD. *Angle Orthod.* **2019**, *89*, 903–909. [CrossRef] [PubMed]
65. Kim, H.; Shim, E.; Park, J.; Kim, Y.J.; Lee, U.; Kim, Y. Web-Based Fully Automated Cephalometric Analysis by Deep Learning. *Comput. Methods Programs Biomed.* **2020**, *194*, 105513. [CrossRef]
66. Grau, V.; Alcañiz, M.; Juan, M.C.; Monserrat, C.; Knoll, C. Automatic Localization of Cephalometric Landmarks. *J. Biomed. Inf.* **2001**, *34*, 146–156. [CrossRef] [PubMed]
67. Yao, J.; Zeng, W.; He, T.; Zhou, S.; Zhang, Y.; Guo, J.; Tang, W. Automatic Localization of Cephalometric Landmarks Based on Convolutional Neural Network. *Am. J. Orthod. Dentofac. Orthop.* **2022**, *161*, e250–e259. [CrossRef] [PubMed]
68. Nishimoto, S.; Sotsuka, Y.; Kawai, K.; Ishise, H.; Kakibuchi, M. Personal Computer-Based Cephalometric Landmark Detection with Deep Learning, Using Cephalograms on the Internet. *J. Craniofacial Surg.* **2019**, *30*, 91–95. [CrossRef] [PubMed]
69. Kunz, F.; Stellzig-Eisenhauer, A.; Zeman, F.; Boldt, J. Artificial Intelligence in Orthodontics: Evaluation of a Fully Automated Cephalometric Analysis Using a Customized Convolutional Neural Network. *J. Orofac. Orthop.* **2020**, *81*, 52–68. [CrossRef]
70. Yu, H.J.; Cho, S.R.; Kim, M.J.; Kim, W.H.; Kim, J.W.; Choi, J. Automated Skeletal Classification with Lateral Cephalometry Based on Artificial Intelligence. *J. Dent. Res.* **2020**, *99*, 249–256. [CrossRef]
71. Lee, J.H.; Yu, H.J.; Kim, M.J.; Kim, J.W.; Choi, J. Automated Cephalometric Landmark Detection with Confidence Regions Using Bayesian Convolutional Neural Networks. *BMC Oral Health* **2020**, *20*, 270. [CrossRef]
72. Nishimoto, S. Locating Cephalometric Landmarks with Multi-Phase Deep Learning. *J. Dent. Health Oral. Res.* **2023**, *4*, 1–13. [CrossRef]
73. Palomo, J.M.; Yang, C.Y.; Hans, M.G. Clinical Application of Three-Dimensional Craniofacial Imaging in Orthodontics. *J. Med. Sci.* **2005**, *25*, 269.
74. Kazimierczak, N.; Kazimierczak, W.; Serafin, Z.; Nowicki, P.; Lemanowicz, A.; Nadolska, K.; Janiszewska-Olszowska, J. Correlation Analysis of Nasal Septum Deviation and Results of AI-Driven Automated 3D Cephalometric Analysis. *J. Clin. Med.* **2023**, *12*, 6621. [CrossRef] [PubMed]
75. Ed-Dhahraouy, M.; Riri, H.; Ezzahmouly, M.; Bourzgui, F.; El Moutaoukkil, A. A New Methodology for Automatic Detection of Reference Points in 3D Cephalometry: A Pilot Study. *Int. Orthod.* **2018**, *16*, 328–337. [CrossRef] [PubMed]

76. Gupta, A.; Kharbanda, O.P.; Sardana, V.; Balachandran, R.; Sardana, H.K. A Knowledge-Based Algorithm for Automatic Detection of Cephalometric Landmarks on CBCT Images. *Int. J. Comput. Assist. Radiol. Surg.* **2015**, *10*, 1737–1752. [CrossRef]
77. Ma, Q.; Kobayashi, E.; Fan, B.; Nakagawa, K.; Sakuma, I.; Masamune, K.; Suenaga, H. Automatic 3D Landmarking Model Using Patch-Based Deep Neural Networks for CT Image of Oral and Maxillofacial Surgery. *Int. J. Med. Robot. Comput. Assist. Surg.* **2020**, *16*, e2093. [CrossRef]
78. Montúfar, J.; Romero, M.; Scougall-Vilchis, R.J. Hybrid Approach for Automatic Cephalometric Landmark Annotation on Cone-Beam Computed Tomography Volumes. *Am. J. Orthod. Dentofac. Orthop.* **2018**, *154*, 140–150. [CrossRef]
79. Gupta, A.; Kharbanda, O.P.; Sardana, V.; Balachandran, R.; Sardana, H.K. Accuracy of 3D Cephalometric Measurements Based on an Automatic Knowledge-Based Landmark Detection Algorithm. *Int. J. Comput. Assist. Radiol. Surg.* **2016**, *11*, 1297–1309. [CrossRef]
80. Kim, M.-J.; Liu, Y.; Oh, S.H.; Ahn, H.-W.; Kim, S.-H.; Nelson, G. Evaluation of a Multi-Stage Convolutional Neural Network-Based Fully Automated Landmark Identification System Using Cone-Beam Computed Tomographysynthesized Posteroanterior Cephalometric Images. *Korean J. Orthod.* **2021**, *51*, 77–85. [CrossRef]
81. Muraev, A.A.; Tsai, P.; Kibardin, I.; Oborotistov, N.; Shirayeva, T.; Ivanov, S.; Ivanov, S.; Guseynov, N.; Aleshina, O.; Bosykh, Y.; et al. Frontal Cephalometric Landmarking: Humans vs Artificial Neural Networks. *Int. J. Comput. Dent.* **2020**, *23*, 139–148.
82. Bao, H.; Zhang, K.; Yu, C.; Li, H.; Cao, D.; Shu, H.; Liu, L.; Yan, B. Evaluating the Accuracy of Automated Cephalometric Analysis Based on Artificial Intelligence. *BMC Oral. Health* **2023**, *23*, 191. [CrossRef]
83. de Queiroz Tavares Borges Mesquita, G.; Vieira, W.A.; Vidigal, M.T.C.; Travençolo, B.A.N.; Beaini, T.L.; Spin-Neto, R.; Paranhos, L.R.; de Brito Júnior, R.B. Artificial Intelligence for Detecting Cephalometric Landmarks: A Systematic Review and Meta-Analysis. *J. Digit. Imaging* **2023**, *36*, 1158–1179. [CrossRef] [PubMed]
84. Schwendicke, F.; Chaurasia, A.; Arsiwala, L.; Lee, J.H.; Elhennawy, K.; Jost-Brinkmann, P.G.; Demarco, F.; Krois, J. Deep Learning for Cephalometric Landmark Detection: Systematic Review and Meta-Analysis. *Clin. Oral. Investig.* **2021**, *25*, 4299–4309. [CrossRef] [PubMed]
85. Londono, J.; Ghasemi, S.; Hussain Shah, A.; Fahimipour, A.; Ghadimi, N.; Hashemi, S.; Khurshid, Z.; Dashti, M. Evaluation of Deep Learning and Convolutional Neural Network Algorithms Accuracy for Detecting and Predicting Anatomical Landmarks on 2D Lateral Cephalometric Images: A Systematic Review and Meta-Analysis. *Saudi Dent. J.* **2023**, *35*, 487–497. [CrossRef] [PubMed]
86. Jihed, M.; Dallel, I.; Tobji, S.; Amor, A. Ben The Impact of Artificial Intelligence on Contemporary Orthodontic Treatment Planning—A Systematic Review and Meta-Analysis. *Sch. J. Dent. Sci.* **2022**, *9*, 70–87. [CrossRef]
87. Junaid, N.; Khan, N.; Ahmed, N.; Abbasi, M.S.; Das, G.; Maqsood, A.; Ahmed, A.R.; Marya, A.; Alam, M.K.; Heboyan, A. Development, Application, and Performance of Artificial Intelligence in Cephalometric Landmark Identification and Diagnosis: A Systematic Review. *Healthcare* **2022**, *10*, 2454. [CrossRef] [PubMed]
88. Rauniyar, S.; Jena, S.; Sahoo, N.; Mohanty, P.; Dash, B.P. Artificial Intelligence and Machine Learning for Automated Cephalometric Landmark Identification: A Meta-Analysis Previewed by a Systematic Review. *Cureus* **2023**, *15*, e40934. [CrossRef]
89. Serafin, M.; Baldini, B.; Cabitza, F.; Carrafiello, G.; Baselli, G.; Del Fabbro, M.; Sforza, C.; Caprioglio, A.; Tartaglia, G.M. Accuracy of Automated 3D Cephalometric Landmarks by Deep Learning Algorithms: Systematic Review and Meta-Analysis. *Radiol. Medica* **2023**, *128*, 544–555. [CrossRef]
90. Baccetti, T.; Franchi, L.; McNamara, J.A. The Cervical Vertebral Maturation (CVM) Method for the Assessment of Optimal Treatment Timing in Dentofacial Orthopedics. *Semin. Orthod.* **2005**, *11*, 119–129. [CrossRef]
91. McNamara, J.A.; Bookstein, F.L.; Shaughnessy, T.G. Skeletal and Dental Changes Following Functional Regulator Therapy on Class II Patients. *Am. J. Orthod.* **1985**, *88*, 91–110. [CrossRef]
92. Durka-Zając, M.; Derwich, M.; Mituś-Kenig, M.; Łoboda, M.; Pawłowska, E. Analysis of Dental Maturation in Relation to Sagittal Jaw Relationships. *Pol. J. Radiol.* **2017**, *82*, 32–37. [CrossRef]
93. Flores-Mir, C.; Nebbe, B.; Major, P.W. Use of Skeletal Maturation Based on Hand-Wrist Radiographic Analysis as a Predictor of Facial Growth: A Systematic Review. *Angle Orthod.* **2004**, *74*, 118–124. [PubMed]
94. Khanagar, S.B.; Al-Ehaideb, A.; Vishwanathaiah, S.; Maganur, P.C.; Patil, S.; Naik, S.; Baeshen, H.A.; Sarode, S.S. Scope and Performance of Artificial Intelligence Technology in Orthodontic Diagnosis, Treatment Planning, and Clinical Decision-Making—A Systematic Review. *J. Dent. Sci.* **2021**, *16*, 482–492. [CrossRef] [PubMed]
95. Kim, D.W.; Kim, J.; Kim, T.; Kim, T.; Kim, Y.J.; Song, I.S.; Ahn, B.; Choo, J.; Lee, D.Y. Prediction of Hand-Wrist Maturation Stages Based on Cervical Vertebrae Images Using Artificial Intelligence. *Orthod. Craniofac Res.* **2021**, *24*, 68–75. [CrossRef] [PubMed]
96. Uysal, T.; Sari, Z.; Ramoglu, S.I.; Basciftci, F.A. Relationships between Dental and Skeletal Maturity in Turkish Subjects. *Angle Orthod.* **2004**, *74*, 657–664. [CrossRef] [PubMed]
97. Jourieh, A.; Khan, H.; Mheissen, S.; Assali, M.; Alam, M.K. The Correlation between Dental Stages and Skeletal Maturity Stages. *Biomed. Res. Int.* **2021**, *2021*, 9986498. [CrossRef]
98. Morris, J.M.; Park, J.H. Correlation of Dental Maturity with Skeletal Maturity from Radiographic Assessment. *J. Clin. Pediatr. Dent.* **2012**, *36*, 309–314. [CrossRef] [PubMed]
99. Szemraj, A.; Wojtaszek-Słomińska, A.; Racka-Pilszak, B. Is the Cervical Vertebral Maturation (CVM) Method Effective Enough to Replace the Hand-Wrist Maturation (HWM) Method in Determining Skeletal Maturation?—A Systematic Review. *Eur. J. Radiol.* **2018**, *102*, 125–128. [CrossRef]

100. Nguyen, T.; Hermann, A.L.; Ventre, J.; Ducarouge, A.; Pourchot, A.; Marty, V.; Regnard, N.E.; Guermazi, A. High Performance for Bone Age Estimation with an Artificial Intelligence Solution. *Diagn. Interv. Imaging* **2023**, *104*, 330–336. [CrossRef]
101. Eng, D.K.; Khandwala, N.B.; Long, J.; Fefferman, N.R.; Lala, S.V.; Strubel, N.A.; Milla, S.S.; Filice, R.W.; Sharp, S.E.; Towbin, A.J.; et al. Artificial Intelligence Algorithm Improves Radiologist Performance in Skeletal Age Assessment: A Prospective Multicenter Randomized Controlled Trial. *Radiology* **2021**, *301*, 692–699. [CrossRef]
102. Amasya, H.; Cesur, E.; Yıldırım, D.; Orhan, K. Validation of Cervical Vertebral Maturation Stages: Artificial Intelligence vs Human Observer Visual Analysis. *Am. J. Orthod. Dentofac. Orthop.* **2020**, *158*, e173–e179. [CrossRef]
103. Zhou, J.; Zhou, H.; Pu, L.; Gao, Y.; Tang, Z.; Yang, Y.; You, M.; Yang, Z.; Lai, W.; Long, H. Development of an Artificial Intelligence System for the Automatic Evaluation of Cervical Vertebral Maturation Status. *Diagnostics* **2021**, *11*, 2200. [CrossRef] [PubMed]
104. Mathew, R.; Palatinus, S.; Padala, S.; Alshehri, A.; Awadh, W.; Bhandi, S.; Thomas, J.; Patil, S. Neural Networks for Classification of Cervical Vertebrae Maturation: A Systematic Review. *Angle Orthod.* **2022**, *92*, 796–804. [CrossRef] [PubMed]
105. Radwan, M.T.; Sin, Ç.; Akkaya, N.; Vahdettin, L. Artificial Intelligence-Based Algorithm for Cervical Vertebrae Maturation Stage Assessment. *Orthod. Craniofac Res.* **2023**, *26*, 349–355. [CrossRef] [PubMed]
106. Reddy, N.E.; Rayan, J.C.; Annapragada, A.V.; Mahmood, N.F.; Scheslinger, A.E.; Zhang, W.; Kan, J.H. Bone Age Determination Using Only the Index Finger: A Novel Approach Using a Convolutional Neural Network Compared with Human Radiologists. *Pediatr. Radiol.* **2020**, *50*, 516–523. [CrossRef] [PubMed]
107. Amasya, H.; Yildirim, D.; Aydogan, T.; Kemaloglu, N.; Orhan, K. Cervical Vertebral Maturation Assessment on Lateral Cephalometric Radiographs Using Artificial Intelligence: Comparison of Machine Learning Classifier Models. *Dentomaxillofacial Radiol.* **2020**, *49*, 20190441. [CrossRef] [PubMed]
108. Rana, S.S.; Nath, B.; Chaudhari, P.K.; Vichare, S. Cervical Vertebral Maturation Assessment Using Various Machine Learning Techniques on Lateral Cephalogram: A Systematic Literature Review. *J. Oral. Biol. Craniofac. Res.* **2023**, *13*, 642–651. [CrossRef]
109. Seo, H.; Hwang, J.; Jeong, T.; Shin, J. Comparison of Deep Learning Models for Cervical Vertebral Maturation Stage Classification on Lateral Cephalometric Radiographs. *J. Clin. Med.* **2021**, *10*, 3591. [CrossRef]
110. Kök, H.; Acilar, A.M.; İzgi, M.S. Usage and Comparison of Artificial Intelligence Algorithms for Determination of Growth and Development by Cervical Vertebrae Stages in Orthodontics. *Prog. Orthod.* **2019**, *20*, 41. [CrossRef]
111. Mohammad-Rahimi, H.; Motamadian, S.R.; Nadimi, M.; Hassanzadeh-Samani, S.; Minabi, M.A.S.; Mahmoudinia, E.; Lee, V.Y.; Rohban, M.H. Deep Learning for the Classification of Cervical Maturation Degree and Pubertal Growth Spurts: A Pilot Study. *Korean J. Orthod.* **2022**, *52*, 112–122. [CrossRef]
112. Tajmir, S.H.; Lee, H.; Shailam, R.; Gale, H.I.; Nguyen, J.C.; Westra, S.J.; Lim, R.; Yune, S.; Gee, M.S.; Do, S. Artificial Intelligence-Assisted Interpretation of Bone Age Radiographs Improves Accuracy and Decreases Variability. *Skelet. Radiol.* **2019**, *48*, 275–283. [CrossRef]
113. Wang, X.D.; Zhang, J.N.; Gan, Y.H.; Zhou, Y.H. Current Understanding of Pathogenesis and Treatment of TMJ Osteoarthritis. *J. Dent. Res.* **2015**, *94*, 666–673. [CrossRef] [PubMed]
114. Derwich, M.; Mitus-Kenig, M.; Pawlowska, E. Interdisciplinary Approach to the Temporomandibular Joint Osteoarthritis—Review of the Literature. *Medicina* **2020**, *56*, 225. [CrossRef] [PubMed]
115. Crincoli, V.; Cortelazzi, R.; De Biase, C.; Cazzolla, A.P.; Campobasso, A.; Dioguardi, M.; Piancino, M.G.; Mattia, L.; Di Comite, M. The Loss of Symmetry in Unilateral Bony Syngnathia: Case Report and Literature Review. *Symmetry* **2022**, *14*, 2008. [CrossRef]
116. Andrade, N.N.; Mathai, P.; Aggarwal, N. Facial Asymmetry. In *Oral and Maxillofacial Surgery for the Clinician*; Springer Nature: Singapore, 2021; pp. 1549–1576.
117. Choi, E.; Kim, D.; Lee, J.Y.; Park, H.K. Artificial Intelligence in Detecting Temporomandibular Joint Osteoarthritis on Orthopantomogram. *Sci. Rep.* **2021**, *11*, 10246. [CrossRef]
118. de Dumast, P.; Mirabel, C.; Cevidanes, L.; Ruellas, A.; Yatabe, M.; Ioshida, M.; Ribera, N.T.; Michoud, L.; Gomes, L.; Huang, C.; et al. A Web-Based System for Neural Network Based Classification in Temporomandibular Joint Osteoarthritis. *Comput. Med. Imaging Graph.* **2018**, *67*, 45–54. [CrossRef]
119. Bianchi, J.; de Oliveira Ruellas, A.C.; Gonçalves, J.R.; Paniagua, B.; Prieto, J.C.; Styner, M.; Li, T.; Zhu, H.; Sugai, J.; Giannobile, W.; et al. Osteoarthritis of the Temporomandibular Joint Can Be Diagnosed Earlier Using Biomarkers and Machine Learning. *Sci. Rep.* **2020**, *10*, 8012. [CrossRef]
120. Shoukri, B.; Prieto, J.C.; Ruellas, A.; Yatabe, M.; Sugai, J.; Styner, M.; Zhu, H.; Huang, C.; Paniagua, B.; Aronovich, S.; et al. Minimally Invasive Approach for Diagnosing TMJ Osteoarthritis. *J. Dent. Res.* **2019**, *98*, 1103–1111. [CrossRef]
121. Ito, S.; Mine, Y.; Yoshimi, Y.; Takeda, S.; Tanaka, A.; Onishi, A.; Peng, T.Y.; Nakamoto, T.; Nagasaki, T.; Kakimoto, N.; et al. Automated Segmentation of Articular Disc of the Temporomandibular Joint on Magnetic Resonance Images Using Deep Learning. *Sci. Rep.* **2022**, *12*, 221. [CrossRef]
122. Bianchi, J.; Ruellas, A.; Prieto, J.C.; Li, T.; Soroushmehr, R.; Najarian, K.; Gryak, J.; Deleat-Besson, R.; Le, C.; Yatabe, M.; et al. Decision Support Systems in Temporomandibular Joint Osteoarthritis: A Review of Data Science and Artificial Intelligence Applications. *Semin. Orthod.* **2021**, *27*, 78–86. [CrossRef]
123. Almăşan, O.; Leucuța, D.C.; Hedeşiu, M.; Mureşanu, S.; Popa, Ș.L. Temporomandibular Joint Osteoarthritis Diagnosis Employing Artificial Intelligence: Systematic Review and Meta-Analysis. *J. Clin. Med.* **2023**, *12*, 942. [CrossRef]
124. Ozsari, S.; Güzel, M.S.; Yılmaz, D.; Kamburoğlu, K. A Comprehensive Review of Artificial Intelligence Based Algorithms Regarding Temporomandibular Joint Related Diseases. *Diagnostics* **2023**, *13*, 2700. [CrossRef] [PubMed]

125. Jha, N.; Lee, K.S.; Kim, Y.J. Diagnosis of Temporomandibular Disorders Using Artificial Intelligence Technologies: A Systematic Review and Meta-Analysis. *PLoS ONE* **2022**, *17*, e0272715. [CrossRef] [PubMed]
126. Xu, L.; Chen, J.; Qiu, K.; Yang, F.; Wu, W. Artificial Intelligence for Detecting Temporomandibular Joint Osteoarthritis Using Radiographic Image Data: A Systematic Review and Meta-Analysis of Diagnostic Test Accuracy. *PLoS ONE* **2023**, *18*, e0288631. [CrossRef] [PubMed]
127. Al-Ani, M.H.; Mageet, A.O. Extraction Planning in Orthodontics. *J. Contemp. Dent. Pract.* **2018**, *19*, 619–623. [CrossRef] [PubMed]
128. Peck, S. Extractions, Retention and Stability: The Search for Orthodontic Truth. *Eur. J. Orthod.* **2017**, *39*, 109–115. [CrossRef]
129. Del Real, A.; Del Real, O.; Sardina, S.; Oyonarte, R. Use of Automated Artificial Intelligence to Predict the Need for Orthodontic Extractions. *Korean J. Orthod.* **2022**, *52*, 102–111. [CrossRef]
130. Ribarevski, R.; Vig, P.; Dryland Vig, K.; Weyant, R.; O'Brien, K. Consistency of Orthodontic Extraction Decisions. *Eur. J. Orthod.* **1996**, *18*, 77–80. [CrossRef]
131. Proffit, W.R. Forty-Year Review of Extraction Frequencies at a University Orthodontic Clinic. *Angle Orthod.* **1994**, *64*, 407–414. [CrossRef]
132. Jackson, T.H.; Guez, C.; Lin, F.C.; Proffit, W.R.; Ko, C.C. Extraction Frequencies at a University Orthodontic Clinic in the 21st Century: Demographic and Diagnostic Factors Affecting the Likelihood of Extraction. *Am. J. Orthod. Dentofac. Orthop.* **2017**, *151*, 456–462. [CrossRef]
133. Evrard, A.S.; Tepedino, M.; Cattaneo, P.M.; Cornelis, M.A. Which Factors Influence Orthodontists in Their Decision to Extract? A Questionnaire Survey. *J. Clin. Exp. Dent.* **2019**, *11*, e432–e438. [CrossRef]
134. Chambers, D.W.; Thakkar, D. Consistency of Orthodontists' Clinical Decisions: A Systematic Review, Meta-Analysis, and Theory Development. *Am. J. Orthod. Dentofac. Orthop.* **2022**, *161*, 497–509. [CrossRef] [PubMed]
135. Saghafi, N.; Heaton, L.J.; Bayirli, B.; Turpin, D.L.; Khosravi, R.; Bollen, A.M. Influence of Clinicians' Experience and Gender on Extraction Decision in Orthodontics. *Angle Orthod.* **2017**, *87*, 641–650. [CrossRef] [PubMed]
136. Baumrind, S.; Korn, E.L.; Boyd, R.L.; Maxwell, R. The Decision to Extract: Part 1--Interclinician Agreement. *Am. J. Orthod. Dentofac. Orthop.* **1996**, *109*, 297–309. [CrossRef] [PubMed]
137. Konstantonis, D.; Anthopoulou, C.; Makou, M. Extraction Decision and Identification of Treatment Predictors in Class I Malocclusions. *Prog. Orthod.* **2013**, *14*, 47. [CrossRef] [PubMed]
138. Evangelista, K.; de Freitas Silva, B.S.; Yamamoto-Silva, F.P.; Valladares-Neto, J.; Silva, M.A.G.; Cevidanes, L.H.S.; de Luca Canto, G.; Massignan, C. Accuracy of Artificial Intelligence for Tooth Extraction Decision-Making in Orthodontics: A Systematic Review and Meta-Analysis. *Clin. Oral. Investig.* **2022**, *26*, 6893–6905. [CrossRef] [PubMed]
139. Liu, J.; Chen, Y.; Li, S.; Zhao, Z.; Wu, Z. Machine Learning in Orthodontics: Challenges and Perspectives. *Adv. Clin. Exp. Med.* **2021**, *30*, 1065–1074. [CrossRef] [PubMed]
140. Choi, H.I.; Jung, S.K.; Baek, S.H.; Lim, W.H.; Ahn, S.J.; Yang, I.H.; Kim, T.W. Artificial Intelligent Model with Neural Network Machine Learning for the Diagnosis of Orthognathic Surgery. *J. Craniofacial Surg.* **2019**, *30*, 1986–1989. [CrossRef]
141. Takada, K. Artificial Intelligence Expert Systems with Neural Network Machine Learning May Assist Decision-Making for Extractions in Orthodontic Treatment Planning. *J. Evid. Based Dent. Pract.* **2016**, *16*, 190–192. [CrossRef]
142. Jung, S.K.; Kim, T.W. New Approach for the Diagnosis of Extractions with Neural Network Machine Learning. *Am. J. Orthod. Dentofac. Orthop.* **2016**, *149*, 127–133. [CrossRef]
143. Li, P.; Kong, D.; Tang, T.; Su, D.; Yang, P.; Wang, H.; Zhao, Z.; Liu, Y. Orthodontic Treatment Planning Based on Artificial Neural Networks. *Sci. Rep.* **2019**, *9*, 2037. [CrossRef]
144. Xie, X.; Wang, L.; Wang, A. Artificial Neural Network Modeling for Deciding If Extractions Are Necessary Prior to Orthodontic Treatment. *Angle Orthod.* **2010**, *80*, 262–266. [CrossRef] [PubMed]
145. Georgalis, K.; Woods, M.G. A Study of Class III Treatment: Orthodontic Camouflage vs Orthognathic Surgery. *Aust. Orthod. J.* **2015**, *31*, 138–148. [CrossRef] [PubMed]
146. Raposo, R.; Peleteiro, B.; Paço, M.; Pinho, T. Orthodontic Camouflage versus Orthodontic-Orthognathic Surgical Treatment in Class II Malocclusion: A Systematic Review and Meta-Analysis. *Int. J. Oral. Maxillofac. Surg.* **2018**, *47*, 445–455. [CrossRef] [PubMed]
147. Hong, M.; Kim, I.; Cho, J.H.; Kang, K.H.; Kim, M.; Kim, S.J.; Kim, Y.J.; Sung, S.J.; Kim, Y.H.; Lim, S.H.; et al. Accuracy of Artificial Intelligence-Assisted Landmark Identification in Serial Lateral Cephalograms of Class III Patients Who Underwent Orthodontic Treatment and Two-Jaw Orthognathic Surgery. *Korean J. Orthod.* **2022**, *52*, 287–297. [CrossRef] [PubMed]
148. Shin, W.S.; Yeom, H.G.; Lee, G.H.; Yun, J.P.; Jeong, S.H.; Lee, J.H.; Kim, H.K.; Kim, B.C. Deep Learning Based Prediction of Necessity for Orthognathic Surgery of Skeletal Malocclusion Using Cephalogram in Korean Individuals. *BMC Oral. Health* **2021**, *21*, 130. [CrossRef] [PubMed]
149. Kim, Y.H.; Park, J.B.; Chang, M.S.; Ryu, J.J.; Lim, W.H.; Jung, S.K. Influence of the Depth of the Convolutional Neural Networks on an Artificial Intelligence Model for Diagnosis of Orthognathic Surgery. *J. Pers. Med.* **2021**, *11*, 356. [CrossRef]
150. Lee, K.S.; Ryu, J.J.; Jang, H.S.; Lee, D.Y.; Jung, S.K. Deep Convolutional Neural Networks Based Analysis of Cephalometric Radiographs for Differential Diagnosis of Orthognathic Surgery Indications. *Appl. Sci.* **2020**, *10*, 2124. [CrossRef]
151. Jeong, S.H.; Yun, J.P.; Yeom, H.G.; Lim, H.J.; Lee, J.; Kim, B.C. Deep Learning Based Discrimination of Soft Tissue Profiles Requiring Orthognathic Surgery by Facial Photographs. *Sci. Rep.* **2020**, *10*, 16235. [CrossRef]

152. Chung, M.; Lee, J.; Song, W.; Song, Y.; Yang, I.H.; Lee, J.; Shin, Y.G. Automatic Registration between Dental Cone-Beam CT and Scanned Surface via Deep Pose Regression Neural Networks and Clustered Similarities. *IEEE Trans. Med. Imaging* **2020**, *39*, 3900–3909. [CrossRef]
153. Knoops, P.G.M.; Papaioannou, A.; Borghi, A.; Breakey, R.W.F.; Wilson, A.T.; Jeelani, O.; Zafeiriou, S.; Steinbacher, D.; Padwa, B.L.; Dunaway, D.J.; et al. A Machine Learning Framework for Automated Diagnosis and Computer-Assisted Planning in Plastic and Reconstructive Surgery. *Sci. Rep.* **2019**, *9*, 13597. [CrossRef]
154. Salazar, D.; Rossouw, P.E.; Javed, F.; Michelogiannakis, D. Artificial Intelligence for Treatment Planning and Soft Tissue Outcome Prediction of Orthognathic Treatment: A Systematic Review. *J. Orthod.* **2023**. [CrossRef] [PubMed]
155. Patcas, R.; Bernini, D.A.J.; Volokitin, A.; Agustsson, E.; Rothe, R.; Timofte, R. Applying Artificial Intelligence to Assess the Impact of Orthognathic Treatment on Facial Attractiveness and Estimated Age. *Int. J. Oral. Maxillofac. Surg.* **2019**, *48*, 77–83. [CrossRef]
156. Lo, L.J.; Yang, C.T.; Ho, C.T.; Liao, C.H.; Lin, H.H. Automatic Assessment of 3-Dimensional Facial Soft Tissue Symmetry Before and After Orthognathic Surgery Using a Machine Learning Model: A Preliminary Experience. *Ann. Plast. Surg.* **2021**, *86*, S224–S228. [CrossRef] [PubMed]
157. Seo, J.; Yang, I.H.; Choi, J.Y.; Lee, J.H.; Baek, S.H. Three-Dimensional Facial Soft Tissue Changes After Orthognathic Surgery in Cleft Patients Using Artificial Intelligence-Assisted Landmark Autodigitization. *J. Craniofacial Surg.* **2021**, *32*, 2695–2700. [CrossRef] [PubMed]
158. Lin, H.H.; Chiang, W.C.; Yang, C.T.; Cheng, C.T.; Zhang, T.; Lo, L.J. On Construction of Transfer Learning for Facial Symmetry Assessment before and after Orthognathic Surgery. *Comput. Methods Programs Biomed.* **2021**, *200*, 105928. [CrossRef] [PubMed]
159. Xu, L.; Mei, L.; Lu, R.; Li, Y.; Li, H.; Li, Y. Predicting Patient Experience of Invisalign Treatment: An Analysis Using Artificial Neural Network. *Korean J. Orthod.* **2022**, *52*, 268–277. [CrossRef]
160. Park, Y.S.; Choi, J.H.; Kim, Y.; Choi, S.H.; Lee, J.H.; Kim, K.H.; Chung, C.J. Deep Learning–Based Prediction of the 3D Post-torthodontic Facial Changes. *J. Dent. Res.* **2022**, *101*, 1372–1379. [CrossRef]
161. Park, J.H.; Kim, Y.J.; Kim, J.; Kim, J.; Kim, I.H.; Kim, N.; Vaid, N.R.; Kook, Y.A. Use of Artificial Intelligence to Predict Outcomes of Nonextraction Treatment of Class II Malocclusions. *Semin. Orthod.* **2021**, *27*, 87–95. [CrossRef]
162. Woo, H.; Jha, N.; Kim, Y.J.; Sung, S.J. Evaluating the Accuracy of Automated Orthodontic Digital Setup Models. *Semin. Orthod.* **2023**, *29*, 60–67. [CrossRef]
163. Tanikawa, C.; Yamashiro, T. Development of Novel Artificial Intelligence Systems to Predict Facial Morphology after Orthognathic Surgery and Orthodontic Treatment in Japanese Patients. *Sci. Rep.* **2021**, *11*, 15853. [CrossRef]
164. Cassi, D.; Battistoni, G.; Magnifico, M.; Di Blasio, C.; Pedrazzi, G.; Di Blasio, A. Three-Dimensional Evaluation of Facial Asymmetry in Patients with Hemifacial Microsomia Using Stereophotogrammetry. *J. Cranio-Maxillofac. Surg.* **2019**, *47*, 179–184. [CrossRef]
165. Khanagar, S.B.; Alfouzan, K.; Awawdeh, M.; Alkadi, L.; Albalawi, F.; Alghilan, M.A. Performance of Artificial Intelligence Models Designed for Diagnosis, Treatment Planning and Predicting Prognosis of Orthognathic Surgery (OGS)—A Scoping Review. *Appl. Sci.* **2022**, *12*, 5581. [CrossRef]
166. Alam, M.K.; Abutayyem, H.; Kanwal, B.; Shayeb, M.A.L. Future of Orthodontics—A Systematic Review and Meta-Analysis on the Emerging Trends in This Field. *J. Clin. Med.* **2023**, *12*, 532. [CrossRef] [PubMed]
167. Portnoy, J.; Waller, M.; Elliott, T. Telemedicine in the Era of COVID-19. *J. Allergy Clin. Immunol. Pract.* **2020**, *8*, 1489–1491. [CrossRef] [PubMed]
168. Tsichlaki, A.; Chin, S.Y.; Pandis, N.; Fleming, P.S. How Long Does Treatment with Fixed Orthodontic Appliances Last? A Systematic Review. *Am. J. Orthod. Dentofac. Orthop.* **2016**, *149*, 308–318. [CrossRef] [PubMed]
169. Caruso, S.; Caruso, S.; Pellegrino, M.; Skafi, R.; Nota, A.; Tecco, S. A Knowledge-Based Algorithm for Automatic Monitoring of Orthodontic Treatment: The Dental Monitoring System. Two Cases. *Sensors* **2021**, *21*, 1856. [CrossRef] [PubMed]
170. Roisin, L.-C.; Brézulier, D.; Sorel, O. Remotely-Controlled Orthodontics: Fundamentals and Description of the Dental Monitoring System. *J. Dentofac. Anom. Orthod.* **2016**, *19*, 408. [CrossRef]
171. Hansa, I.; Katyal, V.; Semaan, S.J.; Coyne, R.; Vaid, N.R. Artificial Intelligence Driven Remote Monitoring of Orthodontic Patients: Clinical Applicability and Rationale. *Semin. Orthod.* **2021**, *27*, 138–156. [CrossRef]
172. Strunga, M.; Urban, R.; Surovková, J.; Thurzo, A. Artificial Intelligence Systems Assisting in the Assessment of the Course and Retention of Orthodontic Treatment. *Healthcare* **2023**, *11*, 683. [CrossRef]
173. Hannequin, R.; Ouadi, E.; Racy, E.; Moreau, N. Clinical Follow-up of Corticotomy-Accelerated Invisalign Orthodontic Treatment with Dental Monitoring. *Am. J. Orthod. Dentofac. Orthop.* **2020**, *158*, 878–888. [CrossRef]
174. Sangalli, L.; Savoldi, F.; Dalessandri, D.; Visconti, L.; Massetti, F.; Bonetti, S. Remote Digital Monitoring during the Retention Phase of Orthodontic Treatment: A Prospective Feasibility Study. *Korean J. Orthod.* **2022**, *52*, 123–130. [CrossRef] [PubMed]
175. Hansa, I.; Semaan, S.J.; Vaid, N.R. Clinical Outcomes and Patient Perspectives of Dental Monitoring®GoLive®with Invisalign®—A Retrospective Cohort Study. *Prog. Orthod.* **2020**, *21*, 16. [CrossRef] [PubMed]
176. Sangalli, L.; Savoldi, F.; Dalessandri, D.; Bonetti, S.; Gu, M.; Signoroni, A.; Paganelli, C. Effects of Remote Digital Monitoring on Oral Hygiene of Orthodontic Patients: A Prospective Study. *BMC Oral. Health* **2021**, *21*, 435. [CrossRef] [PubMed]

177. Homsi, K.; Snider, V.; Kusnoto, B.; Atsawasuwan, P.; Viana, G.; Allareddy, V.; Gajendrareddy, P.; Elnagar, M.H. In-Vivo Evaluation of Artificial Intelligence Driven Remote Monitoring Technology for Tracking Tooth Movement and Reconstruction of 3-Dimensional Digital Models during Orthodontic Treatment. *Am. J. Orthod. Dentofac. Orthop.* **2023**, *164*, 690–699. [CrossRef] [PubMed]
178. Sangalli, L.; Alessandri-Bonetti, A.; Dalessandri, D. Effectiveness of Dental Monitoring System in Orthodontics: A Systematic Review. *J. Orthod.* **2023**. [CrossRef] [PubMed]
179. van Leeuwen, K.G.; de Rooij, M.; Schalekamp, S.; van Ginneken, B.; Rutten, M.J.C.M. How Does Artificial Intelligence in Radiology Improve Efficiency and Health Outcomes? *Pediatr. Radiol.* **2022**, *52*, 2087–2093. [CrossRef] [PubMed]
180. Tolle, K.M.; Tansley, D.S.W.; Hey, A.J.G. The Fourth Paradigm: Data-Intensive Scientific Discovery. *Proc. Proc. IEEE* **2011**, *99*, 1334–1337. [CrossRef]
181. Dania, D.; Walter, F.W.; Matthew, P.L.; Tarik, A.; Nina, K.; Bibb, A.; Christopher, J.R.; Bernardo, C.B.; Kimberly, D.; James, A.B.; et al. Implementation of Clinical Artificial Intelligence in Radiology: Who Decides and How? *Radiology* **2022**, *305*, 555–563. [CrossRef]
182. Waller, J.; O'connor, A.; Rafaat, E.; Amireh, A.; Dempsey, J.; Martin, C.; Umair, M. Applications and Challenges of Artificial Intelligence in Diagnostic and Interventional Radiology. *Pol. J. Radiol.* **2022**, *87*, 113–117. [CrossRef]
183. The Lancet. AI in Medicine: Creating a Safe and Equitable Future. *Lancet* **2023**, *402*, 503. [CrossRef]
184. van Leeuwen, K.G.; Schalekamp, S.; Rutten, M.J.C.M.; van Ginneken, B.; de Rooij, M. Artificial Intelligence in Radiology: 100 Commercially Available Products and Their Scientific Evidence. *Eur. Radiol.* **2021**, *31*, 3797–3804. [CrossRef] [PubMed]

Disclaimer/Publisher's Note: The statements, opinions and data contained in all publications are solely those of the individual author(s) and contributor(s) and not of MDPI and/or the editor(s). MDPI and/or the editor(s) disclaim responsibility for any injury to people or property resulting from any ideas, methods, instructions or products referred to in the content.

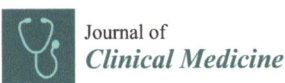

Article

Influence of the Tube Angle on the Measurement Accuracy of Peri-Implant Bone Defects in Rectangular Intraoral X-ray Imaging

Petra Rugani *, Katharina Weingartner and Norbert Jakse

Department of Dental Medicine and Oral Health, Division of Oral Surgery and Orthodontics, Medical University of Graz, Billrothgasse 4, 8010 Graz, Austria
* Correspondence: petra.rugani@medunigraz.at; Tel.: +43-316-385-13486

Abstract: Background: Intraoral radiography in the right-angle technique is the standard procedure to examine the peri-implant bone level in implant follow-up and implant-related studies. For the implementation of the right-angle or parallel technique, mostly ready-made image receptor holders are used. The aim of this experimental study is to analyze changes in the measurement of standardized peri-implant defects caused by a deviation in the position of the image receptor. Methods: Eleven Xive® implants (Dentsply Sirona, Bensheim, Germany) were placed in bovine bone, and peri-implant defects of varying depths were created. The preparations were fixed in a specially made test stand, and intraoral radiographs were taken using the right-angle technique with standard film holders at various horizontal and vertical projection angles. Defect measurement was carried out with the imaging software Sidexis 4 V 4.3 (Dentsply Sirona, Bensheim, Germany). Results: With increasing angular deviation, larger deviations between the measured and the real extent of the defect occurred. Vertical tilting caused significant distortion, while horizontal rotation showed less effect. Conclusion: Intraoral radiography only provides a valid representation of the peri-implant bone level for follow-up or as a tool in implant-related studies if a reproducible projection direction is assured.

Keywords: peri-implant bone level; intra-oral radiography; implantology

Citation: Rugani, P.; Weingartner, K.; Jakse, N. Influence of the Tube Angle on the Measurement Accuracy of Peri-Implant Bone Defects in Rectangular Intraoral X-ray Imaging. *J. Clin. Med.* **2024**, *13*, 391. https://doi.org/10.3390/jcm13020391

Academic Editors: James Kit-Hon Tsoi and Erich Sorantin

Received: 25 November 2023
Revised: 20 December 2023
Accepted: 6 January 2024
Published: 10 January 2024

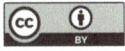

Copyright: © 2024 by the authors. Licensee MDPI, Basel, Switzerland. This article is an open access article distributed under the terms and conditions of the Creative Commons Attribution (CC BY) license (https://creativecommons.org/licenses/by/4.0/).

1. Introduction

Intraoral radiography using the right-angle technique is the standard procedure to examine the peri-implant bone level. It is indispensable for implant follow-up and also serves as a basis for the assessment of peri-implant bone loss and, thus, the diagnosis of peri-implantitis. It is also the preferred technique to analyze peri-implant bone level in implant-related studies [1,2]. Peri-implant inflammation is the main cause of loss of previously osseointegrated dental implants, with a prevalence of 22% (2131 patients, 8893 implants) [3]. While in peri-implant mucositis, the inflammatory cell infiltrate is limited to the supracrestal soft tissue interface, in peri-implantitis, it is spread to the bony implant site [4]. This is a serious complication that, if left untreated, will progress, leading to pain and other signs of inflammation, and may ultimately result in implant loss. Part of standardized implant aftercare is to recognize, classify, and treat early signs of peri-implant inflammation to prevent the progression to more advanced stages. Taking an intraoral radiograph to evaluate the crestal bone level is part of the strategy. It is recommended to take an intraoral radiograph using the right-angle or parallel technique at the time of installation of the prosthetic component as a baseline and to repeat this examination at regular intervals [5]. In the case of manifest peri-implantitis, the type of bone loss, i.e., whether it is an intraosseous defect or a supra-alveolar manifestation, or whether there are mixed forms [6], can already be estimated. Furthermore, the peri-implant bone level or the development and progression of peri-implantitis can be influenced by a wide variety of variables [2], including implant surface, abutment connection, prosthetic concepts, hygiene ability, etc. Consequently, radiographic imaging of the peri-implant bone is a common research method in studies in the field of implantology [7,8]. A clear depiction of the crestal bone level and the verification of the existence and/or progression of bone loss in periodically repeated radiographs with the same projection geometry are essential for the comparison to earlier images or other implants. Particularly in scientific studies, this is of utmost importance [9–11].

In daily dental practice, intraoral radiographs represent the standard tool to assess the crestal bone level around dental implants. The spatial relationship between the beam source, object, and image receiver essentially determines the two-dimensional radiograph formation during the recording. The projection of three-dimensional defects onto two-dimensional image receptors is associated with typical misrepresentations. These include:

- Image enlargement through projection magnification;
- tilting of the examination objects, misinterpretation of the edges of the examination object/sites on the image; and
- an inaccurate evaluation method for distance measurements within the image [12].

In order to obtain representations that are as accurate as possible, it is recommended to reduce the influence of these factors as much as possible. Images are taken using standardized film holders in combination with a right-angle or parallel technique [13]. The image receptor is aligned via the film holder at a defined angle to an indicator ring, onto which the tube is placed flush. This means that the central beam is always perpendicular to the image receptor axis. In addition, the holder should be aligned with the patient's bite on a bite plate so that the image receptor is positioned parallel to the tooth or implant axis [1]. Even if this is not often the case, at least a reproducible alignment of the central beam with the object axis should be achieved for the correct assessment of changes in the crestal bone level. Since reference values such as the implant length are often known, measurements can also be made, and thus a quantitative analysis of changes over time can be carried out. These measurements usually take place in the submillimeter range [14]. A weakness of this method is the uncertainty of how the film holder is placed and deflected by the patient's bite, which is not a constant parameter and can be different with each examination. Being able to estimate the dimensions of such deviations is important for assessing the accuracy of the image. Since calculating geometric distortions cannot be established in everyday life, guideline values are of great importance [1].

The aim of this experimental study is to assess the effect of deflection of the right-angle holder on the measurement results of standardized peri-implant defects.

2. Materials and Methods

Uncooked bovine ribs were used for the implantation because they have the same properties as a human jawbone. The ribs were encased in SnowWhite plaster to ensure stability. As a next step, eleven Xive® implants (Dentsply Sirona, Bensheim, Germany) with a diameter of 3.8 mm and a length of 11 mm were placed in the bones. The implantation was carried out according to the protocol specified by the manufacturer. All drilling was carried out with a fixed drill bit, which ensured that the identical axis could be maintained exactly every time. (Figure 1a) Subsequently, implants were placed. Insertion torque exceeded 25 Ncm for all implants.

After implant insertion, a circumferential defect was created using a trephine bur in the implant axis. Eleven defects with depths of 2, 2.5, 3, 4, 5, 6, 7, 8, 9, 10, and 11 mm were created. (Figure 1b) Water cooling was applied throughout the complete drilling process.

To ensure accurate and repeatable measurements with exactly defined parameters, a test environment was created (Figure 2a).

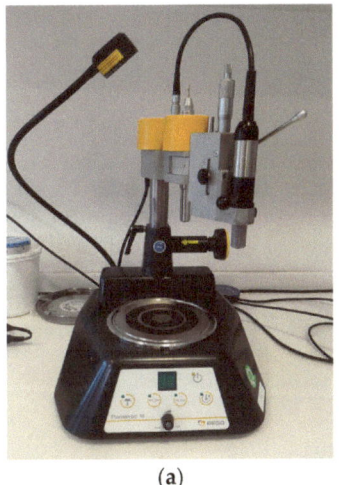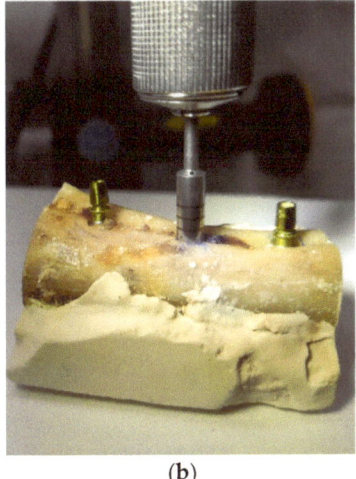

Figure 1. Implant placement and defect creation (**a**) Drill press to maintain the exact drilling direction. (**b**) Creation of defect around a previously inserted implant with the trephine bur.

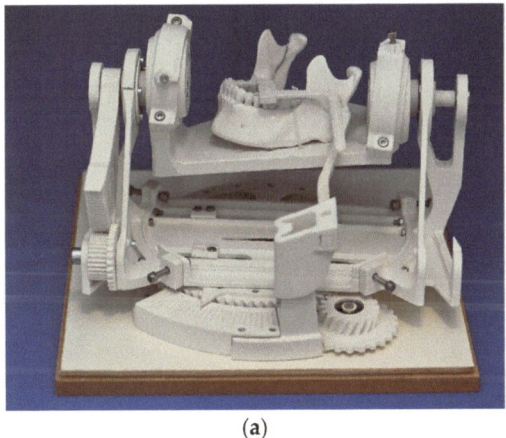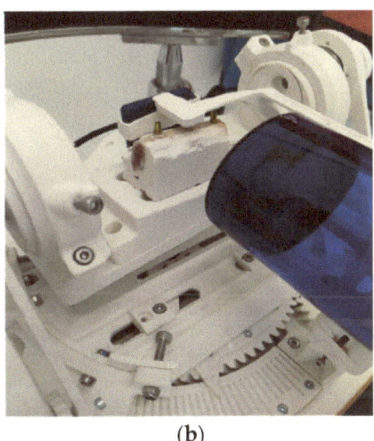

Figure 2. Experimental setting (**a**) test stand. (**b**) Prepared bovine ribs and positioned radiographic film rigidly fixated to the radiation tube.

The mechanics contained here made it possible to change the angle between the radiation tube and the test objects in precise, predefined steps. By this, a biangular deviation in the vertical and horizontal directions was imitated. (Figure 2b) The displacement of the angle was minus 15 degrees to plus 15 degrees in steps of 5 degrees in the vertical plane and minus 8 degrees to plus 8 degrees in steps of 3 degrees in the horizontal plane. The test stand was designed by a technical engineer (Konrad Felix Fellner e.U., Graz, Austria) in the programs Rhino V4® (Robert McNeel & Associates, Seattle, Washington, DC, USA) and Solidworks 2017® (Dassault Systèmes SolidWorks Corporation, Waltham, MA, USA).

The individual parts were manufactured through 3D printing using the Fused Filament Fabrication additive process. Polyactic acid 3D printing filament (PLA) was chosen as the material because of its good physical properties and easy availability. PLA is largely resistant to most common solvents and does not affect X-rays. The used cylinder head screws and ball bearings were kept outside the region of interest. The characteristics of the test stand were:

- A platform for fixing the objects to be X-rayed
- Adjustment options for adjusting the object to the respective axis pivot points
- Two independently rotatable axes
- Angle markings for referencing, measurement, and data collection
- An adjustable holder for the X-ray sensor and X-ray machine

The platform, to which the test object was fixated, was positioned at an angle in the room and held by appropriate components so that it could be moved freely. This changed the projection angle of the rigidly positioned central beam.

The horizontal rotation of the platform allowed seven different settings with the angular positions $-8°$, $-5°$, $-3°$, $0°$, $3°$, $5°$, and $8°$. The vertical axis allowed the angle settings of $-15°$, $-10°$, $-5°$, $0°$, $5°$, $10°$, and $15°$. (Figure 3) The ribs encased in plaster were positioned centrally on the platform to allow free movement in all directions.

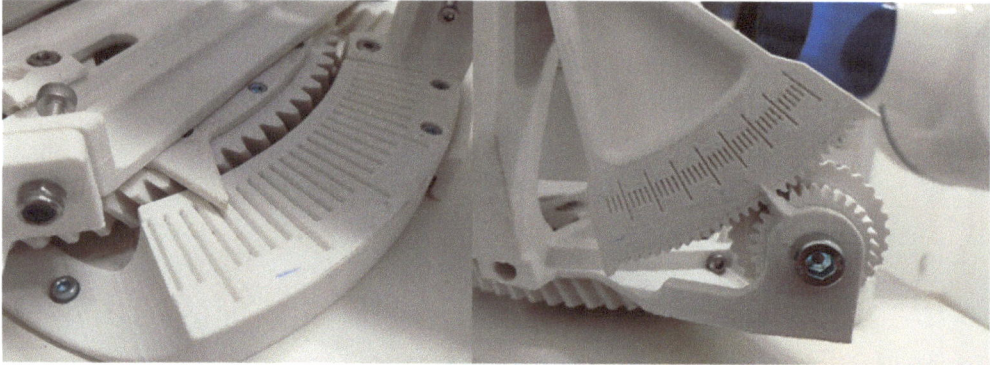

Figure 3. Mechanism to adjust horizontal and vertical angulation.

The X-ray tube (Heliodent Plus, Dentsply Sirona, Bensheim, Germany) was set in a zero-degree position parallel to the holding arm of the digital sensor at a distance of 8 cm from the image receptor. The fixed models were imaged radiographically with a tube current of 7 mA, a tube voltage of 60 kV, and an exposure time of 0.06 s using the right-angle technique.

The Sidexis 4 V 4.3 imaging software (Dentsply Sirona, Charlotte, NC, USA) was used to measure the depiction of the defects on the radiographs. The measurement tool was calibrated based on the implant length of 11 mm.

Every defect was traced individually using the Sidexis measurement tool parallel to the implant axis, starting from the crestal bone edge. Defects were 2 to 11 mm deep. Each defect was pictured 49 times in different directions, ranging from -15 to $+15$ degrees in the vertical dimension and from -8 to $+8$ degrees in the horizontal dimension.

The data were collected in an Excel® spreadsheet. (Microsoft 365, Version 2207 (Build 15427.20194), Microsoft, Redmond, Washington, DC, USA). The deviation of the measuring depth from the true depth of the defect was calculated. Statistical analysis to assess the results included ANOVA and regression analysis using SPSS software (IBM SPSS Statistics 26.0, IBM Corporation, Armonk, NY, USA) at a 5% significance level.

3. Results

Altogether, 539 images were analyzed. The deviation of the measured dimensions of the depicted defects from the known true defect depths was 0.0 to 4.6 mm (mean 0.7 ± 0.7 mm) (Figures 4 and 5).

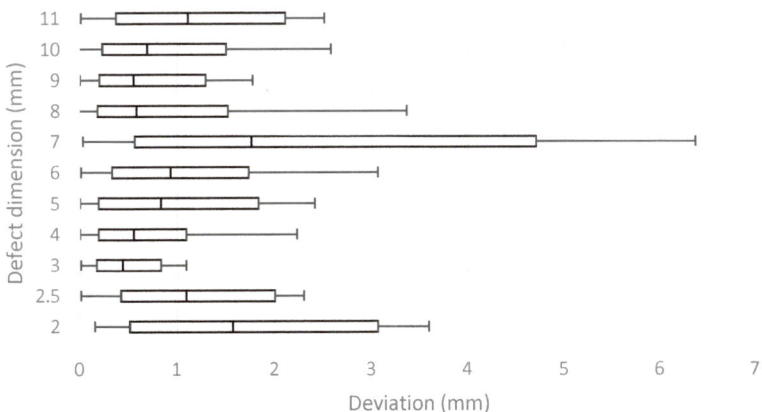

Figure 4. Mean measurement errors of all 11 defects (2.5–11 mm) of all horizontal and vertical deflections.

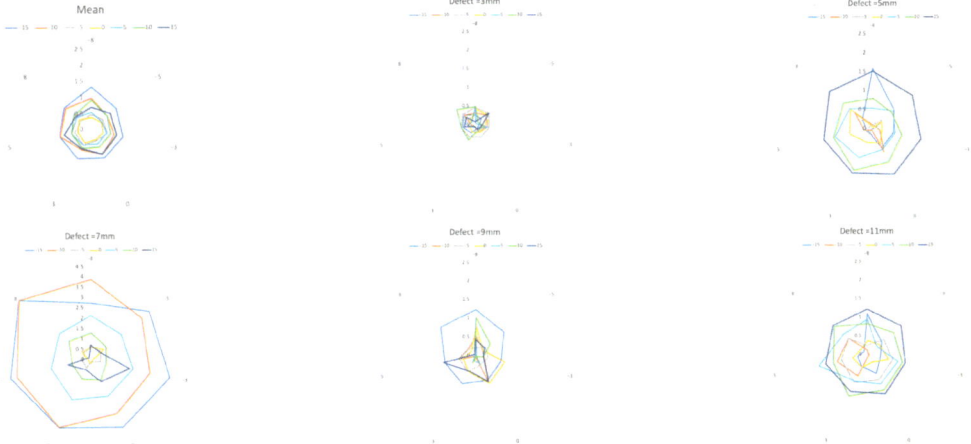

Figure 5. Measurement error due to vertical deviation of the projection. Mean over all defects and defects with 3, 5, 7, 9, and 11 mm. A greater vertical deviation (−15 to 15 degrees, colored lines) of the projection direction led to a larger measurement error. (Each mesh section equals 0.5 mm, with horizontal rotation at the corner points of the mesh.) Note the extreme outliers in the 7 mm defect.

When viewed in terms of the length of each individual defect, the mean results of each defect differed in relation to the correspondent real depth between 7% and 28%, respectively, from 0.34 mm to 1.34 mm (mean 0.70 ± 0.24). This resulted in mean deviations of 15.2% (± 5.0%).

Vertical tilting alone resulted in mean deviations of 0.34 to 1 mm (mean 0.65 ± 0.26 mm) or 7% to 20% (mean 13.9 ± 5.4%) (Table 1). In the horizontal plane, measurements differed from real lengths by 0.34 mm to 0.5 mm (mean 0.42 ± 0.06) or 8% to 10% (mean 8.6 ± 1%) (Table 1).

Table 1. Relative mean deviations in regard to deflection across all 11 defects. (columns—horizontal deflection (−8° to +8°), lines—vertical deflection (−15° to +15°)).

Deflection	−8	−5	−3	0	3	5	8
−15	28%	21%	22%	20%	20%	21%	22%
−10	21%	17%	18%	19%	13%	19%	25%
−5	12%	12%	12%	9%	11%	12%	10%
0	8%	9%	8%	7%	9%	9%	10%
5	9%	7%	10%	9%	9%	13%	11%
10	2%	15%	15%	15%	15%	16%	16%
15	16%	18%	18%	18%	16%	20%	15%

The deeper the defect, the greater the deviation that appeared when the angle changed horizontally and vertically. The smallest deviation from the actual length in the range of seven to 10% was found in the vertical zero-degree position, even with horizontal angular rotation. The more the vertical angle differed from the zero-degree position, the greater the mean deviation. (Table 1, Figure 5) On the other hand, differences barely increased in the horizontal direction, as the rotation increased.

An ANOVA analysis of variance showed that the influence of the vertical tilt was highly significant, but the results for the horizontal twist were not. Furthermore, Pearson's correlation coefficient showed a positive correlation between vertical tilt and measurement error. An exception were the results of the 7 mm defect, some of which showed noticeably high outliers (Table 2).

Table 2. Mostly positive correlation of vertical tilting to measurement deviation.

Defect	2 mm	2.5 mm	3 mm	4 mm	5 mm	6 mm	7 mm	8 mm	9 mm	10 mm	11 mm
PCC *	r = 0.177 p = 0.224	r = 0.857 p < 0.001	r = 0.190 p = 0.192	r = 0.619 p < 0.001	r = 0.734 p < 0.001	r = 0.607 p < 0.001	r = −0.606 p < 0.001	r = 0.803 p < 0.001	r = 0.478 p = 0.519	r = 0.094 p = 0.519	r = 0.827 p < 0.001

* Pearson's correlation coefficient (PCC).

A regression analysis also confirmed a significant connection between vertical tilting and the resulting measurement difference ($p < 0.001$), but none for horizontal rotation ($p = 0.372$).

The largest average deviation of the defects occurred at the −8° horizontal and −15° vertical degree settings. Rotating in the negative degree range brought the defect closer to the radiation source. At the same time, the distance to the image sensor increased. Consequently, distortion was more pronounced and measured lengths, and therefore, the differences to the real lengths were larger in all values of the negative direction of rotation (Figure 6).

The mean range from the shortest to the longest measurement of a defect was 2.61 mm (±1.12 [0.95; 5.06]) or 51% (±25% [18.2%; 93%]) in relation to the depth of the corresponding defects (Figure 7).

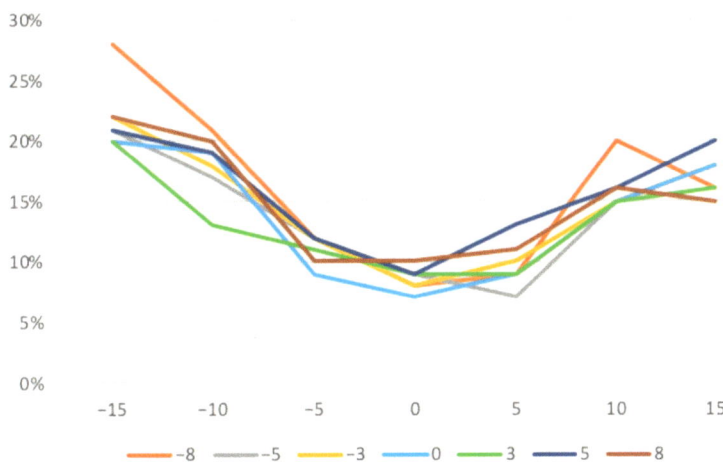

Figure 6. Mean measurement deviations across all defects with horizontal (−8 to +8 degrees) and vertical tilting (−15 to +15 degrees).

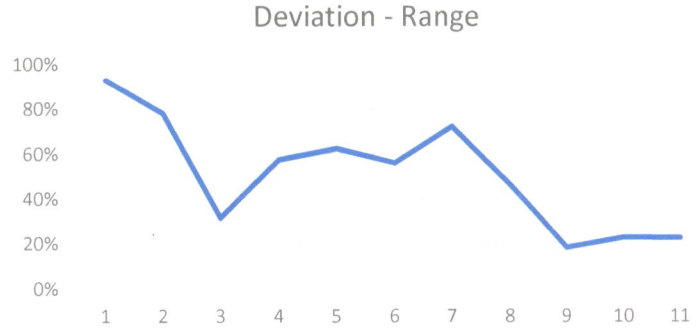

Figure 7. Range of most extreme measurements for all defects in relation to the defect dimension.

4. Discussion

The study demonstrated that tilting of prefabricated right-angle holders led to measurement errors when evaluating peri-implant bone defects in intraoral radiographs. A vertical deflection resulted in a greater length deviation than a horizontal deflection. Although horizontal rotation alone had no real effect on the measurement deviations, an even greater deviation was evident when horizontal rotation was correlated with vertical rotation. The results deviated from the true defect size by an average of 15.2%. The maximum range of deviations occurred in the 7 mm defect, where the shortest and longest measurements differed by 5 mm; the mean range was 2.61 mm (±1.12 [0.95; 5.06]) or 51% (±25% [18.2%; 93%]) of the defect size. Nevertheless, considering the wide distrubtion of measurements with extreme outliers in the 7 mm defect, errors in execution must be considered probable. To the best of our knowledge, there is only one comparable experimental study that calculated a 11.4% distortion if the film holder is tilted 30% in the vertical direction [10,15].

There are several imaging modalities that can be used for radiological diagnostics in dental practice. Since the turn of the millennium, the classic procedures of intraoral radiography and panoramic radiography have been joined by cone-beam-computed tomography (CBCT), which allows in-office cross-sectional diagnostics. Before CBCT was established, this was mainly carried out using computed tomography, for which patients had to be referred to a radiology institute or to a specialized radiologist. The advantages of cross-sectional imaging are apparent. While in two-dimensional imaging, the structures that lie one behind the other in the beam path are superimposed, cross-sectional imaging makes it possible to display the structures separately from one another. In the case of peri-implant defects, this means that the buccal and lingual parts of the peri-implant bone, which can also be affected by an osseous lesion, can potentially also be visualized.

In the case of peri-implant bony defects, this means the three-dimensional extent of the defect and the parts that are located buccaly or orally to the implant, as well as revealing fenestration and dehiscence defects, might be better depicted [16,17]. Studies by Ritter et al. and Steiger-Ronay et al. concluded that measurements of distal and mesial bone levels are equally accurate with intraoral radiography and CBCT [18,19].

Kühl et al. compared the diagnostic capacity of different dental imaging modalities in the depiction of peri-implant defects in a cadaver study [20]. Six implants were inserted into a human edentulous lower jaw. Defects with known depth and three-dimensional configuration were created. Conventional intraoral radiography in parallel technique using a film holder, digital panoramic radiography, cone-beam-computed tomography with a volume of 8×8 and a voxel size of 0.125, and computed tomography with a slice thickness of 0.72 mm were employed. For intraoral radiography, CBCT, and computed tomography, the mandible was fixated in an individualized Plexiglas panel.

In their study, intraoral radiography performed best, with the highest sensitivity and specificity over all defects, even though only the mesial and distal bone surrounding the implant could be depicted. Furthermore, despite superimposition and distortion, panoramic radiography yielded the best results in determining the defect type (two-, three-, or four-wall defect). This was even the case in two-wall defects, where the buccal and oral parts of an implant—areas that are usually not clearly shown on two-dimensional images—are affected (classification of Renvert and Giovannoli 2012 [21]).

On the other hand, panoramic radiography showed the worst sensitivity for 1 mm defects. These small defects were discovered best by CBCT, but CBCT also showed the lowest specificity for 3 mm defects. Computed tomography yielded the lowest overall sensitivity.

Consequently, despite the technology-specific shortcomings of two-dimensional imaging, conventional or digital intraoral radiography is still the gold standard for picturing the peri-implant bone [2,22]. It is a widely accepted technique for the long-term evaluation of marginal bone changes, especially at interproximal sites, of osseointegrated implants [23]. For this, there are several main reasons: First, the high sensitivity and specificity in depicting osseous lesions of all dimensions, as mentioned above, are the most important capacities of intraoral radiography. This is probably due to the high spatial resolution of the technology, with 10 to approximately 25 line pairs per mm (lp/mm), whereas three-dimensional imaging techniques display only 1–2 lp/mm or even less (computed tomography) [24]. Further, the widespread availability and cost-effectiveness of intraoral radiography are supporting its practicability and, consequently, its daily use. The possibility of standardized image acquisition through the use of image holders allows use in the area of years of postoperative follow-up. And last but not least, intraoral radiography is associated with the lowest patient exposure to radiation of all dental imaging modalities [25,26]. In general, the long-cone paralleling technique, supported by positioning devices, is used. For posterior intraoral radiographs with the widely used photo-stimulable phosphor storage, a radiation dose of 1.2 µSv to 2 µSv arises [27].

Despite the low patient doses in dental radiography, the International Commission on Radiological Protection (ICRP) considers the linear non-threshold model when recommending radiation safety guidelines. The cumulative effects of low-dose radiation could trigger cytotoxic alterations and genetic instability in sensitive tissues and organs [28]. Dentoalveolar cone-beam-computed tomography (CBCT) has been advocated as a superior radiologic method but is potentially linked to higher radiation doses of 11–674 µSv [25,29].

The three-dimensional depiction of defects might offer additional information. This could be particularly beneficial in the detection of small defects or the planning of invasive procedures. Nevertheless, it has to be considered that titanium implants cause extensive metal artifacts. The depiction of the implant is increased in size by 12–15%, and consequently, the buccal bone is clearly visible and reduced by about 0.3 mm, which makes the dentist's assessment with respect to implant-bone density and thickness massively difficult [30,31]. This is probably the main difference in imaging defects around implants compared to defects around natural teeth. Therefore, CBCT should not be used routinely to assess peri-implant bone defects [32].

In summary, two-dimensional imaging (e.g., periapical or panoramic radiography in cases with multiple implants) should be the first selection criterion for the assessment and monitoring of bone levels around the implant following its placement and osseointegration [33].

Many factors can influence the peri-implant bone level. The most common cause of crestal bone loss is peri-implantitis. The definition of this infection-related inflammatory disease was not uniform until the World Workshop on the Classification of Periodontal and Peri-implant Diseases and Conditions, which took place in Chicago (USA) in November 2017. The World Workshop was co-sponsored by the American Academy of Periodontology (AAP) and the European Federation of Periodontology (EFP) [34].

Since then, peri-implantitis has been defined by the following triad:

- Bleeding and/or suppuration on gentle probing;
- Increased probing depth compared to previous examinations;
- Bone loss.

If no baseline information is available, the following findings may indicate peri-implantitis:

- Bleeding and/or suppuration on gentle probing;
- Probing depths of ≥ 6 mm;
- Bone level ≥ 3 mm apical to the most coronal section of the intraosseous implant portion.

But even before this classification, all definitions included, in varying degrees, the loss of the alveolar jawbone. In the case of manifest peri-implantitis, the intraoral radiograph is used, among other things, not only to diagnose the disease but also to assess the further course or the success of the therapy. It is recommended to perform a baseline radiograph at the timepoint of installation of the prosthetic component as an initial reference to which further images are compared in follow-up [35].

Other possible factors influencing the peri-implant crestal bone level are mechanical stress, especially in the case of occlusal miscontact or bruxism, or inflammatory stimuli due to the materials used or the nature of the implant-abutment connection [36–38].

The therapeutic protocol, such as the time of implantation, the healing time, and the healing conditions, may also have an impact [14,36]. These factors are scientifically investigated in controlled clinical studies. In these studies, the intraoral right-angle radiograph is often used as a diagnostic method, and ready-made image holders might have been used. The results are mostly in the millimeter, not infrequently even in the submillimeter range [8,39].

A recent study demonstrated high inter-observer consistency in bitewing images of high quality [40]. The high spatial resolution and low radiation dose are ideal for the necessary repeated recordings over many months and years. Furthermore, the quality of cross-sectional imaging is substantially limited around dental implants due to metal-related extinction or beam-hardening artefacts. For this reason and also due to lower spatial resolution and higher radiation dose, cross-sectional cone-beam-computed tomography is not routinely used to examine the peri-implant bone. On the other hand, the superiority of CBCT in the assessment of peri-implant bone defects was demonstrated in a dog study [41]. Especially vestibular dehiscences could not be visualized on the intraoral radiographs.

Intraoral radiographs are summation images with the typical associated shortcomings: The superimposition of all objects between the radiation source and the image receptor, since the beam of rays spreads out in a cone shape, the magnified depiction of the imaged object, and the image distortion, or unequal magnification in spots, owing to the oblique position of the object. The extent of magnification is directly connected with the position of the image receptor and its distance to the radiation source, or with the ratio of the film-focus distance to the focus-object distance. This aspect was not particularly addressed in the experimental setting of the presented study because the film focus distance was a fixed value. In the oral cavity, the possible causes of a tilted object or film position as a cause of distortion are varied. In the maxilla, a strong inclination of the palate and/or a low palate, and in the mandible, interference with the floor of the mouth may force the image receptor out of its ideal position [1].

Furthermore, uncertainties in the determination of the crestal reference point for length measurements might cause measurement errors. The depiction of the crestal level of the peri-implant bone could be ambiguous due to the superimposition of bone images corresponding to the crest on the buccal and the lingual sides that may not coincide.

Consequently, the correct recognition of the reference points at the interface between the alveolar bone and the implant might be difficult [1].

In order to at least minimize the importance of these influencing factors, identical recording conditions are crucial to ensuring that the images are comparable. Commercially available image receptor holders are intended to ensure these reproducible conditions. The radiographic film or sensor is rigidly fixed in these holders, thereby achieving a constant right angle to the central beam of the radiation source if the X-ray tube is positioned correctly on the holder. In addition, the holder has a bite block that is used to position it in relation to the depicted object. When the patient bites down on the block, the sensor should align itself parallel to this object, usually a tooth or an implant.

The key problem is that the final bite position of each individual patient is not exactly determined by the design of such holders. Deviations in the contact surface or twisting or tilting of the holder are easily possible in the daily routine and may be different each time. For example, anatomic obstacles such as the tongue or the hard palate may prevent the holder from aligning itself perpendicular to the object. This intended position is also not reached if the patient does not close the mouth completely, for example, due to pain or gagging. If the contact area is small and the position of the bite block is therefore unstable, the risk of tilting is even greater.

About 20–30 years ago, the distortion of intraoral radiographs showing periodontal defects was a common topic in scientific papers [42–48]. Back then, in vivo comparison with measurements of defects during periodontal surgeries was the gold standard to examine the accuracy of measurements on intraoral radiographs [43]. The horizontal and vertical angulation differences of the central beam from the orthoradial projection and radiographic magnification were calculated, for example, by interpreting the depiction of the wires placed in known distances from the film holder [49,50]. It has to be considered that many factors may cause biases when interpreting in vivo measurements. Defects are irregularly shaped, and reference structures are not always clearly shown. The deflection of the central beam is not known but calculated. These factors add up to deviations that can additionally occur when interpreting the images.

The experimental setting of the presented study, with uniform defects of known length and fixed deflections of the central beam, ruled out some of these uncontrollable influences.

The results demonstrated that deviations in the tenth of a millimeter range can easily occur if the image holder is twisted or tilted, even under these idealized conditions. The limitations of this study are due to its experimental setting. Measurement errors might even be greater in real-life situations, where additional factors like the local anatomy might exert an additional influence. These factors might lead to inconsistencies in the technical parameters of the image acquisition, like the film-focus distance or even the more pronounced tilting of the image holder. Real-life peri-implant defects come in various configurations, and the identification of a reference point might be difficult [49]. Furthermore, deviations in the interpretation of the radiographs might occur. These aspects were not addressed in this study, which means that the magnitude of the measurement errors could be underestimated.

Therefore, results obtained with the use of pre-fabricated right-angle image holders to assess the peri-implant bone level have to be interpreted with caution. The lack of reproducibility of the measurement conditions is even more relevant than the deviation of the measurement compared to the actual defect size. As part of studies, the production of individually adapted image holders might assure identical alignment of the image receptor at each radiographic examination [51–54]. The bite block is individually adjusted using silicone or plastic materials.

However, there are a few points to consider when making such holders with individualized bite blocks.

Soft and flexible materials, such as silicone, may be more susceptible to incorrect positioning, especially if they are only supported on one side. These inaccuracies can mean that a better representation of the crestal bone level cannot be achieved with such holders [1].

Designing bite blocks with a larger support or that cross the dental arch might help increase the accuracy of the method. Sadek et al. demonstrated in a study comparing two images taken at three-month intervals in vivo that measurements using individual X-ray positioning stents provided more precise and reproducible images than those fabricated with conventional film holders [55].

5. Conclusions

The assessment of the peri-implant bone level with intraoral radiographs may be biased if ready-made image holders are used. Vertical tilting of the image holder may result in distortion of images in the tenths of a millimeter range. The use of individualized film holders may produce comparable results over a longer period of time and thus ensure comparability between implants in scientific studies on the influence of various biological or technical parameters on bone healing or the peri-implant bone level.

Author Contributions: Conceptualization, P.R. and K.W.; methodology, P.R. and K.W.; validation, P.R., K.W., and N.J.; formal analysis, P.R. and N.J.; investigation, P.R. and K.W.; resources, N.J.; data curation, P.R. and K.W.; writing—original draft preparation, P.R.; writing—review and editing, K.W.; visualization, P.R. and K.W.; supervision, N.J.; project administration, P.R. All authors have read and agreed to the published version of the manuscript.

Funding: This research received no external funding.

Institutional Review Board Statement: Not applicable.

Informed Consent Statement: Not applicable.

Data Availability Statement: The data that support the findings of this study are available from the corresponding author upon reasonable request.

Acknowledgments: Statistical evaluation by Irene Mischak, Medical University of Graz.

Conflicts of Interest: The authors declare no conflicts of interest.

References

1. Fernández-Formoso, N.; Rilo, B.; Mora, M.J.; Martínez-Silva, I.; Santana, U. A paralleling technique modification to deter- mine the bone crest level around dental implants. *Dento Maxillo Facial Radiol.* **2011**, *40*, 385–389. [CrossRef] [PubMed]
2. Naveau, A.; Shinmyouzu, K.; Moore, C.; Avivi-Arber, L.; Jokerst, J.; Koka, S. Etiology and Measurement of Peri-Implant Crestal Bone Loss (CBL). *J. Clin. Med.* **2019**, *8*, 166. [CrossRef] [PubMed]
3. Derks, J.; Tomasi, C. Peri-implant health and disease. A systematic review of current epidemiology. *J. Clin. Periodontol.* **2015**, *42* (Suppl. S16), S158–S171. [CrossRef] [PubMed]
4. Lindhe, J.; Meyle, J.; Group D of the European Workshop on Periodontology. Peri-implant diseases: Consensus Report of the Sixth European Workshop on Periodontology. *J. Clin. Periodontol.* **2008**, *35* (Suppl. S8), 282–285. [CrossRef] [PubMed]

5. Berglundh, T.; Armitage, G.; Araujo, M.G.; Avila-Ortiz, G.; Blanco, J.; Camargo, P.M.; Chen, S.; Cochran, D.; Derks, J.; Figuero, E.; et al. Peri-implant diseases and conditions: Consensus report of workgroup 4 of the 2017 World Workshop on the Classification of Periodontal and Peri-Implant Diseases and Conditions. *J. Clin. Periodontol.* **2018**, *45* (Suppl. S20), S286–S291. [CrossRef]
6. Schwarz, F.; Herten, M.; Sager, M.; Bieling, K.; Sculean, A.; Becker, J. Comparison of natu- rally occuring and ligature-induced peri- implantitis bone defects in humans and dogs. *Clin. Oral Implant. Res.* **2007**, *18*, 161–170. [CrossRef]
7. Gil, J.; Sandino, C.; Cerrolaza, M.; Pérez, R.; Herrero-Climent, M.; Rios-Carrasco, B.; Rios-Santos, J.V.; Brizuela, A. Influence of Bone-Level Dental Implants Placement and of Cortical Thickness on Osseointegration: In Silico and In Vivo Analyses. *J. Clin. Med.* **2022**, *11*, 1027. [CrossRef]
8. Kim, S.Y.; Dodson, T.B.; Do, D.T.; Wadhwa, G.; Chuang, S.K. Factors Associated With Crestal Bone Loss Following Dental Implant Placement in a Longitudinal Follow-up Study. *J. Oral Implantol.* **2015**, *41*, 579–585. [CrossRef]
9. Yadav, R.; Agrawal, K.K.; Rao, J.; Anwar, M.; Alvi, H.A.; Singh, K.; Himanshu, D. Crestal Bone Loss under Delayed Loading of Full Thickness Versus Flapless Surgically Placed Dental Implants in Controlled Type 2 Diabetic Patients: A Parallel Group Randomized Clinical Trial. *J. Prosthodont. Off. J. Am. Coll. Prosthodont.* **2018**, *27*, 611–617. [CrossRef]
10. Puisys, A.; Auzbikaviciute, V.; Vindasiute-Narbute, E.; Zukauskas, S.; Vaicekauskas, K.; Razukevicus, D. Crestal bone stability after flapless placement of sloped implants with immediate temporization in edentulous mandible. A prospective comparative clinical trial. *Clin. Exp. Dent. Res.* **2021**, *7*, 131–136. [CrossRef]
11. de Siqueira, R.A.C.; Savaget Gonçalves Junior, R.; Dos Santos, P.G.F.; de Mattias Sartori, I.A.; Wang, H.L.; Fontão, F.N.G.K. Effect of different implant placement depths on crestal bone levels and soft tissue behavior: A 5-year randomized clinical trial. *Clin. Oral Implant. Res.* **2020**, *31*, 282–293. [CrossRef] [PubMed]
12. Schulze, R.K.; d'Hoedt, B. Mathematical analysis of projection errors in "paralleling technique" with respect to implant geometry. *Clin. Oral Implant. Res.* **2001**, *12*, 364–371. [CrossRef] [PubMed]
13. Van Steenberghe, D.; Quirynen, M. Reproducibility and detection threshold of peri-implant diagnostics. *Adv. Dent. Res.* **1993**, *7*, 191–195. [CrossRef]
14. Pardal-Peláez, B.; Flores-Fraile, J.; Pardal-Refoyo, J.L.; Montero, J. Implant loss and crestal bone loss in early loading versus delayed and immediate loading in edentulous mandibles. A systematic review and meta-analysis. *J. Clin. Exp. Dent.* **2021**, *13*, e397–e405. [CrossRef] [PubMed]
15. Preus, H.R.; Torgersen, G.R.; Koldsland, O.C.; Hansen, B.F.; Aass, A.M.; Larheim, T.A.; Sandvik, L. A new digital tool for radiographic bone level measurements in longitudinal studies. *BMC Oral Health* **2015**, *15*, 107. [CrossRef]
16. Costa, J.A.; Mendes, J.M.; Salazar, F.; Pacheco, J.J.; Rompante, P.; Câmara, M.I. Analysis of peri-implant bone defects by using cone beam computed tomography (CBCT): An integrative review. *Oral Radiol.* **2023**, *39*, 455–466. [CrossRef]
17. Jacobs, R.; Vranckx, M.; Vanderstuyft, T.; Quirynen, M.; Salmon, B. CBCT vs other imaging modalities to assess peri-implant bone and diagnose complications: A systematic review. *Eur. J. Oral Implantol.* **2018**, *11* (Suppl. S1), 77–92.
18. Ritter, L.; Elger, M.C.; Rothamel, D.; Fienitz, T.; Zinser, M.; Schwarz, F.; Zöller, J.E. Accuracy of peri-implant bone evaluation using cone beam CT, digital intra-oral radiographs and histology. *Dento Maxillo Facial Radiol.* **2014**, *43*, 20130088. [CrossRef]
19. Steiger-Ronay, V.; Krcmaric, Z.; Schmidlin, P.R.; Sahrmann, P.; Wiedemeier, D.B.; Benic, G.I. Assessment of peri-implant defects at titanium and zirconium dioxide implants by means of periapical radiographs and cone beam computed tomography: An in-vitro examination. *Clin. Oral Implant. Res.* **2018**, *29*, 1195–1201. [CrossRef]
20. Kühl, S.; Zürcher, S.; Zitzmann, N.U.; Filippi, A.; Payer, M.; Dagassan-Berndt, D. Detection of peri-implant bone defects with different radiographic techniques-a human cadaver study. *Clin. Oral Implant. Res.* **2016**, *27*, 529–534. [CrossRef] [PubMed]
21. Renvert, S.; Giovannoli, J.L. Diagnostik. In *Periimplantitis*, 1st ed.; Renvert, S., Giovannoli, J.L., Eds.; Quintessenz: Berlin, Germany, 2012; Volume 1.
22. De Bruyn, H.; Vandeweghe, S.; Ruyffelaert, C.; Cosyn, J.; Sennerby, L. Radiographic evaluation of modern oral implants with emphasis on crestal bone level and relevance to peri-implant health. *Periodontology 2000* **2013**, *62*, 256–270. [CrossRef] [PubMed]
23. Salvi, G.E.; Lang, N.P. Diagnostic parameters for monitoring peri-implant conditions. *Int. J. Oral Maxillofac. Implant.* **2004**, *19*, 116–127.
24. Devlin, H.; Yuan, J. Object position and image magnification in dental panoramic radiography: A theoretical analysis. *Dentomaxillo-Facial Radiol.* **2013**, *42*, 29951683. [CrossRef]
25. Harris, D.; Horner, K.; Gröndahl, K.; Jacobs, R.; Helmrot, E.; Benic, G.I.; Bornstein, M.M.; Dawood, A.; Quirynen, M.E.A.O. Guidelines for the use of diagnostic imaging in implant dentistry 2011. A consensus workshop organized by the European Association for Osseointegration at the Medical University of Warsaw. *Clin. Oral Implant. Res.* **2012**, *23*, 1243–1253. [CrossRef] [PubMed]
26. Horner, K.; Shelley, A.M. Preoperative radiological evaluation of missing single teeth: A review. *Eur. J. Oral Implantol.* **2016**, *9* (Suppl. S1), S69–S88.
27. Ludlow, J.B.; Davies-Ludlow, L.E.; White, S.C. Patient risk related to common dental radiographic examinations: The impact of 2007 International Commission on Radiological Protection recommendations regarding dose calculation. *J. Am. Dent. Assoc.* **2008**, *139*, 1237–1243. [CrossRef]

28. Shetty, A.; Almeida, F.T.; Ganatra, S.; Senior, A.; Pacheco-Pereira, C. Evidence on radiation dose reduction using rectangular collimation: A systematic review. *Int. Dent. J.* **2019**, *69*, 84–97. [CrossRef]
29. European Commission, Directorate-General for Energy. Cone Beam CT for Dental and Maxillofacial Radiology: Evidence-Based Guidelines, Publications Office. 2012. Available online: https://op.europa.eu/en/publication-detail/-/publication/ec5936c7-5 a29-4a93-9b3a-01a5d78d7b2e (accessed on 1 November 2023).
30. Benic, G.I.; Sancho-Puchades, M.S.; Jung, R.E.; Deyhle, H.; Hämmerle, C.H.F. In vitro assessment of artifacts induced by titanium dental implants in cone beam computed tomography. *Clin. Oral Implant. Res.* **2013**, *24*, 378–383. [CrossRef]
31. Schulze, R.K.; Berndt, D.; d'Hoedt, B. On cone-beam computed tomography artifacts induced by titanium implants. *Clin. Oral Implant. Res.* **2010**, *21*, 100–107. [CrossRef]
32. Lee, C.; Lee, S.S.; Kim, J.E.; Symkhampha, K.; Lee, W.J.; Huh, K.H.; Yi, W.J.; Heo, M.S.; Choi, S.C.; Yeom, H.Y. A dose monitoring system for dental radiography. *Imaging Sci. Dent.* **2016**, *46*, 103–108. [CrossRef]
33. Kim, M.J.; Lee, S.S.; Choi, M.; Yong, H.S.; Lee, C.; Kim, J.E.; Heo, M.S. Developing evidence-based clinical imaging guidelines of justification for radiographic examination after dental implant installation. *BMC Med. Imaging* **2020**, *20*, 102. [CrossRef] [PubMed]
34. Caton, J.G.; Armitage, G.; Berglundh, T.; Chapple, I.L.C.; Jepsen, S.; Kornman, K.S.; Mealey, B.L.; Papapanou, P.N.; Sanz, M.; Tonetti, M.S. A new classification scheme for periodontal and peri-implant diseases and conditions-Introduction and key changes from the 1999 classification. *J. Clin. Periodontol.* **2018**, *45* (Suppl. S20), S1–S8. [CrossRef] [PubMed]
35. Ramanauskaite, A.; Juodzbalys, G. Diagnostic Principles of Peri-Implantitis: A Systematic Review and Guidelines for Peri-Implantitis Diagnosis Proposal. *J. Oral Maxillofac. Res.* **2016**, *7*, e8. [CrossRef] [PubMed]
36. Artzi, Z.; Shlafstein, R. Monitoring crestal bone level of single- and two-stage implant placement modes up to final prosthetic delivery: An observational study. *Quintessence Int.* **2021**, *52*, 236–246. [CrossRef]
37. Sasada, Y.; Cochran, D.L. Implant-Abutment Connections: A Review of Biologic Consequences and Peri-implantitis Implications. *Int. J. Oral Maxillofac. Implant.* **2017**, *32*, 1296–1307. [CrossRef]
38. Schwarz, F.; Hegewald, A.; Becker, J. Impact of implant-abutment connection and positioning of the machined collar/microgap on crestal bone level changes: A systematic review. *Clin. Oral Implant. Res.* **2014**, *25*, 417–425. [CrossRef]
39. Urdaneta, R.A.; Daher, S.; Lery, J.; Emanuel, K.; Chuang, S.K. Factors associated with crestal bone gain on single-tooth locking-taper implants: The effect of nonsteroidal anti-inflammatory drugs. *Int. J. Oral Maxillofac. Implant.* **2011**, *26*, 1063–1078.
40. Hellén-Halme, K.; Lith, A.; Shi, X.Q. Reliability of marginal bone level measurements on digital panoramic and digital intraoral radiographs. *Oral Radiol.* **2020**, *36*, 135–140. [CrossRef]
41. Song, D.; Shujaat, S.; de Faria Vasconcelos, K.; Huang, Y.; Politis, C.; Lambrichts, I.; Jacobs, R. Diagnostic accuracy of CBCT versus intraoral imaging for assessment of peri-implant bone defects. *BMC Med. Imaging* **2021**, *21*, 23. [CrossRef]
42. Eickholz, P.; Kim, T.S.; Benn, D.K.; Staehle, H.J. Validity of radiographic measurement of interproximal bone loss. *Oral Surg. Oral Med. Oral Pathol. Oral Radiol. Endod.* **1998**, *85*, 99–106. [CrossRef]
43. Eickholz, P.; Hausmann, E. Accuracy of radiographic assessment of interproximal bone loss in intrabony defects using linear measurements. *Eur. J. Oral Sci.* **2000**, *108*, 70–73. [CrossRef] [PubMed]
44. Hämmerle, C.H.; Ingold, H.P.; Lang, N.P. Evaluation of clinical and radiographic scoring methods before and after initial periodontal therapy. *J. Clin. Periodontol.* **1990**, *17*, 255–263. [CrossRef]
45. Hou, G.L.; Lin, C.H.; Hung, C.C.; Yang, Y.S.; Shieh, T.Y.; Lin, I.C.; Tsai, C.C. The consistency and reliability of periodontal bone level measurements using digital scanning radiographic image analysis--a pilot study. *Kaohsiung J. Med. Sci.* **2000**, *16*, 566–573.
46. Shrout, M.K.; Hildebolt, C.F.; Vannier, M.W. Alignment errors in bitewing radiographs using uncoupled positioning devices. *Dento Maxillo Facial Radiol.* **1993**, *22*, 33–37. [CrossRef] [PubMed]
47. Potter, B.J.; Shrout, M.K.; Harrell, J.C. Reproducibility of beam alignment using different bite-wing radiographic techniques. *Oral Surg. Oral Med. Oral Pathol. Oral Radiol. Endod.* **1995**, *79*, 532–535. [CrossRef] [PubMed]
48. Janssen, P.T.; van Palenstein Helderman, W.H.; van Aken, J. The effect of in-vivo-occurring errors in the reproducibility of radiographs on the use of the subtraction technique. *J. Clin. Periodontol.* **1989**, *16*, 53–58. [CrossRef] [PubMed]
49. Schulz, A.; Müller, H.P.; Topoll, H.H.; Lange, D.E. Abweichungen des Zentralstrahls bei standardisierten Bissflügelaufnahmen [Deviations of the central ray in standardized bite-wing radiographs]. *Dtsch. Zahnärztliche Z.* **1991**, *46*, 505–508.
50. Kim, T.S.; Benn, D.K.; Eickholz, P. Accuracy of computer-assisted radiographic measurement of interproximal bone loss in vertical bone defects. *Oral Surg. Oral Med. Oral Pathol. Oral Radiol. Endod.* **2002**, *94*, 379–387. [CrossRef]
51. Linkevicius, T.; Puisys, A.; Linkevicius, R.; Alkimavicius, J.; Gineviciute, E.; Linkeviciene, L. The influence of submerged healing abutment or subcrestal implant placement on soft tissue thickness and crestal bone stability. A 2-year randomized clinical trial. *Clin. Implant. Dent. Relat. Res.* **2020**, *22*, 497–506. [CrossRef]
52. Glibert, M.; Vervaeke, S.; Jacquet, W.; Vermeersch, K.; Östman, P.O.; De Bruyn, H. A randomized controlled clinical trial to assess crestal bone remodeling of four different implant designs. *Clin. Implant Dent. Relat. Res.* **2018**, *20*, 455–462. [CrossRef] [PubMed]
53. van Eekeren, P.; Tahmaseb, A.; Wismeijer, D. Crestal bone changes in macrogeometrically similar implants with the implant-abutment connection at the crestal bone level or 2.5 mm above: A prospective randomized clinical trial. *Clin. Oral Implant. Res.* **2016**, *27*, 1479–1484. [CrossRef] [PubMed]

54. Sugita, R.; Jones, A.A.; Kotsakis, G.A.; Cochran, D.L. Radiographic evaluation of a novel bone adhesive for maintenance of crestal bone around implants in canine oversized osteotomies. *J. Periodontol.* **2022**, *93*, 924–932. [CrossRef] [PubMed]
55. Sadek, S.A.; Abbas, H.M.; Alfelali, M.; Almahdali, A. Using acrylic customized X-ray positioning stents for long-term follow-up studies. *Saudi Dent. J.* **2020**, *32*, 120–128. [CrossRef] [PubMed]

Disclaimer/Publisher's Note: The statements, opinions and data contained in all publications are solely those of the individual author(s) and contributor(s) and not of MDPI and/or the editor(s). MDPI and/or the editor(s) disclaim responsibility for any injury to people or property resulting from any ideas, methods, instructions or products referred to in the content.

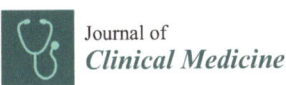

Article

The Diagnostic Value of CEUS in Assessing Non-Ossified Thyroid Cartilage Invasion in Patients with Laryngeal Squamous Cell Carcinoma

Milda Pucėtaitė [1,*], Davide Farina [2], Silvija Ryškienė [1], Dalia Mitraitė [1], Rytis Tarasevičius [3], Saulius Lukoševičius [1], Evaldas Padervinskis [4] and Saulius Vaitkus [4]

[1] Department of Radiology, Medical Academy, Lithuanian University of Health Sciences, A. Mickevičiaus Str. 9, 44307 Kaunas, Lithuania; silvija.ryskiene@lsmu.lt (S.R.); dalia.mitraite@lsmu.lt (D.M.)
[2] Department of Radiological Sciences, University of Brescia, Piazzale Spedali Civili 1, 25123 Brescia, Italy; davide.farina@unibs.it
[3] Department of Radiology, Lithuanian University of Health Sciences Kaunas Clinics, Eivenių 2, 50009 Kaunas, Lithuania
[4] Department of Otorhinolaryngology, Medical Academy, Lithuanian University of Health Sciences, A. Mickevičiaus Str. 9, 44307 Kaunas, Lithuania; evaldas.padervinskis@lsmu.lt (E.P.); saulius.vaitkus@lsmu.lt (S.V.)
* Correspondence: milda.pucetaite@lsmu.lt

Abstract: Background: Accurate assessment of thyroid cartilage invasion in squamous cell carcinoma (SCC) of the larynx remains a challenge in clinical practice. The aim of this study was to assess the diagnostic performance of contrast-enhanced ultrasound (CEUS), contrast-enhanced computed tomography (CECT), and magnetic resonance imaging (MRI) in the detection of non-ossified thyroid cartilage invasion in patients with SCC. **Methods:** CEUS, CECT, and MRI scans of 27 male patients with histologically proven SCC were evaluated and compared. A total of 31 cases were assessed via CEUS and CECT. The MR images of five patients and six cases were excluded (one patient had two suspected sites), leaving twenty-five cases for analysis via MRI. **Results:** CEUS showed the highest accuracy and specificity compared with CECT and MRI (87.1% vs. 64.5% and 76.0% as well as 84.0% vs. 64.0% and 72.7%, respectively). The sensitivity and negative predictive value of CEUS and MRI were the same (100%). CEUS yielded four false-positive findings. However, there were no statistically significant differences among the imaging modalities ($p > 0.05$). **Conclusions:** CEUS showed better diagnostic performance than CECT and MRI. Therefore, CEUS has the potential to accurately assess non-ossified thyroid cartilage invasion and guide appropriate treatment decisions, hopefully leading to improved patient outcomes.

Keywords: non-ossified thyroid cartilage; CEUS; CECT; MRI; laryngeal cancer

1. Introduction

Imaging of the local spread of laryngeal cancer plays an important role in choosing a suitable treatment strategy, such as organ-sparing therapy, radical surgery, or combined therapy. The decision regarding which treatment strategy to employ affects the effectiveness of treatment and quality of life [1–3]. The role of imaging is more crucial in discriminating between T3 and T4 stages than between T1 and T2 stages according to the tumor-node-metastasis (TNM) classification. As reported in the review by Deganello et al. [4], patients with T4 stage tumors have a higher risk of developing lymph node metastases, which also affects both prognosis and treatment planning. Therefore, radiologists often face great challenges in evaluating subtle findings.

Both contrast-enhanced computed tomography (CECT) and magnetic resonance imaging (MRI) are the main and most widely used modalities for laryngeal imaging; most

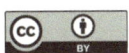

guidelines leave the choice between the two techniques up to local protocols and scanner availability. In CECT, one of the most controversial issues in the assessment of the tumor invasion of non-ossified thyroid cartilage is a similar post-contrast density of the tumor and the non-ossified thyroid cartilage [5]. In these cases, dual-energy computed tomography (DECT) or MRI may provide added value. In particular, the study published by Becker et al. [6] demonstrated that the application of revised MRI criteria led to an overall statistically significant improvement in the assessment of thyroid cartilage invasion. However, none of the cross-sectional techniques outperform the others on the specific issue of non-ossified thyroid cartilage [5–10].

Contrast-enhanced ultrasound (CEUS) can be used to assess and quantify microcirculation in normal and pathological conditions with a good acoustic window [11]. Moreover, it has been widely used in clinical practice to diagnose hepatic and renal pathologies [12,13]. In a recent publication, CEUS showed potential in assessing non-ossified thyroid cartilage invasion [14]. Non-ossified thyroid cartilage and adjacent laryngeal cancer are well visualized on CEUS due to the differences between non-enhancing non-ossified thyroid cartilage and enhancing adjacent laryngeal cancer. Therefore, the detection of enhancement along the course of a thyroid lamina contacting a tumor suggests infiltration. However, there is currently a lack of studies and data that can strongly support the use of CEUS as an additional imaging modality in the diagnostic algorithms for determining the local spread of laryngeal cancer more accurately.

Therefore, the purpose of this study was to assess the diagnostic value of CEUS, compared with that of CECT and MRI, in the detection of non-ossified thyroid cartilage invasion in SCC of the larynx.

2. Materials and Methods

2.1. Patients

Between 2021 and 2023, a prospective comparative study was carried out at the Hospital of Lithuanian University of Health Sciences Kaunas Clinics. A total of 38 patients with histopathologically proven SCC of the larynx were enrolled in this study. The inclusion criteria were as follows: an available CECT scan demonstrating pathological infiltration adjacent to the non-ossified tract of the thyroid cartilage or its clear infiltration; no history of previous laryngeal–hypopharyngeal surgery or chemoradiation; and having undergone surgery planned after multidisciplinary team discussion. Eleven patients were excluded because they refused surgical treatment or did not attend further consultations or undergo further surgery.

All 27 male patients meeting the inclusion criteria were subjected to CEUS and MRI. Informed consent was obtained from all participants before the study. The study was conducted according to the guidelines of the Declaration of Helsinki. Ethical approval was obtained from Kaunas Regional Biomedical Research Ethics Committee (protocol No. 2021-BE-10-00016; dated 2021).

2.2. CECT Examination

Multislice CT examinations were performed using an Aquilion ONE TSX-301 scanner (Toshiba, Tokyo, Japan) with the following parameters: 120 kVp; specific effective mAs for each patient based on the patient's size and tissue thickness; collimation, 128 × 0.625 mm; field of view, 260 mm; and matrix, 512 × 512. The patients were asked to assume a supine position, breathe quietly, and avoid coughing and swallowing. The field of view was from the skull base to the aortic arch. Scanning was performed without and with intravenous contrast media (65–100 mL) with a 50 mL saline flush to obtain contrast-enhanced images with a 60–80 s delay after administration; the concentration of iodine in the contrast agent was 320–370 mg/mL. Images were reconstructed for axial (parallel to the plane of the true vocal cords), sagittal, and coronal (perpendicular to the plane of the true vocal cords) planes with soft tissue and bone algorithms (2 mm in thickness).

2.3. CEUS Examination

CEUS examination was performed using a Philips Epiq 7 (expert-class) US system (Philips Healthcare, Best, The Netherlands) with a 5–12-MHz linear transducer. The patients were asked to assume the supine position with their necks extended. The larynx and its surrounding structures were evaluated in the transverse and longitudinal sections. The distance between the area of lesion contact to the non-ossified thyroid cartilage seen via CECT and the upper border of the thyroid lamina was measured via CECT and then used as a reference to target the same area through CEUS.

CEUS examination was performed by administering an intravenous bolus of SonoVue (Bracco SpA, Milan, Italy) (5 mL, followed by saline flush) [14]. The scan was performed with a frequency of 12 MHz and a mechanical index of 0.8. The patients were asked to refrain from swallowing and coughing during the examination. Dynamic perfusion of the tumor and peritumoral tissues was observed and recorded in the hard drive of the device for about 1 min. If there was more than one suspected site of invasion, the CEUS procedure was repeated after 10 min.

2.4. MRI Examination

MRI examination was performed using a Philips Ingenia 3.0T scanner (Philips Healthcare, Best, The Netherlands) with dedicated head–neck 20-channel parallel imaging array coils. The patients were imaged in the supine position and asked to breathe quietly and refrain from swallowing and coughing during the scanning. Axial images were captured parallel to the plane of the true vocal cords; coronal images were obtained perpendicular to this plane. The MRI protocol employed is specified in Table 1.

Table 1. MRI protocol.

Sequence	Plane	Slice Thickness, mm	Repetition Time, ms	Time to Echo, ms	Field of View, mm
High-resolution T2-weighted turbo spin echo Dixon	Axial, coronal, sagittal	2.5–3	2888	80	190–210
High-resolution T1-weighted turbo spin echo Dixon	Axial	2.1–2.5	634	8	190–210
DWI and ADC	Axial	2	14,439; 220	66	250
Contrast-enhanced high-resolution T1-weighted turbo spin echo Dixon	Axial, coronal	2.1–2.5	634	8	190–210

DWI, diffusion-weighted imaging; ADC, apparent diffusion coefficient.

2.5. Image Analysis

The analysis of CEUS images was performed by two radiologists with >4 and >20 years of experience, respectively. The findings from the CECT and MRI examinations were interpreted by one head-and-neck radiologist with >20 years of experience in head-and-neck imaging. The radiologists were not blinded to the clinical and CECT information during the analysis of CEUS and MRI images.

2.5.1. CEUS Imaging

CEUS images were evaluated and interpreted by both radiologists during examination and post-processing. The non-ossified thyroid cartilage was considered infiltrated by a tumor when contrast enhancement was observed (Figure 1). When the cases were evaluated, there was no disagreement between the radiologists.

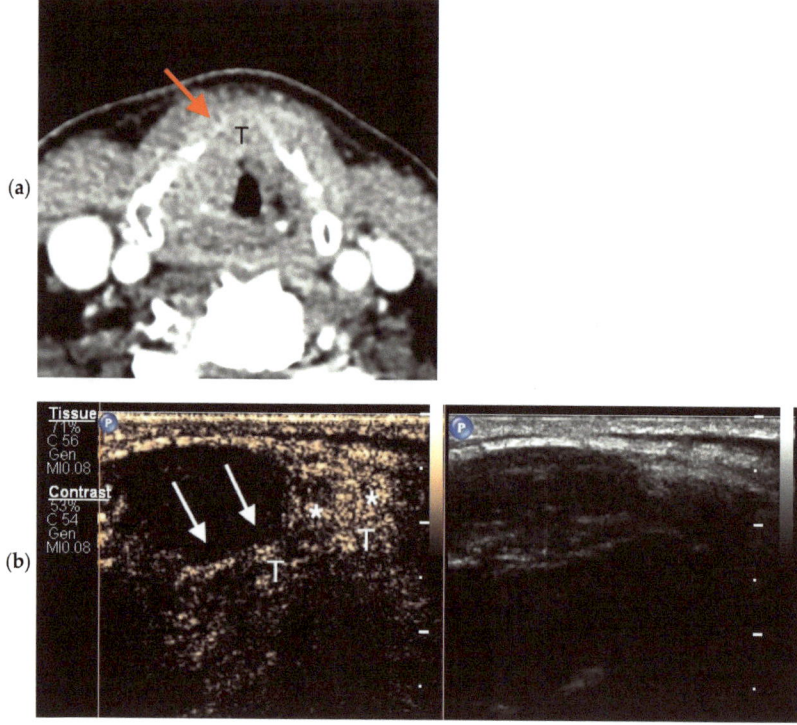

Figure 1. True-positive findings through axial CECT and CEUS. (**a**) In this CECT image, a partial bilateral ossification of the thyroid cartilage with a similar tissue density between the tumor (T) and the non-ossified thyroid cartilage (red arrow) can be seen; (**b**) CEUS image taken after intravenous contrast material administration showing the enhancement of the tumor (T) with invasion of the right anterior part of the non-ossified thyroid cartilage (asterisks); the adjacent hypoechogenic cartilage is non-invaded (white arrows).

2.5.2. Cross-Sectional Imaging

CECT and MRI images were evaluated and interpreted according to previous articles [6,7,9,15].

In CECT images, non-ossified thyroid cartilage invasion was positive when the following criteria were met: a focal cartilage defect in close proximity to the tumor was found; replacement of the cartilage by soft tissue with enhancement matching that adjacent to the cartilage occurred; and the lesion was in direct contact with the thyroid cartilage and densities were indistinguishable (Figure 2). Findings obtained via CECT were considered negative if the densities between the tumor/pathologic infiltration and the non-ossified cartilage were distinguishable.

When conducting MRI, thyroid cartilage invasion was diagnosed when the thyroid lamina showed abnormal signal intensity matching the signal of the tumor in T2-weighted image (T2WI), T1-weighted image (T1WI) (before and after contrast administration), DWI, and ADC map (Figure 3). When the thyroid lamina showed a T2WI signal, enhancement, and an ADC value higher than those of the tumor, the abnormal signal was classified as inflammation.

2.6. Histologic Examination

A pathologist with >20 years of experience evaluated the surgical specimens according to the existing guidelines described elsewhere [16]. To ensure precise correspondence between radiological findings and pathology, the suspected area of invasion was indicated by radiologists on an anatomical sketch of the larynx that accompanied each specimen.

2.7. Statistical Analysis

The IBM SPSS Statistics 20.0 (IBM Corp. in Armonk, NY, USA) statistical software package was used in this study. Sensitivity, specificity, accuracy, negative predictive value (NPV), and positive predictive value (PPV) of CEUS, CECT, and MRI in evaluating non-ossified laryngeal cartilage involvement were assessed by comparing results with histopathological findings [17,18]. Accuracy was calculated according to the following formula:

$$\text{Accuracy} = \frac{TP + TN}{TP + TN + FP + FN}$$

where TP is true positive; TN denotes true negative; FP denotes false positive; and FN denotes false negative.

McNemar's test was used to compare the accuracy of imaging modalities. A p value of <0.05 was considered statistically significant.

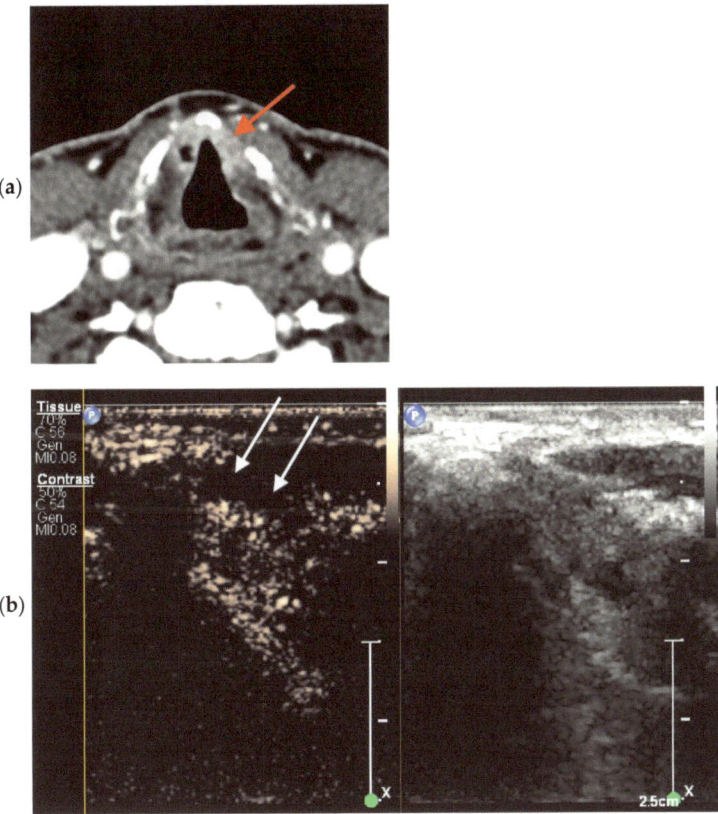

Figure 2. Bilateral glottic cancer adjacent to the non-ossified thyroid cartilage lamina. (**a**) Axial CECT findings on the left side were false-positive for tumor invasion (red arrow). (**b**) CEUS image of the left side at the same level as (**a**) in the transverse plane shows true-negative findings, i.e., non-enhanced non-ossified cartilage (white arrows).

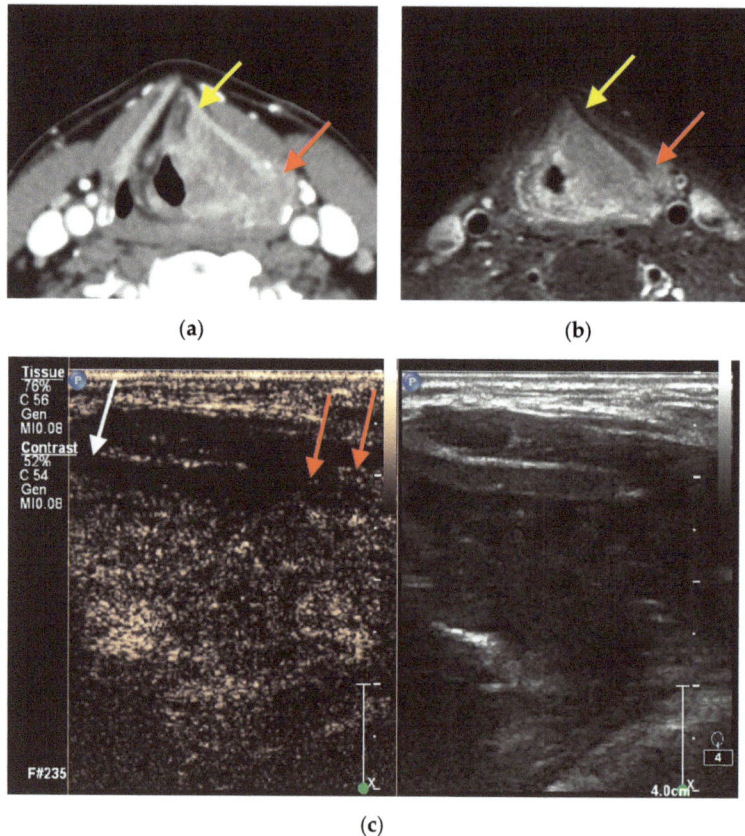

Figure 3. Supraglottic squamous cell carcinoma on the left side. (**a**) Axial CECT represents two sites, namely, sites that were false-positive anteriorly (yellow arrow) and true-positive posteriorly (red arrow), whereas MRI (**b**) contrast-enhanced high-resolution T1-weighted turbo spin echo Dixon and CEUS (**c**) findings were true-negative anteriorly (white arrow) and true-positive posteriorly (red arrows), respectively.

3. Results

In this prospective study, 27 male patients with a mean age of 63 years (SD, 8.7; range, 46–84 years) were enrolled.

Overall, there were 31 cases, as four patients had two suspected sites of non-ossified thyroid cartilage invasion. All 31 cases were assessed using CEUS and CECT. The MR images of five patients (corresponding to 6 cases, as one patient had two suspected sites) were non-diagnostic due to major artifacts, leaving 25 cases for analysis via MRI.

There were 14 cases (51.9%) of glottic SCC and 13 cases (48.1%) of transglottic SCC with the majority showing a G2 degree of differentiation (85.2%). The patients' distribution by pT staging is shown in Table 2.

In six cases (19.4%), histological proof of non-ossified thyroid cartilage invasion was obtained. The diagnostic performance of imaging studies is shown in Table 3. There were no statistically significant differences among the modalities ($p > 0.05$). CEUS and MRI showed a NPV of 100%. CEUS had four false-positive findings (Figure 4); however, the PPV was higher than those of CECT and MRI (60% vs. 30.8% and 33.3%, respectively).

Table 2. Distribution of the patients according to pT staging.

pT Group	n (%)
pTis	1 (3.7)
pT1	7 (25.9)
pT2	7 (25.9)
pT3	8 (29.6)
pT4	4 (14.8)

Staging was performed according to the American Joint Committee on Cancer/Union for International Cancer Control (AJCC/UICC), 8th Edition, guidelines.

Table 3. Diagnostic performance of CEUS, CECT, and MRI in the assessment of non-ossified thyroid cartilage invasion.

Imaging Modality	TP, n	TN, n	FP, n	FN, n	Sensitivity, % (95% CI)	Specificity, % (95% CI)	Accuracy, % (95% CI)	PPV, %	NPV, %
CEUS (n = 31)	6	21	4	0	100.0 (54.1–100.0)	84.0 (63.2–95.5)	87.1 (70.2–96.4)	60.0	100.0
CECT (n = 31)	4	16	9	2	66.7 (22.3–95.7)	64.0 (42.5–82.0)	64.5 (45.4–80.8)	30.8	88.9
MRI (n = 25)	3	16	6	0	100.0 (29.2–100.0)	72.7 (49.8–89.3)	76.0 (54.9–90.6)	33.3	100.0

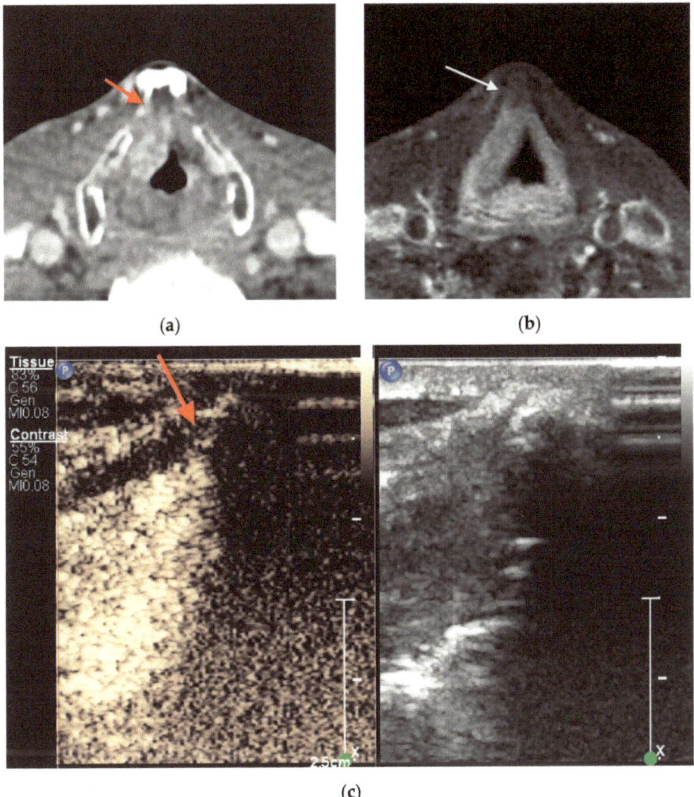

Figure 4. Supraglottic squamous cell carcinoma on the right side anteriorly adjacent to non-ossified cartilage inner lamina. (**a**) Axial CECT and (**c**) CEUS findings were false positive (red arrow) for tumor invasion of the thyroid cartilage, whereas MRI findings, as shown in (**b**), in axial contrast-enhanced high-resolution T1-weighted turbo spin echo Dixon images were true negative (white arrow).

There were no statistically significant differences between these imaging modalities ($p > 0.05$). CEUS, contrast-enhanced ultrasound; CECT, contrast-enhanced computed tomography; MRI, magnetic resonance imaging; TP, true positive; TN, true negative; FP, false positive; FN, false negative; PPV, positive predictive value; NPV, negative predictive value.

4. Discussion

In the current study, we aimed at evaluating the diagnostic performance of CEUS, CECT, and MRI in detecting non-ossified thyroid cartilage tumor invasion, taking postoperative histopathological examination as the gold standard. Our results show that based on the presence of enhancement, CEUS allows for the discrimination of invaded (i.e., enhancing) from normal (i.e., non-enhancing) non-ossified thyroid cartilage. CEUS, CECT, and MRI evaluation demonstrated high accuracy (87.1%, 64.5%, and 76%, respectively) with minor differences. Moreover, CEUS was slightly superior to other modalities employed in this study in detecting non-ossified thyroid cartilage tumor invasion.

The detection of laryngeal cartilage invasion can significantly influence the choice of optimal treatment strategy and the prognosis of SCC of the larynx. Currently, the choice of optimal treatment strategy is controversial. However, in the case of thyroid cartilage invasion or its suspicion, transoral laryngeal microsurgery (TOLMS) should be ruled out due to possible non-radical tumor removal, and in such cases, open partial horizontal laryngectomy (OPHL), total laryngectomy, or non-surgical treatments should be considered [2,3,19–21]. In addition, deep tumor invasion into the thyroid cartilage leads to negative outcomes through treatment with radiation therapy [21]. Therefore, for the selection of an optimal treatment plan avoiding complications and incomplete resection as well as improving disease control and survival, an accurate clinical and radiological assessment of local spread, especially the most controversial invasion of the cartilage, is necessary.

Cross-sectional imaging with multi-slice CT or MRI is designed to map deep tumor spread to the submucosal soft tissues and cartilaginous framework. CECT examination can be quickly performed, is widely available, and allows volumetric acquisition with a submillimetric voxel size: the short acquisition time minimizes the risk of motion artifacts, while the high spatial resolution allows the detection of subtle areas of tumor invasion of soft tissue spaces and cartilage [9,22,23].

MRI has higher contrast resolution, which is boosted by the possibility of combining different pulse sequences. In the literature, this potential has mainly been exploited to assess cartilage invasion [6,24], and MRI is reported to have significantly higher sensitivity than CECT for cartilage invasion [22]. A recent meta-analysis of studies involving patients with laryngo–hypopharyngeal cancer reported pooled sensitivities of 88% for MRI and 66% for CT, with specificities of 81% and 90%, respectively, in the detection of cartilage invasion [22]. Expectedly, CT's performance was more heterogeneous than that of MRI, as it differed when taking into account which type of cartilage was involved: when only thyroid cartilage was analyzed, the sensitivity was 69%, which was close to that in our study (66%), but the specificity was higher (86% vs. 64%). Based on the results of the above-mentioned meta-analysis and our current study, we can assume that the diagnosis of thyroid cartilage invasion poses significant challenges that are better handled by MRI than CT.

However, most studies evaluating the diagnostic performance of imaging techniques in the detection of cartilage invasion tend to focus—intentionally or unintentionally—on the ossified cartilage. This occurs for several reasons: first, because, in most cases, invasion involves the ossified parts, and second, because CT and MRI better visualize the invasion of ossified cartilage, manifesting with a panel of findings including sclerosis, erosion, or destruction with cartilage replacement by tumor tissue [5]. This is mainly due to the lack of differences in density in CT images between the tumor and the non-ossified thyroid cartilage and because of the overlapping features of the tumor and non-neoplastic changes such as reactive inflammation, edema, and fibrosis in MRI images [22,24]. Peritumoral inflammation is another potential confounding factor at the interface between a tumor and cartilage, although the combination of different sequences may improve differentiation when conducting MRI.

DECT is another promising imaging modality that has been analyzed in recent years. One research group [25] used DECT to evaluate the spectral attenuation curves of tumor tissue and non-ossified thyroid cartilage. Virtual monochromatic images (VMIs) of different energy levels showed that tumor tissue density dropped in higher-kiloelectron-volt VMIs, while the non-ossified cartilage maintained high attenuation, allowing distinguishment between the two. However, this study did not directly evaluate non-ossified cartilage invasion by tumor tissue.

US was also previously investigated for its possible role in solving the problem of thyroid cartilage invasion. Indeed, US seemed to uniquely take a place among cross-sectional modalities for evaluating non-ossified cartilage invasion, as the larynx is a superficial structure, and because it best visualizes the non-ossified parts, which present the most diagnostic challenges when conducting CT and MRI scans [14,26,27]. One study involving 62 patients with laryngeal or hypopharyngeal cancer showed that US and CECT had sensitivities of 98% and 91%, respectively, and equal specificities of 75% [26]. The authors speculated that clear visualization of the fat plane between the tumor and the cartilage as well as independent movement of the thyroid cartilage and adjacent tumor tissues contributed to the higher sensitivity of US [26]. The results of the previously mentioned studies prompted the cited researchers to further analyze the possibilities of US examination by incorporating CEUS.

Our study aligns with the study by Hu et al. [14] in terms of showing a higher accuracy of CEUS than CECT (90% and 83%, respectively) in detecting thyroid cartilage invasion, even though there were the following relevant differences in the methodological part: In our study, the exact site of possible non-ossified thyroid cartilage invasion as indicated by CECT examination was further investigated using CEUS and MRI and postoperative histopathological examination. Moreover, the radiologist who carried out the CEUS and MRI examinations and the pathologist were not blinded to the CECT findings. To the best of our knowledge, this is the first study comparing CEUS, CECT, and MRI regarding the specific topic of non-ossified cartilage invasion. Although we did not observe statistically significant differences among the three imaging modalities ($p > 0.05$), based on the promising results, we suggest that CEUS may be considered a usable imaging modality complementary to CECT and MRI for the assessment of non-ossified thyroid cartilage in the non-infrequent event of equivocal CECT and/or MRI findings. One of the limitations of this study is its small sample size. A second limitation is that the CECT and MRI images were assessed by a single expert/observer. Moreover, in our practice, in some cases, matching the suspected site seen in CECT images to the site observed in CEUS images was difficult due to the small region of interest. In the future, this issue could be solved by fusing CECT with US, and this should be performed by a head-and-neck radiologist due to their comprehensive knowledge of laryngeal anatomy and CECT imaging. Moreover, only one region of interest can be investigated at a time; therefore, we reinjected a contrast agent for the evaluation of another site of tumor invasion, leading to the extended examination time.

5. Conclusions

CEUS showed slightly higher diagnostic values in the detection of non-ossified thyroid cartilage invasion in laryngeal and hypopharyngeal cancer than CECT and MRI. This may result in CEUS being an important problem-solving tool in routine clinical practice that can be used to confidently assess non-ossified thyroid cartilage invasion and guide appropriate treatment decisions, hopefully leading to improved patient outcomes. Further studies are needed to increase the number of observations and confirm the evidence obtained.

Author Contributions: Conceptualization M.P.; methodology, M.P., S.V. and S.R.; statistical analysis, R.T.; investigation, M.P., S.V., D.M., S.R. and E.P.; data curation, M.P. and R.T.; writing—original draft preparation, M.P.; writing—review and editing, D.F. and S.R.; visualization, M.P., S.R. and D.M.; supervision S.V.; consulting, D.F.; project administration, S.L. All authors have read and agreed to the published version of the manuscript.

Funding: This research received no external funding.

Institutional Review Board Statement: The current study was conducted according to the guidelines of the Declaration of Helsinki. Ethical approval was obtained from Kaunas Regional Biomedical Research Ethics Committee (protocol No. 2021-BE-10-00016; dated 2021).

Informed Consent Statement: Informed consent was obtained from all subjects involved in the study.

Data Availability Statement: The data that support the findings of this study are available from the corresponding author upon reasonable request. The data are not publicly available due to privacy or ethical restrictions.

Conflicts of Interest: The authors declare no conflicts of interest.

References

1. Shoushtari, S.T.; Gal, J.; Chamorey, E.; Schiappa, R.; Dassonville, O.; Poissonnet, G.; Aloi, D.; Barret, M.; Safta, I.; Saada, E.; et al. Salvage vs. Primary Total Laryngectomy in Patients with Locally Advanced Laryngeal or Hypopharyngeal Carcinoma: Oncologic Outcomes and Their Predictive Factors. *J. Clin. Med.* **2023**, *12*, 1305. [CrossRef]
2. Connor, S. Laryngeal cancer: How does the radiologist help? *Cancer Imaging* **2007**, *7*, 93–103. [CrossRef]
3. Hermans, R. Staging of laryngeal and hypopharyngeal cancer: Value of imaging studies. *Eur. Radiol.* **2006**, *16*, 2386–2400. [CrossRef]
4. Deganello, A.; Ruaro, A.; Gualtieri, T.; Berretti, G.; Rampinelli, V.; Borsetto, D.; Russo, S.; Boscolo-Rizzo, P.; Ferrari, M.; Bussu, F. Central Compartment Neck Dissection in Laryngeal and Hypopharyngeal Squamous Cell Carcinoma: Clinical Considerations. *Cancers* **2023**, *15*, 804. [CrossRef] [PubMed]
5. Dadfar, N.; Seyyedi, M.; Forghani, R.; Curtin, H.D. Computed Tomography Appearance of Normal Nonossified Thyroid Cartilage Implication for Tumor Invasion Diagnosis. *J. Comput. Assist. Tomogr.* **2015**, *39*, 240–243. [CrossRef] [PubMed]
6. Becker, M.; Zbären, P.; Casselman, J.W.; Kohler, R.; Dulguerov, P.; Becker, C.D. Neoplastic invasion of laryngeal cartilage: Reassessment of criteria for diagnosis at MR imaging. *Radiology* **2008**, *249*, 551–559. [CrossRef]
7. Becker, M.; Burkhardt, K.; Dulguerov, P.; Allal, A. Imaging of the larynx and hypopharynx. *Eur. J. Radiol.* **2008**, *66*, 460–479. [CrossRef]
8. Dankbaar, J.W.; Oosterbroek, J.; Jager, E.A.; de Jong, H.W.; Raaijmakers, C.P.; Willems, S.M.; Terhaard, C.H.; Philippens, M.E.; Pameijer, F.A. Detection of cartilage invasion in laryngeal carcinoma with dynamic contrast-enhanced CT. *Laryngoscope Investig. Otolaryngol.* **2017**, *2*, 373–379. [CrossRef]
9. Kuno, H.; Onaya, H.; Fujii, S.; Ojiri, H.; Otani, K.; Satake, M. Primary staging of laryngeal and hypopharyngeal cancer: CT, MR imaging and dual-energy CT. *Eur. J. Radiol.* **2014**, *83*, e23–e35. [CrossRef]
10. Li, B.; Bobinski, M.; Gandour-Edwards, R.; Farwell, D.G.; Chen, A.M. Overstaging of cartilage invasion by multidetector CT scan for laryngeal cancer and its potential effect on the use of organ preservation with chemoradiation. *Br. J. Radiol.* **2011**, *84*, 64–69. [CrossRef] [PubMed]
11. Tamas-Szora, A.; Badea, A.F.; Opincariu, I.; Badea, R.I. Noninvasive Evaluation of Microcirculation under Normal and Pathological Conditions Using Contrast-Enhanced Ultrasonography (CEUS). In *Microcirculation Revisited—From Molecules to Clinical Practice*; InTech: Vienna, Austria, 2016.
12. D'Onofrio, M.; Crosara, S.; De Robertis, R.; Canestrini, S.; Mucelli, R.P. Contrast-enhanced ultrasound of focal liver lesions. *Am. J. Roentgenol.* **2015**, *205*, W56–W66. [CrossRef] [PubMed]
13. Furrer, M.A.; Spycher, S.C.; Büttiker, S.M.; Gross, T.; Bosshard, P.; Thalmann, G.N.; Schneider, M.P.; Roth, B. Comparison of the Diagnostic Performance of Contrast-enhanced Ultrasound with That of Contrast-enhanced Computed Tomography and Contrast-enhanced Magnetic Resonance Imaging in the Evaluation of Renal Masses: A Systematic Review and Meta-analysis. *Eur. Urol. Oncol.* **2020**, *3*, 464–473. [CrossRef] [PubMed]
14. Hu, Q.; Zhu, S.Y.; Liu, R.C.; Zheng, H.Y.; Lun, H.M.; Wei, H.M.; Weng, J.J. Contrast-enhanced ultrasound for the preoperative assessment of laryngeal carcinoma: A preliminary study. *Acta Radiol.* **2021**, *62*, 1016–1024. [CrossRef] [PubMed]
15. Maroldi, R.; Ravanelli, M.; Farina, D. Magnetic resonance for laryngeal cancer. *Curr. Opin. Otolaryngol. Head Neck Surg.* **2014**, *22*, 131–139. [CrossRef] [PubMed]
16. Westra, W.H. *Surgical Pathology Dissection: An Illustrated Guide*, 2nd ed.; Springer: New York, NY, USA, 2003; pp. 38–42.
17. Šimundić, A.M. Measures of Diagnostic Accuracy: Basic Definitions. *EJIFCC* **2009**, *19*, 203–211. [PubMed]
18. Baratloo, A.; Hosseini, M.; Negida, A.; El Ashal, G. Part 1: Simple Definition and Calculation of Accuracy, Sensitivity and Specificity. *Emergency* **2015**, *3*, 48–49.

19. Scherl, C.; Mantsopoulos, K.; Semrau, S.; Fietkau, R.; Kapsreiter, M.; Koch, M.; Traxdorf, M.; Grundtner, P.; Iro, H. Management of advanced hypopharyngeal and laryngeal cancer with and without cartilage invasion. *Auris Nasus Larynx* **2017**, *44*, 333–339. [CrossRef]
20. Chiesa-Estomba, C.M.; Ravanelli, M.; Farina, D.; Remacle, M.; Simo, R.; Peretti, G.; Sjogren, E.; Sistiaga-Suarez, J.A.; Gónzalez-García, J.A.; Larruscain, E.; et al. Imaging checklist for preoperative evaluation of laryngeal tumors to be treated by transoral microsurgery: Guidelines from the European Laryngological Society. *Eur. Arch. Oto-Rhino-Laryngol.* **2020**, *277*, 1707–1714. [CrossRef]
21. Obid, R.; Redlich, M.; Tomeh, C. *The Treatment of Laryngeal Cancer. Oral and Maxillofacial Surgery Clinics of North America*; W.B. Saunders: Philadelphia, PA, USA, 2019; Volume 31, pp. 1–11.
22. Cho, S.J.; Lee, J.H.; Suh, C.H.; Kim, J.Y.; Kim, D.; Bin Lee, J.; Lee, M.K.; Chung, S.R.; Choi, Y.J.; Baek, J.H. Comparison of diagnostic performance between CT and MRI for detection of cartilage invasion for primary tumor staging in patients with laryngo-hypopharyngeal cancer: A systematic review and meta-analysis. *Eur. Radiol.* **2020**, *30*, 3803–3812. [CrossRef]
23. Juliano, A.; Moonis, G. Computed Tomography Versus Magnetic Resonance in Head and Neck Cancer: When to Use What and Image Optimization Strategies. *Magn. Reson. Imaging Clin. N. Am.* **2018**, *26*, 63–84. [CrossRef] [PubMed]
24. Becker, M.; Monnier, Y.; de Vito, C. MR Imaging of Laryngeal and Hypopharyngeal Cancer. *Magn. Reson. Imaging Clin. N. Am.* **2022**, *30*, 53–72. [CrossRef] [PubMed]
25. Forghani, R.; Levental, M.; Gupta, R.; Lam, S.; Dadfar, N.; Curtin, H. Different spectral Hounsfield unit curve and high-energy virtual monochromatic image characteristics of squamous cell carcinoma compared with nonossified thyroid cartilage. *Am. J. Neuroradiol.* **2015**, *36*, 1194–1200. [CrossRef]
26. Dhoot, N.M.; Choudhury, B.; Kataki, A.C.; Kakoti, L.; Ahmed, S.; Sharma, J. Effectiveness of ultrasonography and computed to-mography in assessing thyroid cartilage invasion in laryngeal and hypopharyngeal cancers. *J. Ultrasound* **2017**, *20*, 205–211. [CrossRef] [PubMed]
27. Xia, C.-X.; Zhu, Q.; Zhao, H.-X.; Yan, F.; Li, S.-L.; Zhang, S.-M. Usefulness of ultrasonography in assessment of laryngeal carcinoma. *Br. J. Radiol.* **2013**, *86*, 20130343. [CrossRef] [PubMed]

Disclaimer/Publisher's Note: The statements, opinions and data contained in all publications are solely those of the individual author(s) and contributor(s) and not of MDPI and/or the editor(s). MDPI and/or the editor(s) disclaim responsibility for any injury to people or property resulting from any ideas, methods, instructions or products referred to in the content.

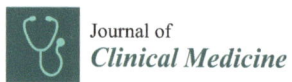

Review

CT and MR Appearance of Teeth: Analysis of Anatomy and Embryology and Implications for Disease

Zachary Abramson [1,*], Chris Oh [2], Martha Wells [3], Asim F. Choudhri [4] and Matthew T. Whitehead [5,6]

1. Clinical Radiology, Radiologist, Body Imaging, Department of Diagnostic Imaging, St. Jude Children's Research Hospital, 262 Danny Thomas Place, Memphis, TN 38105, USA
2. Quantum Radiology, 790 Church St., Suite 400, Marietta, GA 30060, USA; coh@quantumrad.com
3. Department of Surgery, St. Jude Children's Research Hospital, Memphis, TN 38105, USA; martha.wells@stjude.org
4. Department of Radiology, Le Bonheur Children's Hospital, University of Tennessee Health Science Center, 50 N. Dunlap St., Memphis, TN 38103, USA; achoudhri@uthsc.edu
5. Department of Radiology, Perelman School of Medicine, University of Pennsylvania, Philadelphia, PA 19104, USA; whiteheadm@chop.edu
6. Division of Neuroradiology, Children's Hospital of Philadelphia, Philadelphia, PA 19104, USA
* Correspondence: zachary.abramson@stjude.org; Tel.: +1-901-595-2085

Abstract: Abnormalities of dental development and anatomy may suggest the presence of congenital or acquired anomalies. The detection of abnormalities, therefore, is an important skill for radiologists to achieve. Knowledge of dental embryology and an understanding of the radiologic appearances of teeth at various stages of maturation are required for the appreciation of abnormal dental development. While many tooth abnormalities are well-depicted on dedicated dental radiographs, the first encounter with a dental anomaly may be by a radiologist on a computed tomographic (CT) or magnetic resonance (MR) exam performed for other reasons. This article depicts normal dental anatomy and development, describing the appearance of the neonatal dentition on CT and MRI, the modalities most often encountered by clinical radiologists. The radiology and dental literature are reviewed, and key concepts are illustrated with supplemental cases from our institution. The value of knowledge of dental development is investigated using the analysis of consecutive MR brain examinations. Finally, the anatomical principles are applied to the diagnosis of odontogenic infection on CT. Through analysis of the literature and case data, the contrast of dental pathology with normal anatomy and development facilitates the detection and characterization of both congenital and acquired dental disease.

Keywords: teeth; embryology; anatomy; computed tomography; magnetic resonance imaging; odontogenic infection

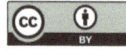

1. Introduction

Abnormalities of dental development and anatomy often suggest the presence of congenital or acquired anomalies [1,2]. The detection of abnormal dental development or anatomy, therefore, is an important skill for radiologists to achieve. Knowledge of dental embryology and an understanding of the radiologic appearances of teeth at various stages of maturation are required for the appreciation of abnormal dental development and anatomy.

While a complete description of the radiologic appearance of teeth at all stages of development from fetal to and throughout adult life is ideal, investigating the neonatal dentition is valuable for several reasons: (1) the variable stages of dental development present in the neonatal period represent most of the developmental stages seen throughout life; (2) these stages also include cellular and mineralized tissues, providing a wide range of imaging appearances helping to demonstrate key radiology principles; (3) abnormalities that appear at this age are more likely associated with other anomalies; (4) understanding early dental development, as seen in the neonatal period, reinforces the appreciation for mature tooth anatomy, which is needed to identify acquired conditions, such as infection.

While many abnormalities of the dentition are well-depicted on dedicated dental radiographs [3], the first encounter with a dental anomaly may be by a radiologist on a computed tomographic (CT) or magnetic resonance (MR) exam performed for other reasons [4–6]. Further, most dental radiographs are interpreted by dental clinicians and not viewed by a radiologist in a medical setting. This review describes normal dental anatomy and development, describing the appearance of the neonatal dentition on CT and MRI, the modalities most-often encountered by clinical radiologists. The radiology and dental literature are reviewed, and key concepts are illustrated with supplemental cases from our institution. We analyze a consecutive series of neonatal brain MR examinations demonstrating the clinical value of knowledge of dental development. Finally, anatomical principles are applied to the diagnosis of odontogenic infection on CT. The focus on imaging modalities more commonly encountered by non-dental specialists is intended to broaden the knowledgebase of providers who may see the patient or patient images prior to referral to a dentist. The information presented in this manuscript provides a foundation for understanding dental imaging at all stages of dental development.

2. Materials and Methods

A combination of journal articles, textbooks and personal educational materials by the authors were used to summarize the anatomy and embryology of developing teeth and their radiologic appearances on CT and MRI. The knowledge and principles learned through this investigation were then applied to a series of patients who underwent neonatal brain MR imaging for a variety of reasons. Consecutive-term neonatal patients who underwent brain MR at our institution were retrospectively analyzed after IRB approval. The review was performed by two neuroradiologists with American Board of Radiology (ABR) subspecialty certificates in neuroradiology with clinical practices focusing on pediatric neuroradiology. Demographic, clinical, and radiological data were compiled in tabular form and descriptive statistics were computed. The application of dental anatomical principles to the diagnosis of odontogenic infection was shown using case examples.

3. Results

3.1. Anatomy of the Dental Arch

In adult humans, a full dental complement comprises 32 teeth, housed in 2 bilaterally symmetric arches [7]. In each quadrant (half an arch) beginning in the midline, humans have two incisors (central and lateral), one canine, two premolars (first and second), and three molars (first, second, and third) (Figure 1). Similar to the adult dentition, the primary dentition is housed in two bilaterally symmetric arches. In a full complement, each quadrant contains (beginning from midline) two incisors (central and lateral), one canine, and two molars (first and second) (Figure 1). By convention, the direction along the arch toward the midline is referred to as mesial, whereas the direction on the arch away from the midline is termed distal.

Several different dental notation systems exist, and not all dental professionals use the same system. Consequently, the best way to refer to teeth mimics the following paradigm: side; arch; tooth (i.e., right maxillary lateral incisor)—in particular when referring to primary dentition. Familiarity with the common numbering system used for adult teeth is also important (Figure 2) [8].

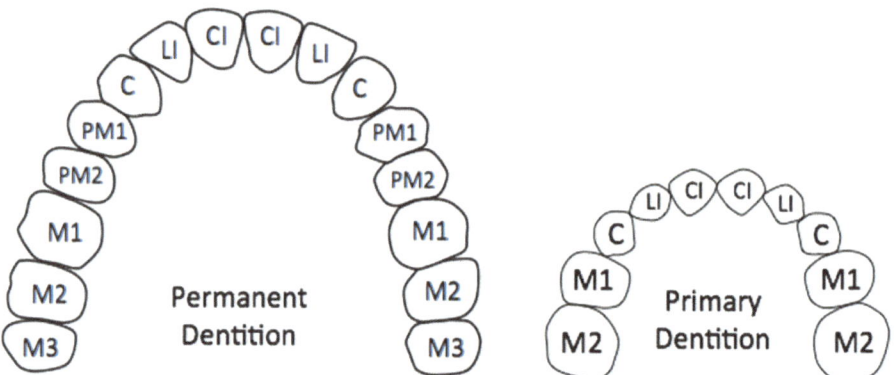

Figure 1. Arrangement of teeth within permanent and primary dental arches.

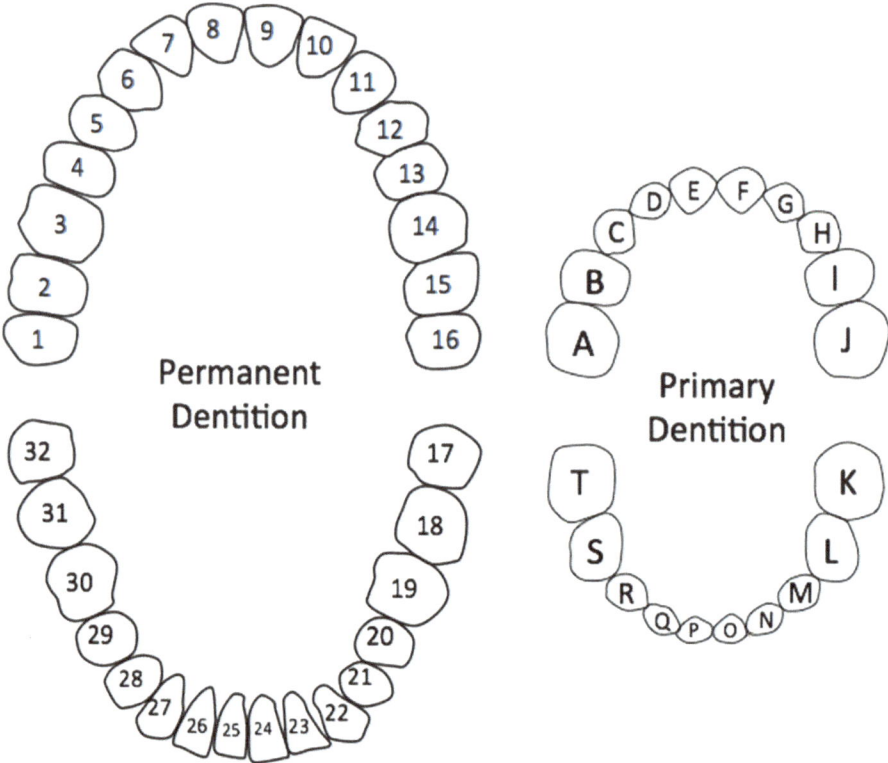

Figure 2. American Dental Association Universal Numbering/Lettering System for permanent and primary dentition.

An abnormal number of teeth can result from missing or supernumerary teeth. The most common supernumerary tooth is located between the two central incisors, termed a mesiodens (Figure 3) [9]. Excluding third molars, the most common congenitally missing permanent teeth are maxillary lateral incisors and mandibular premolars followed by maxillary lateral incisors and maxillary second premolars [9,10]. Congenital absence of primary teeth is very rare and is generally, but not always, followed by agenesis of the succedaneous tooth [11,12]. The general term for less than a full complement of teeth is hypodontia, whereas the term for extra teeth is hyperdontia. Since third molar development is variable, missing third molars is not typically categorized as hypodontia. When few teeth develop, the term 'oligodontia' can be used. Two other processes can lead to confusion in the number of teeth present: fusion and gemination. Fusion occurs when two developing tooth germs partially merge during development (Figure 4). Gemination of a tooth germ results in partial twinning of a tooth germ during development (Figure 5). A useful tip for distinguishing between the two entities is to count the teeth: when a fused or geminated tooth germ is present and counted as one tooth, the total number of teeth will be one shy of the normal complement in the setting of fusion, but normal in gemination [13].

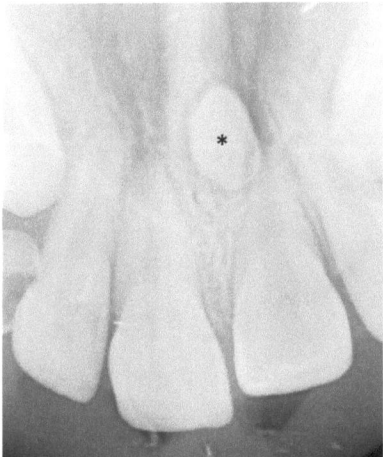

Figure 3. Supernumerary tooth (*) situated in between the roots of the central incisors, termed a mesiodens, shown on a dedicated dental radiograph.

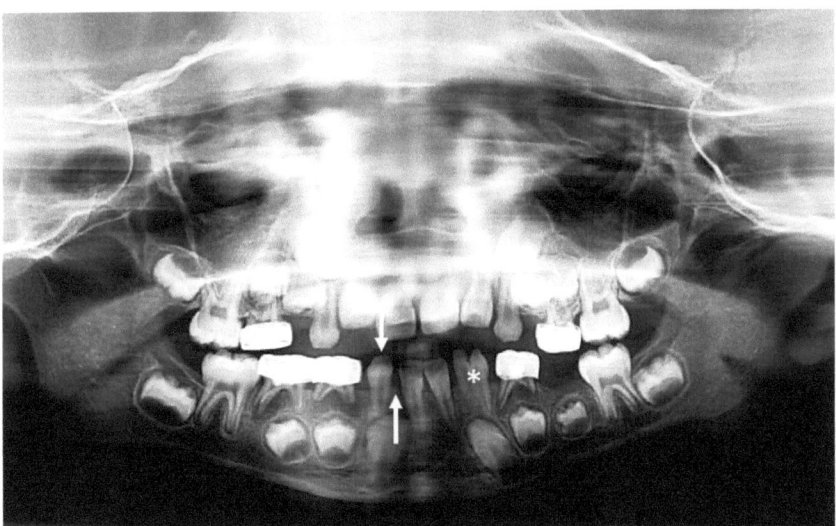

Figure 4. Panoramic radiograph demonstrating congenital absence of right mandibular lateral incisor (up arrow), manifesting as increased space surrounding the right mandibular canine (down arrow). The left mandibular lateral incisor and canine are fused (*). When counted as one tooth, the patient had one less than expected tooth in the lower left quadrant, confirming that this was a fusion of two teeth as opposed to the gemination of a single tooth.

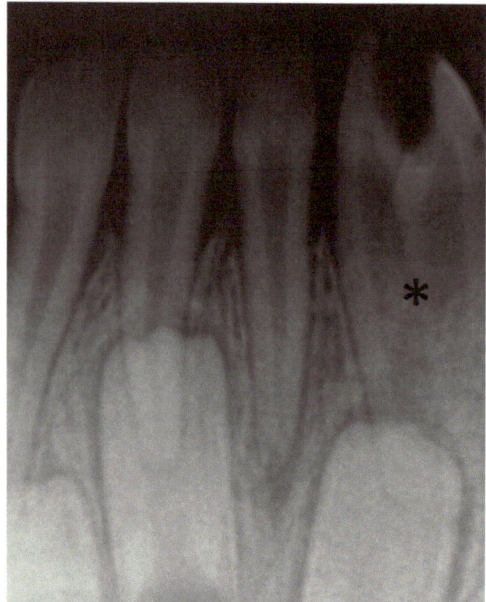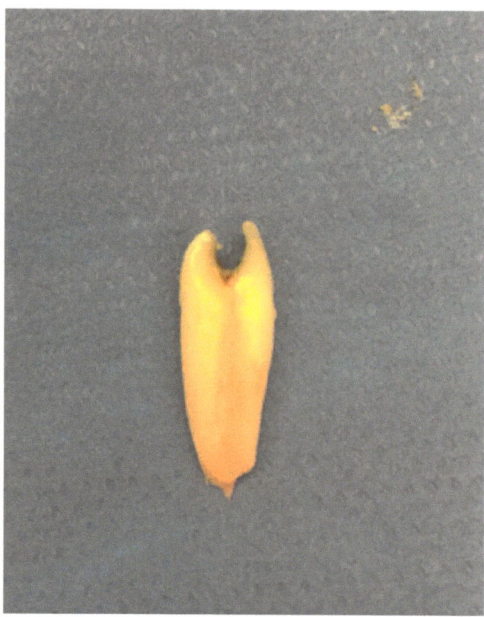

Figure 5. Geminated primary lower lateral incisor shown radiographically (*) and photographically following extraction. When counted as one tooth, the patient had the appropriate number of teeth, confirming this was a geminated tooth as opposed to the fusion of two teeth.

3.1.1. Anatomy of Tooth Structure

The mature tooth is composed of enamel, dentin, and pulp [14]. The tooth can be divided into two segments: the crown and root. The crown contains all three types of tissues whereas the root contains only dentin and pulp (Figure 6). The outer enamel layer of the crown is 96% inorganic and entirely acellular. Within the crown, just underneath the enamel lies the less mineralized dentin (70% inorganic). This layer is also acellular but contains cellular processes from the dentin-producing odontoblasts, which reside in the periphery of the underlying pulp. The pulpal tissue contains blood vessels, connective and lymph tissue, and nociceptive fibers, and has a coronal component (pulp chamber) as well as a root component (pulp canal) [15]. The tip of the root, where nerves and blood vessels enter the pulp, is termed the apex [16]. It is an important structure as it is the last structure to be formed and failure to form a narrow apex may suggest pathology.

3.1.2. Periodontal Tissues

The tissues surrounding the tooth, termed the periodontium, consist of cementum, periodontal ligament, alveolar bone, and gingiva. Cementum is the thin cellular layer surrounding the root, which allows attachment of the periodontal ligament. The periodontal ligament is a thin (200 microns) tissue layer that extends from the alveolar bone to the cementum [17]. The presence of this periodontal ligament space around a focus of very dense but disorganized tissues may suggest odontoma (Figure 7). Alveolar bone houses and supports the teeth within the maxilla and mandible. Finally, the gingiva is the soft tissue covering of the alveolar bone and forms an important tooth–mucosa junction (Figure 6).

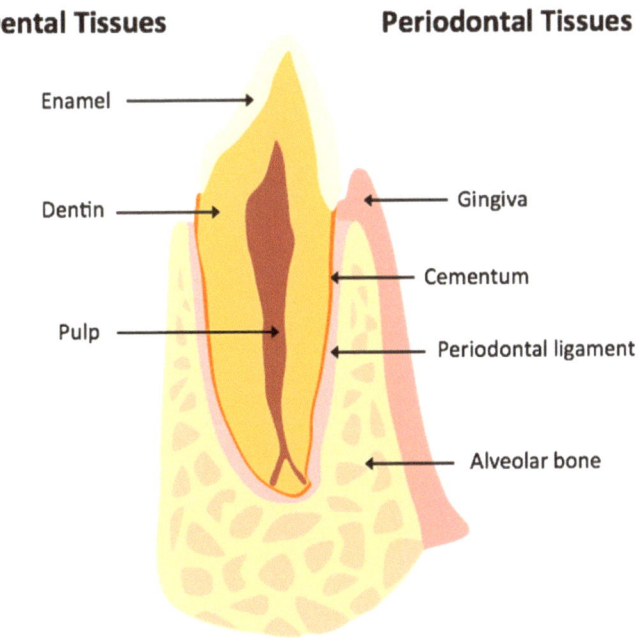

Figure 6. Basic dental and periodontal anatomy.

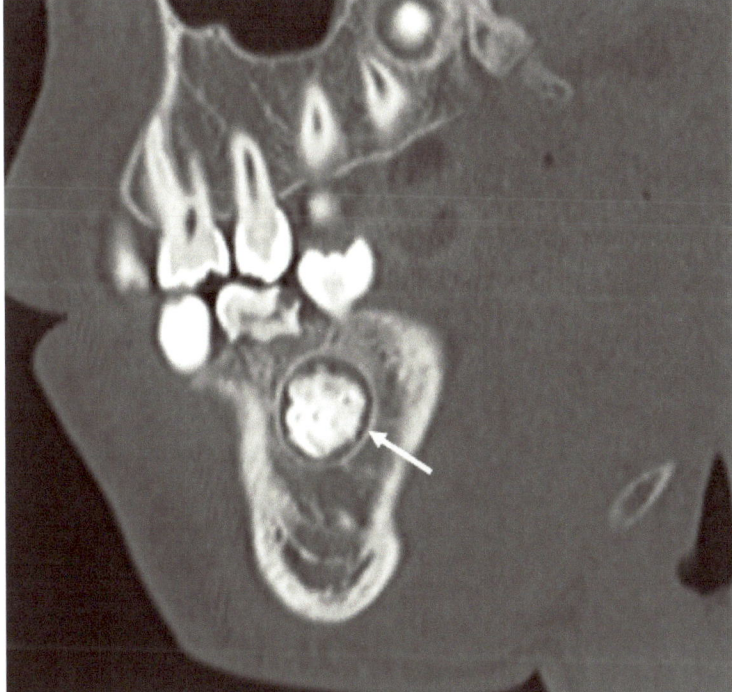

Figure 7. Sagittal section CT demonstrating heterogeneous mineralized tissues with evidence of bone and enamel densities. The uniform surrounding radiolucency (white arrow) suggests the presence of a periodontal ligament space compatible with a diagnosis of an odontoma.

3.2. Dental Development

3.2.1. Initiation of Odontogenesis and Bud Stage

Odontogenesis results from a complex interaction between the specialized oral epithelium termed the dental lamina and the underlying mesenchyme derived from neural crest cells, termed ectomesenchyme [18–20]. It is the mesenchymal cells that first signal the initiation of tooth formation, through a process termed induction. In response to inductive signals, portions of the dental lamina proliferate downwards into the mesenchyme, forming a tuft of epithelial cells with surrounding mesenchyme called a tooth bud or bud stage [21].

3.2.2. Cap Stage

Secondary to unequal epithelial proliferation, the tuft of cells begins to form a cap around densely packed mesenchymal cells. This stage, referred to as the cap stage, marks the beginning of morphodifferentiation and histodifferentiation. A depression forms in the cap of epithelial cells, creating the enamel organ, which will produce the future enamel. The condensing mass of mesenchyme is now referred to as the dental papilla, which will form the future dentin and pulp tissue. The surrounding sac, also composed of mesenchyme, forms the dental follicle, which eventually gives rise to the periodontal tissues [21]. The enamel organ, dental papilla, and dental follicle comprise the tooth germ. A tooth germ may be referred to as a tooth bud, but this should not be confused with the bud stage (Table 1).

Table 1. Key terms in dental development and embryology.

Ectomesenchyme	Mesenchymal Tissue Derived from Neural Crest Cells (Ectoderm)
Tooth germ	A developing tooth containing enamel organ, dental papilla, and dental follicle. Also referred to as tooth anlagen.
Enamel organ	Epithelial-derived structure that helps form the crown of a developing tooth, specifically providing the cells that produce enamel.
Dental papilla	Condensed mass of ectomesenchyme surrounded by enamel organ, which ultimately forms the dentin and pulp of the developing tooth.
Dental follicle	Ectomesenchyme surrounding dental papilla, which becomes cementum and periodontal ligament. Also referred to as dental sac.

3.2.3. Bell Stage

As histodifferentiation and morphodifferentiation continue, the cap assumes a bell shape. The enamel organ contains an inner and outer enamel epithelium and central cellular substances termed stellate reticulum and stratum intermedium, which serve as nutritional support to the enamel epithelium, allowing the enamel organ to separate from the dental lamina. The cells of the stellate reticulum produce glycosaminoglycans, which draw water into the enamel organ, providing further structural support to the enamel organ and contributing to folds to create the appropriate shape of the future crown. Additionally, during this stage, the dental papilla separates into an outer layer of future dentin-secreting cells (odontoblasts) and a central mass of cells that forms the primordium of the future pulp. The follicle at this time is mostly amorphous and increases collagen production (Figure 8A) [21].

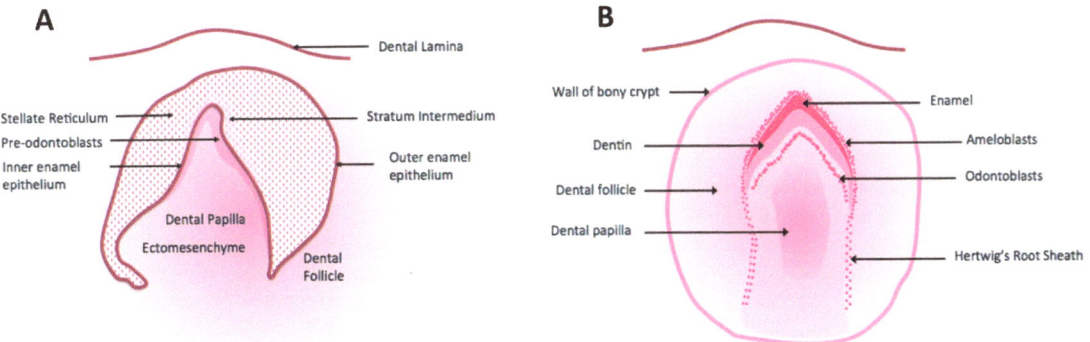

Figure 8. Diagram representation of histology of tooth germ in the bell stage (**A**) and post-apposition maturation stage (**B**). The differentiating features include the collapse of the dental organ and presence of mineralized tissue in the bell stage. The transition between these stages has corresponding imaging findings (see radiological correlations section).

It is at about this time that the primordia for the permanent teeth may arise as extensions of the epithelium associated with the primary tooth germ. Permanent teeth that arise in this fashion are referred to as succedaneous teeth. Non-succedaneous teeth include all permanent molars and are thought to arise separately from posterior extensions of the dental lamina.

3.2.4. Apposition and Maturation

At the end of the bell stage, there is a collapse of the dental organ with loss of the glycosaminoglycan layer and consequent loss of water. This collapse allows for simple diffusion to provide nutrients to the inner enamel epithelium, which is now terminally differentiated. The cells of the inner enamel epithelium, now termed ameloblasts, and the outer cells of the dental papilla, now termed odontoblasts, are primed to secrete the precursors to enamel and dentin, respectively. This next phase is known as the appositional stage, where partially calcified enamel and dentin matrices are secreted and serve as a framework for further calcification. The maturation stage is characterized by completion of calcification (Figure 8B).

3.2.5. Root Formation

As the crown continues calcifying, the roots are still developing. At the edges of the crown, the inner and outer enamel epithelium proliferates downwards, forming a double-layered sheath separating the dental papilla from the surrounding follicle, termed Hertwig's root sheath. Unlike in the enamel organ, there is no stellate reticulum or stratum intermedium in the root sheath and, therefore, no ameloblasts are formed. The odontoblasts of the outer dental papilla interact with the root sheath and are signaled to produce the dentin of the root. The basement membrane of the root sheath subsequently breaks down, and specialized cells of the dental follicle termed cementoblasts produce cementum along the newly exposed dentin surface. While the cementum is forming on the roots, the central cells of the dental papilla form the pulp chamber and canal system. Other specialized cells in the dental follicle go on to form the periodontal ligament attaching to cementum and adjacent alveolar bone [21]. This process continues until the sheath converges at the root apex, which may 2–3 years after the crown of the tooth erupts into the oral cavity [22–24].

3.2.6. Eruption

Eruption sequences are fairly consistent and well-documented in the literature but are beyond the scope of this article [25,26]. All primary tooth germs and first permanent molar tooth germs are detectable by MRI at birth [27]. It is important to note, however, that at birth, none of the teeth are erupted into the oral cavity. An erupted tooth at birth is termed a natal tooth, and a tooth which erupts within the first 30 days of life is termed a neonatal tooth, both of which are abnormal but may or may not be associated with pathology [28,29]. The majority of natal and neonatal teeth ($\geq$90%) are the primary teeth (most commonly the mandibular incisors) and not supernumerary teeth [30]. Another important pearl is that of symmetry. Development tends to be bilaterally symmetric and, to a lesser degree, symmetric among the maxillary and mandibular arches. When correlating cross-sectional findings with radiographs, it should be noted that significant mineralization is required for a developing tooth to appear opaque on X-ray, whereas the unmineralized tooth germ can be visualized much earlier on CT or MRI, as further detailed below.

3.2.7. Post-Maturation Changes

Once a tooth is fully formed, the odontoblasts continue to lay down new dentin, which gradually narrows the pulp chamber and canal. The cessation of continued dentin formation and narrowing of the pulp chamber is a radiologic sign of pulpal necrosis (Figure 9).

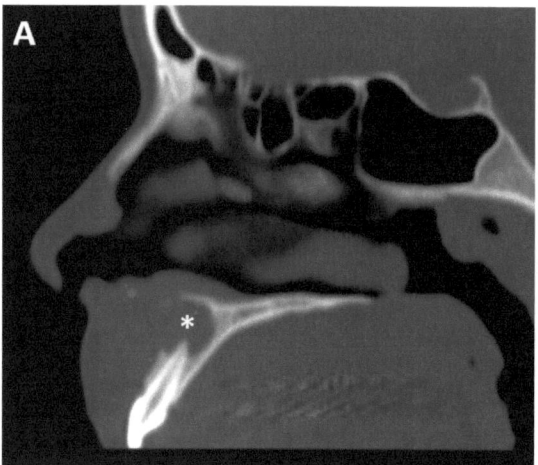
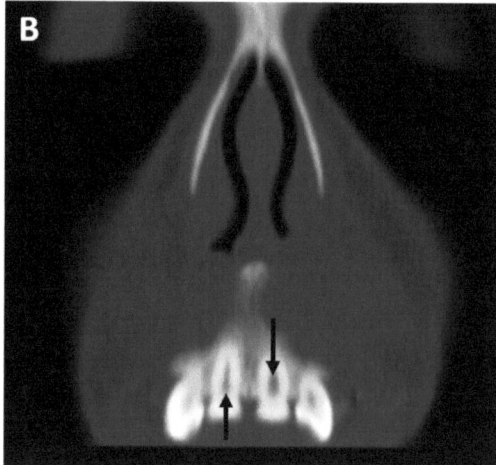

Figure 9. An 18-year-old female with tooth pain. (**A**) Sagittal-reformatted CT shown in bone windows reveals a periapical lucency (asterisk) involving the left maxillary central incisor, compatible with a cyst, granuloma, or abscess, in keeping with a diagnosis of periapical periodontitis. (**B**) Coronal-reformatted CT demonstrating a widened pulp chamber of the left maxillary central incisor (down arrow) relative to the right maxillary central incisor (up arrow), indicative of remote/chronic pulpal necrosis.

3.3. Radiologic Correlations of Embryological Development

Dental arches are readily identified on imaging by the presence of teeth or tooth germs. On axial imaging, the dental arch is U-shaped. Axial sections demonstrate arch asymmetry nicely and can be viewed to quickly screen for missing or supernumerary teeth. Axial imaging also depicts the presence of both primary and secondary teeth on the same image, with secondary teeth arising lingual to the primary dentition (Figure 10). Coronal and sagittal imaging can further detect dental abnormalities, including displacement and associated lesions (Figure 11). Curved-plane coronal CT reformats can be performed to show the entirety of the dental arches in a manner similar to that of panoramic tomography

(Figure 12) [31,32]. When viewing the cross-sectional anatomy of teeth using CT, it is critical to appropriately set the window and level of the image to be able to distinguish the enamel and dentin layers. Wider window levels increase visibility of the dentin–enamel junction (Figure 13) [33]. Three-dimensional CT reconstructions can also be performed of the dental arches (Figure 14) [34–36]. Developmental abnormalities, such as agenesis and supernumerary teeth, can be determined simply by identifying the dental arches and counting teeth and teeth germs. More subtle abnormalities, however, require greater knowledge of the radiologic appearances of the teeth and teeth germs at various stages of development.

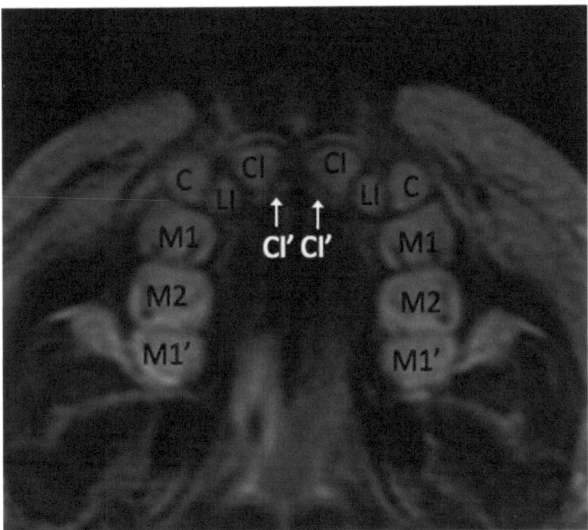

Figure 10. Axial section T2WI MRI: primary maxillary teeth in maturation stage with permanent maxillary central incisors (CI′) and first molars (M1′) in pre-appositional stages.

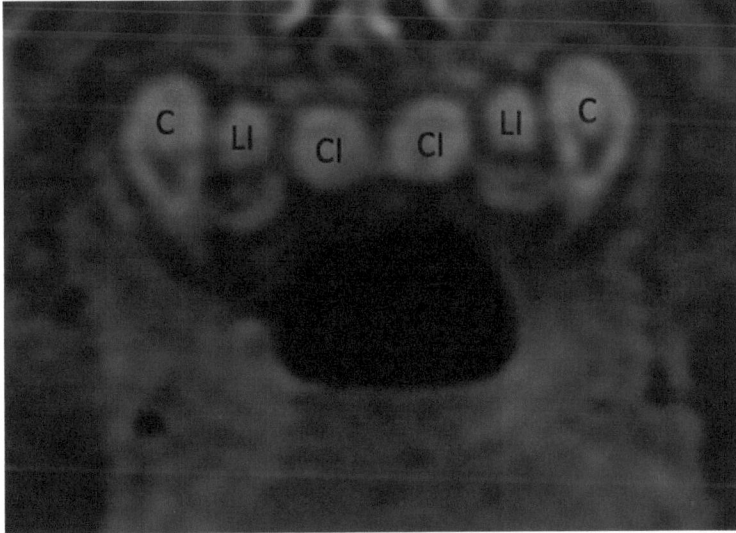

Figure 11. Coronal section T2WI MRI: primary maxillary canines and incisors in maturation stage of development.

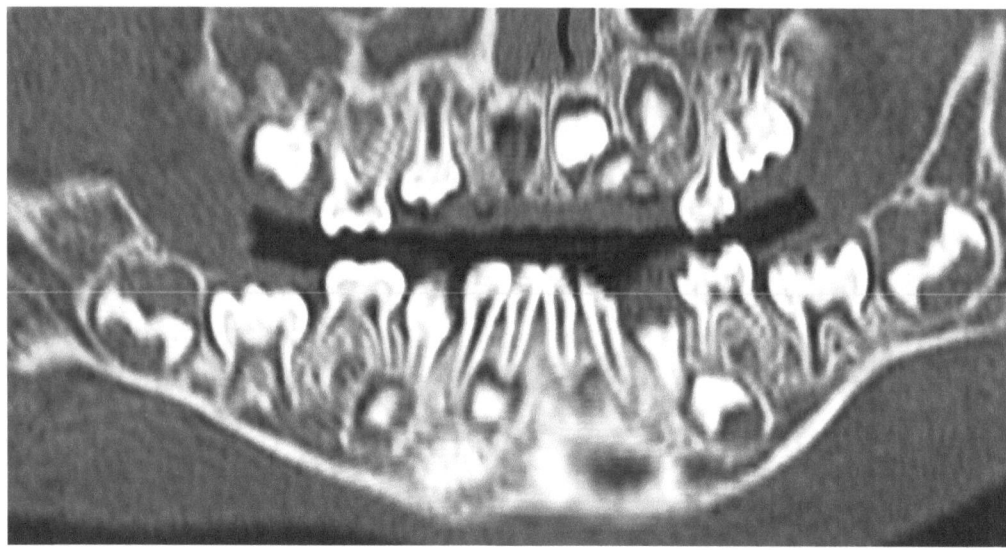

Figure 12. Curved plane coronal CT reconstruction in a 28-month-old child, presented in a manner similar to that of panoramic tomography. The horizontal green line reflects an image processing artifact.

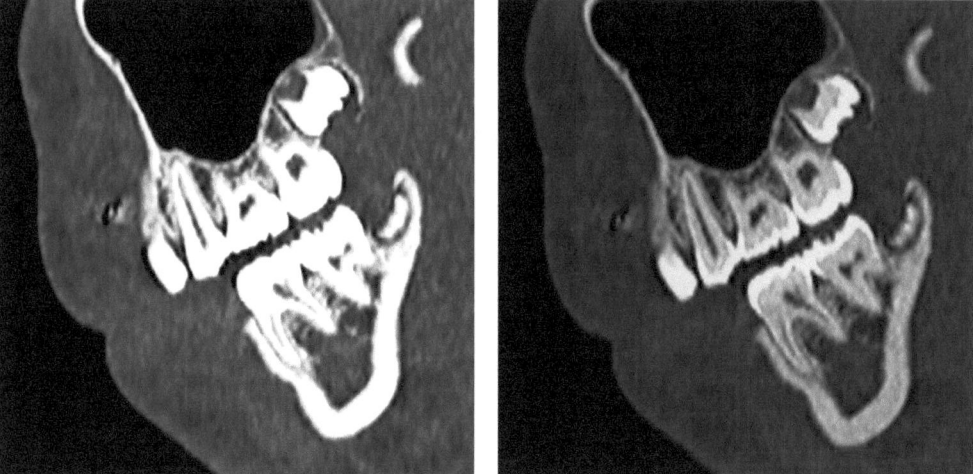

Figure 13. Sagittal section CT shown in bone window and level (**left**). On the **right**, the window has been widened and the level has been increased to allow demonstration of the enamel and dentin components of the dentition.

Visualization of subtle abnormalities can also be hindered by the limitations of imaging modalities. While modern CT scanners acquired images at sub-1 mm resolution, they are often reconstructed at thicker sections (~3 mm) to reduce image noise [37]. MRI, on the other hand, is typically acquired in thick sections with gaps between slices to reduce noise and limit the time on the MR scanner and/or under sedation. Due to these limitations, some abnormalities may be better demonstrated on conventional radiography, which exhibits excellent spatial resolution but suffers from the overlapping of structures inherent to a projection imaging technique in comparison to the cross-sectional techniques emphasized here.

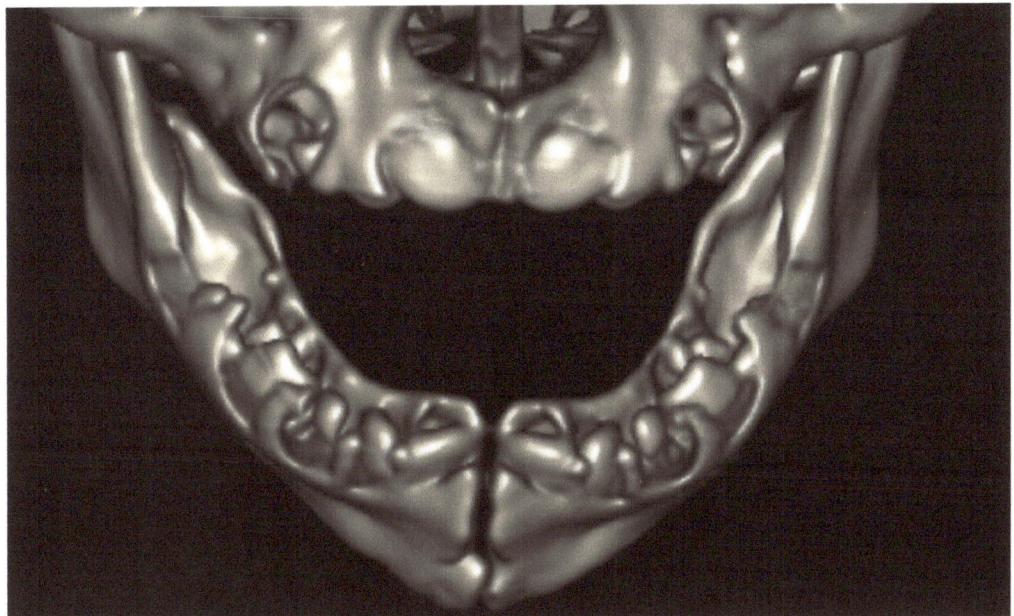

Figure 14. Three-dimensional CT reconstruction of the dental arches in a neonate revealing the numerous bony crypts in which multiple primary teeth are developing.

There are a few radiologic principles that aid interpretation of dental development on MRI and CT:

1. Hydrophilic tissues have greater water content and consequent higher signal on T2-weighted sequences and decreased density on CT;
2. Calcification on MRI presents as hypointense on T2-weighted imaging. On CT, calcification presents as increased density with density greater or equal to bone.

The two simple principles stated above, when combined with the knowledge of dental anatomy and development allow for radiologic–anatomic correlations. Similar to brain imaging, the MR appearance of teeth varies with the stage of development. Analogous to the detection of abnormal myelination on MR, abnormal dental maturation can be readily assessed based on intrinsic T2 properties of developing teeth. Prior to the apposition of enamel and dentin, the developing tooth is largely hydrophilic, which leads to a hyperintense signal on T2-weighted imaging. Following collapse of the enamel organ and apposition of enamel and dentin, the high mineral content largely devoid of water yields the hypo-intense regions on T2-weighted MRI (Figures 15 and 16).

Identification of individual teeth can be aided by the cross-sectional appearance of the developing crown. Incisor crowns, which are described as wedge- or chisel-shaped, are seen as rectangles in the coronal plane and triangular in the sagittal plane. Canine crowns, on the other hand, are pyramidal in shape and are seen as triangular in coronal, sagittal, and axial sections. Molars and premolars, which are box-shaped, are rectangular in cross-sections. Keep in mind that displacements, rotations and abnormal eruption patterns can alter the appearance of crowns on cross-sectional imaging. When this occurs, 3D imaging or curved plane reformats can be employed. Molar crowns can be further identified by the presence of multiple peaks, called cusps. Pre-molars have two cusps, one buccal and one lingual. Molars have between four and five cusps with a central groove running in the mesial–distal direction.

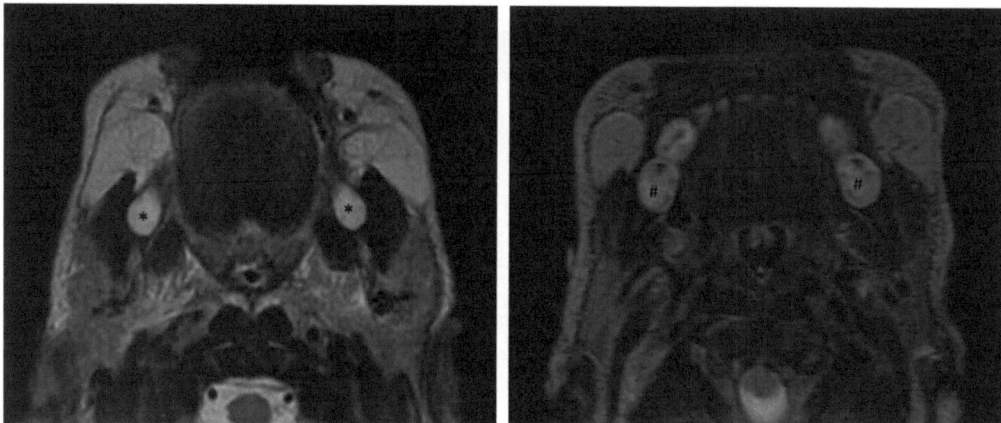

Figure 15. Axial section MRI demonstrating pre-appositional permanent mandibular first molars presenting uniformly hyperintense (*) and post-appositional primary second molars in the same patient presenting with areas of hypointensity/low signal (#).

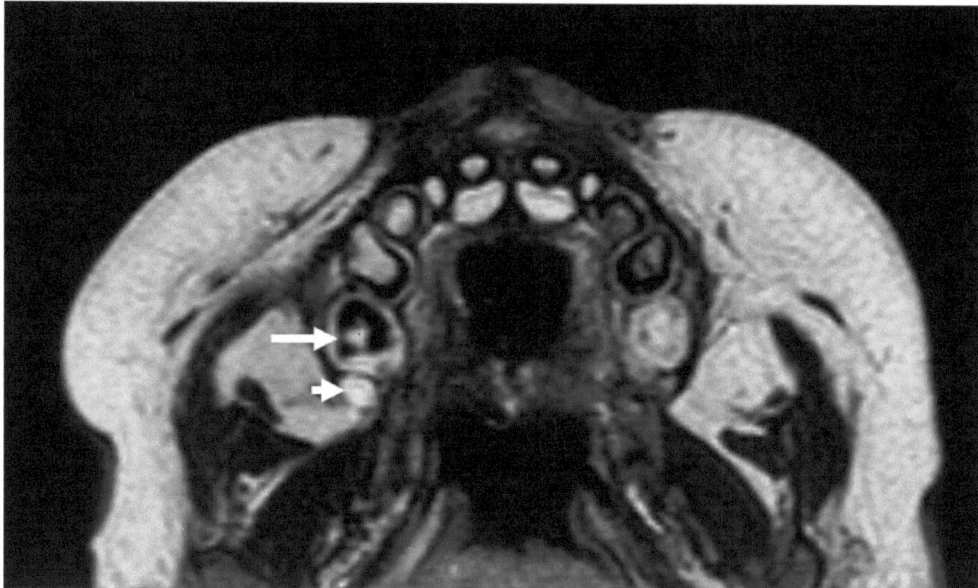

Figure 16. T2-weighted axial MRI through the maxillary dental arch/palate showing a developing primary second molar in the post-appositional phase (long arrow). Note the dark signal corresponding to areas of increased mineralization. Posterior to this tooth germ is a developing first permanent molar tooth germ in the earlier pre-appositional phase without internal areas of dark signal (short arrow).

A closer look at the MRI appearance of a developing tooth germ in a post-appositional stage demonstrates an envelope of partially mineralized, hypo-intense enamel and dentin derived from the enamel organ and outer layer of dental papilla, respectively. This hypointense layer envelops the non-mineralized dental papilla, which demonstrates enhancement and T2 hyperintensity. Surrounding the enamel organ and dental papilla, the dental follicle exhibits similar MR attributes as the dental papilla, as it is composed of the same ectomesenchyme derived from neural crest cells. All tooth germs develop inside a bony crypt. The wall of the crypt is comprised of compact bone, which presents as a hypointense rim surrounding the tooth germ on MRI (Figures 17 and 18).

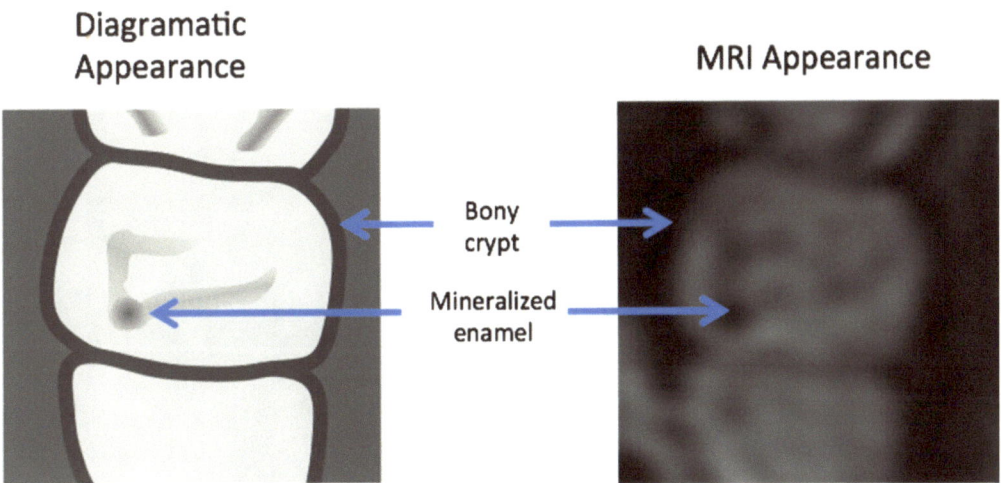

Figure 17. Post-appositional tooth germ anatomy shown diagrammatically (**left**) and as seen on axial MRI (**right**). On MRI, mineralized structures appear hypointense (dark), whereas water/cellular components are hyperintense (bright).

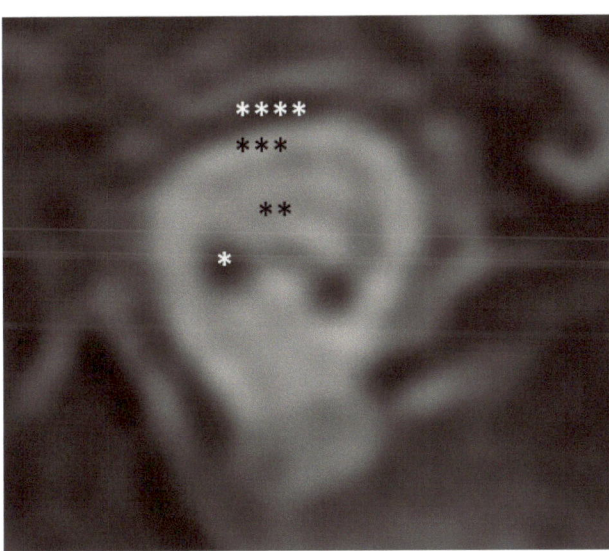

* Mineralized enamel matrix
** Dental papilla
*** Dental follicle
**** Bony crypt

Figure 18. Post-appositional tooth germ anatomy shown on T2-weighted coronal MRI. Note the hypointense (dark) signal corresponding to hypocellular mineralized tissues (bony crypt and enamel).

On CT, post-appositional tooth germs demonstrate hyperdensity of the developing crown (enamel and dentin), with relative hypodensities corresponding to the unmineralized dental papilla and dental follicle. The bony crypt housing the tooth germ, being comprised of bone, is hyperdense on CT (Figure 19). Prior to the convergence of the root sheath, the root apex is open and flared with a "blunderbuss" appearance (Figure 20) [38]. Knowledge of this normal appearance can help differentiate root resorption from a pathologic process vs. normal development. Comparison with the contralateral side is also helpful.

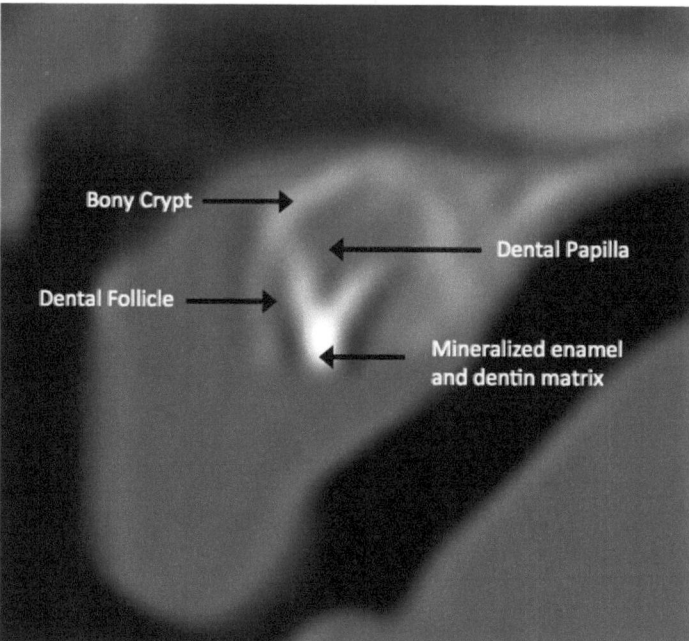

Figure 19. Post-appositional tooth germ anatomy of a central incisor on CT. Note the hyperdense appearance of the mineralized bony crypt and mineralizing crown (enamel and dentin) of the tooth relative to the hypodense appearance of the dental follicle and papilla.

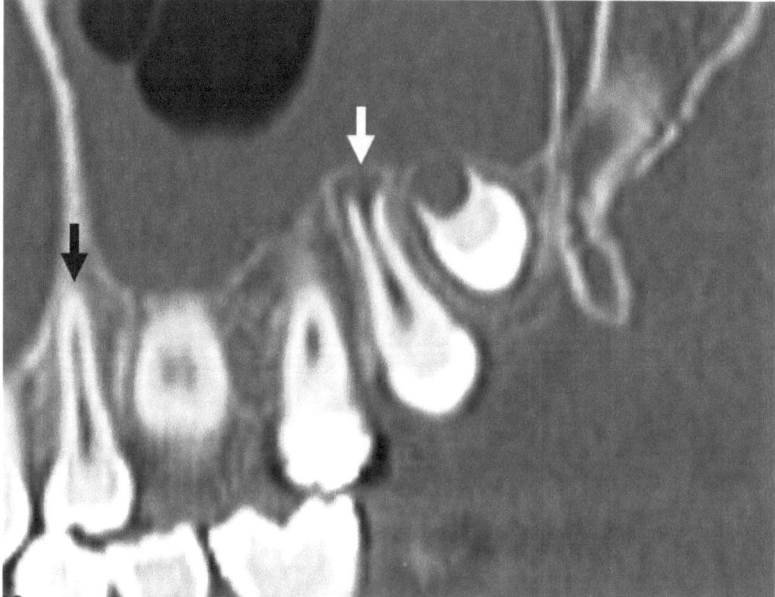

Figure 20. Obliquely reformatted CT demonstrating a mature root apex of the maxillary first premolar (black arrow) and the developing root of maxillary second molar palatal root. Note the flared appearance of the root apex with a "blunderbuss" appearance (white arrow). The increased lucency around the apex should not be mistaken for pathology.

The etiologies of abnormal dental development are variable and it is often not feasible to determine the etiology radiographically. However, understanding the types of abnormalities can occasionally suggest an underlying cause (Figures 21 and 22). A malformation is an abnormality in morphogenesis secondary to an intrinsically abnormal developmental process. A disruption is an alteration to a previously normal developmental process (Figure 23). A deformation is an abnormality in morphogenesis secondary to abnormal forces on a normal developmental process. This is exemplified by space constrictions placed on a developing root resulting in an abnormal curvature termed a dilacerated root (Figure 24) [39].

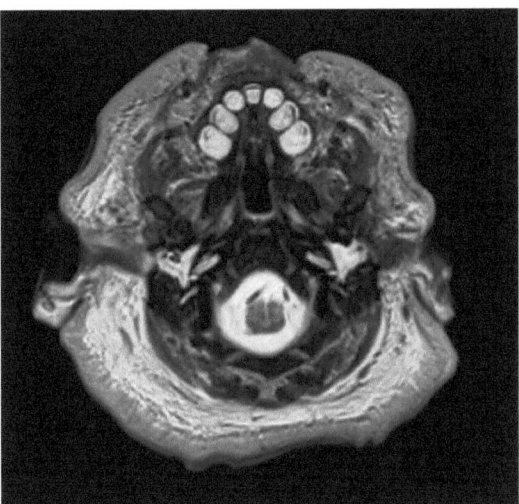

Figure 21. Eight-day old male with holoprosencephaly. Axial T2-weighted MRI demonstrates a single central incisor tooth germ. This appearance is associated with holoprosencephaly the diagnosis and should direct attention to potentially associated abnormalities in the brain.

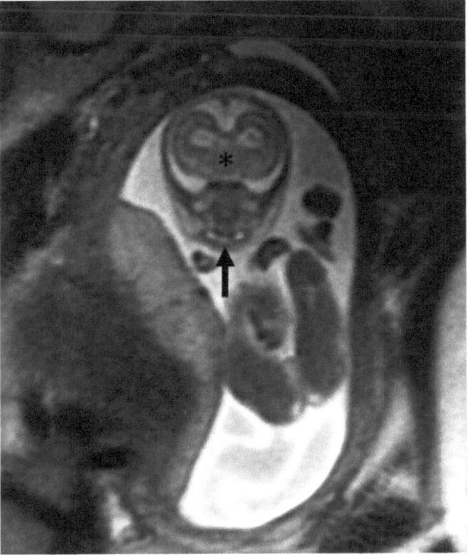

Figure 22. Fetal T2-weighted MRI showing single central incisor of a patient (up arrow) and the failed thalamic separation (*) compatible with holoprosenchephaly.

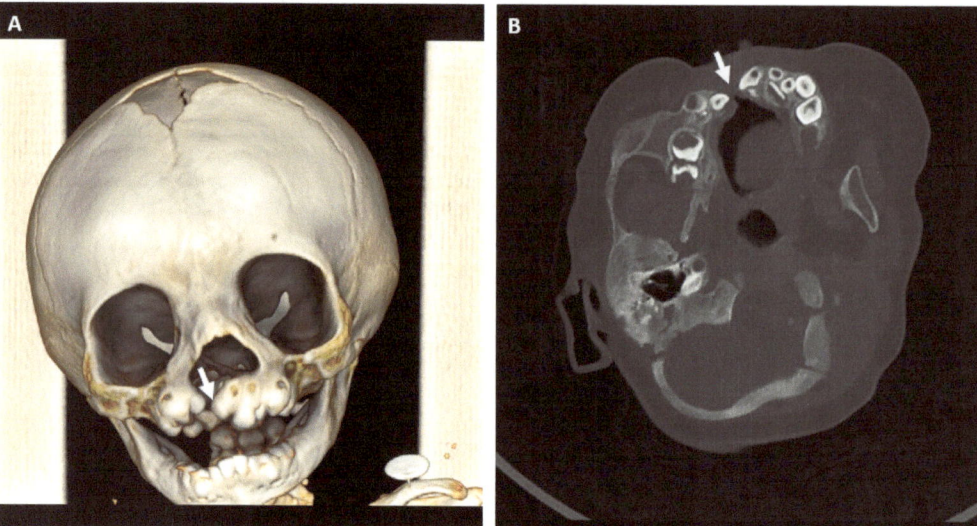

Figure 23. (**A**) Three-dimensional CT reconstruction of a patient with CHARGE syndrome and cleft lip and palate (arrow). (**B**) The presence of a cleft through the dental arch is frequently associated with missing and ectopic teeth (arrow).

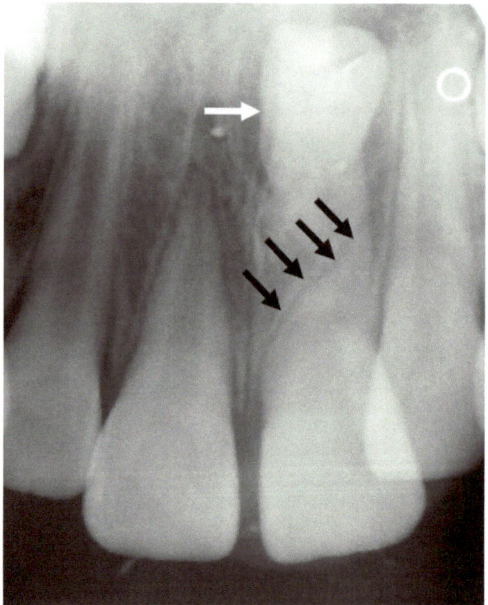

Figure 24. Dedicated dental radiograph demonstrating the presence of an unerupted supernumerary mesiodens (white arrow), which exerted mass effect on the left maxillary central incisor, resulting in a deformation deformity known as a dilacerated root (black arrows).

3.4. Application of Principles to Consecutive MR Exams

The information and principles outlined above were retrospectively applied to a series of fifty patients who underwent neonatal brain magnetic resonance imaging for a variety of reasons. Fifty consecutive-term (≥38 weeks gestation) neonatal patients (mean age 8.7 ± 8.1 days, range 0–27 days, median 6.5 days) who underwent brain MR at our institution were retrospectively analyzed after IRB approval. Review was performed by two neuroradiologists with ABR subspecialty certificates in neuroradiology with clinical practices focusing on pediatric neuroradiology. There were 25 males and 25 females. The most common clinical indications for the MRI examination included seizure (n = 16), hydrocephalus (n = 8), and hypoxic ischemic encephalopathy (n = 7).

Overall, the tooth germs were small, with the maximum size of 4–5 mm in greatest dimension in nearly all patients. All 20 deciduous teeth were visible in every patient. In all 50 patients, the primary teeth were in the early maturation stage of development with little to no root development. Greater mineralization was seen in the crowns (post-appositional phase) of primary first molars when compared to the second molars. Permanent tooth mineralization was not observed in any patient. Except for a single patient, all patients had bilateral pre-appositional-stage permanent mandibular and maxillary central and lateral incisors as well as bilateral maxillary and mandibular permanent first molars developing posterior to the primary second molars. The exception was a child with Down syndrome who had only central maxillary incisors and mandibular molar permanent teeth germs at the time of imaging. In 36 of 50 patients (72%), permanent bilateral maxillary and mandibular canine tooth germs were visible. No premolar, second molar, or third molar tooth germs were visualized.

3.5. Anatomical and Imaging Correlations to Odontogenic Infectious Disease

A thorough understanding of dental maturation not only facilitates diagnosis of disorders of development but can also aid in the diagnosis of pathologic processes of fully formed teeth, the most common of which include odontogenic infections. Odontogenic infection can be categorized into diseases of the tooth (decay) or the periodontal supporting structures (periodontal disease). Many clinical and radiological reports on infectious disease involving the dentition and supporting tissues do not distinguish between decay and periodontal disease. In fact, these are two distinct entities with unique etiologies, pathophysiologies, and treatments. Knowledge of the anatomy and common imaging appearances can assist in distinguishing these two sources of odontogenic infection.

3.5.1. Dental Decay Pathophysiology

Despite its colloquial name, dental decay is an infection like any other, with a bacterial pathogen, the requirement of a susceptible host, and a food substrate [40]. The decay process begins with biofilm formation; bacterial consumption of carbohydrates, resulting in acid production; and demineralization of the outermost tooth structure—enamel. This stage is asymptomatic. As the process continues, the next mineralized layer encountered is the dentin, an inorganic hard tissue produced by living cells located in the soft tissue pulp deep to the dentin. These cells send processes out into the dentin, which can sense temperature and osmotic gradients. This stage is often symptomatic, presenting with sensitivity to sweet or cold food or drink. If the disease goes untreated, the decay will progress to involve the pulp causing pulpitis. Patients with pulpitis often have lingering sensitivity to painful stimuli. At this stage, the pain cannot be localized to a specific tooth, as the pulpal tissue has pain but not proprioceptive fibers. When bacteria exit the apex of the root canal, the surrounding periodontal tissues become inflamed; this condition is called periapical periodontitis. This stage of the disease presents with well-localized pain to palpation of the involved tooth, as the periodontal tissues contain proprioceptive nerve fibers, unlike the pulp. Again, if untreated, spread of infection through the bony cortex can result in a subperiosteal or soft tissue abscess formation and cellulitis with or without systemic involvement.

3.5.2. Dental Decay Radiologic Correlations

While dedicated dental radiographs provide optimal evaluation of the teeth, these are not routinely encountered by radiologists. More likely, a panoramic radiograph or a CT will be obtained. Regardless of the modality, the hallmark image findings of decay are the same—radiolucency of the crown and periapical tissues. During the initial stages of decay resulting in demineralization, the hallmark image finding is lucency of the crown (Figure 25). As demineralization continues, cavitation of the crown may occur, yielding the radiographic appearance of missing coronal tooth structure [6,41].

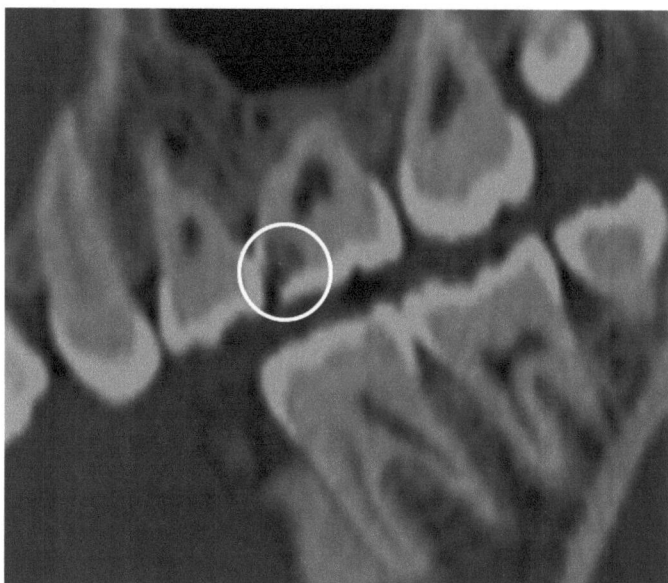

Figure 25. Sagittal section CT demonstrating lucency (white circle) within the enamel and dentin layer of a maxillary first molar, compatible with decay.

Extension of decay into the pulp chamber may occur with or without cavitation resulting in pulpitis. The pulpitis stage cannot be identified radiographically. The progression of bacterial proliferation through the canal and into the periapical periodontal tissues results in a demineralization of the alveolar bone, manifesting as a periapical radiolucency on radiograph or CT (Figure 26) or hyperintensity on T2-weighted MRI [42]. It is important to note that periapical periodontitis can be present without a visible periapical radiolucency [43]. Further, in the case of a tooth treated with root canal therapy, the periapical radiolucency may persist indefinitely even after successful treatment. Importantly, in some cases of periapical infection, the surrounding bone becomes sclerotic in a reactive process called condensing osteitis. In other patients, infection spreads through the outer cortex of the maxilla or mandible and results in a subperiosteal abscess and cellulitis [44].

3.5.3. Periodontal Disease Pathophysiology

Periodontal disease begins with the formation of subgingival plaque (biofilm), which causes gingivitis [45]. The inflamed gingiva creates a deep sulcus (the space between the gum and tooth), which is difficult to clean and is relatively oxygen poor. This local environment is conducive to the proliferation of pathologic bacteria known to cause periodontal disease, specifically, Gram-negative rods, which secrete a lipopolysaccharide endotoxin. This toxin is highly inflammatory and produces a robust host response that leads to the destruction of alveolar bone, periodontal ligament and the gingival attachment to the tooth. This results in an even deeper gingival pocket that is even more difficult to clean. The progressive loss of periodontal support ultimately leads to tooth loss. At any point during this process, an abscess can form within the periodontal tissues, an occurrence that is typically visible clinically.

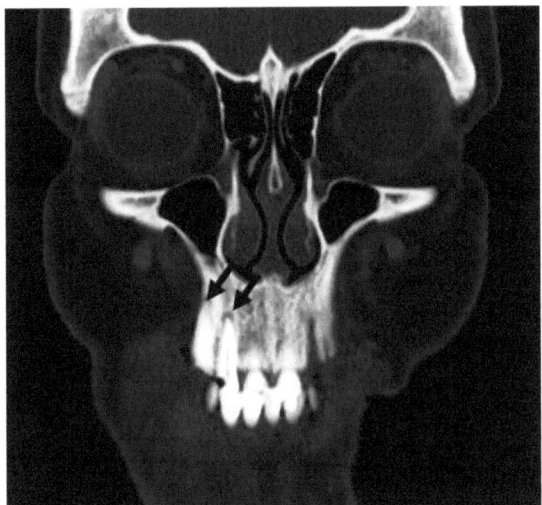

Figure 26. Coronal CT demonstrating periapical radiolucencies (arrows) involving decayed right maxillary lateral incisor and canine, indicative of periapical periodontitis.

3.5.4. Periodontal Disease Radiologic Correlations

The hallmark imaging finding of periodontal disease is bone loss. However, unlike in decay, the bone loss begins at the alveolar crest and progresses inferiorly [46]. There are two general categories of bone loss, horizontal and vertical. Figure 27 demonstrates an example of horizontal bone loss. Depending on the state of the adjacent soft tissues, horizontal bone defects may or may not represent active disease but imply that periodontal tissue destruction has occurred either from present or past disease. A vertical bony defect, on the other hand, suggests active disease. This is because a vertical bony defect is almost always accompanied by a deep gingival sulcus, which is unhygienic and very conducive to periodontal pathogenic bacterial proliferation (Figure 28).

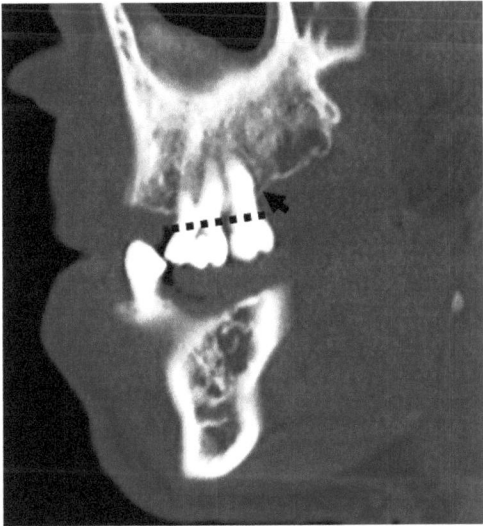

Figure 27. Sagittal section CT demonstrating horizontal bone loss, a sequela of periodontal disease. Note the alveolar crest (arrow) below its normal location at the crown–root junction (dashed line).

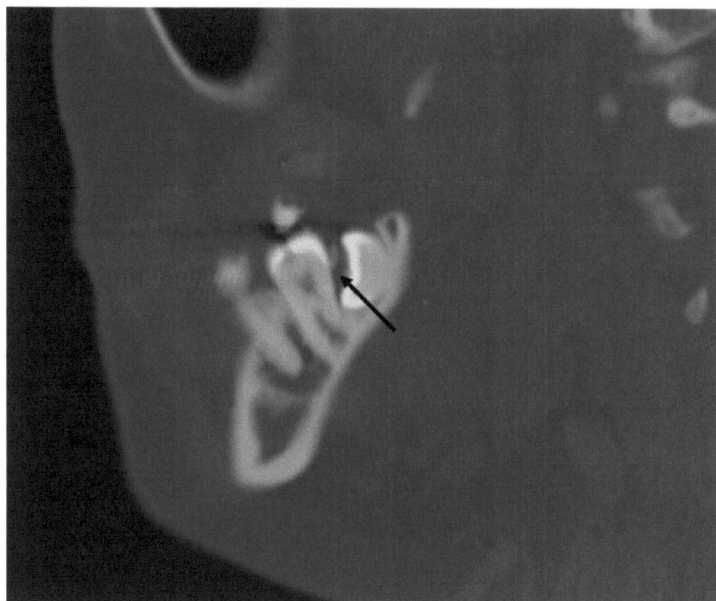

Figure 28. Sagittal section CT showing a vertical bony defect (arrow) posterior to the mandibular second molar, indicative of periodontal disease. In this case, the mesial-angulated third molar is contributing to the vertical bony defect, precluding adequate hygiene.

4. Conclusions

This article reviews normal dental anatomy and development and describes the MRI and CT appearance of developing teeth in the neonatal period. This period is comprised of very active development, with various stages of maturation, resulting in a varied radiologic appearance. Knowledge of normal radiologic appearances of developing and mature teeth can help in the identification of congenital and acquired pathology as well as the prevention of misdiagnosis of normal development as pathologic.

Future Directions

Despite the inclusion of the dentition on several radiologic examinations obtained for non-dental pathology, little is taught in medical school or radiology residency pertaining to the normal appearance of developing teeth. The dissemination of knowledge in a formalized manner is critical to bridging this knowledge gap. Further, opportunistic screening for odontogenic disorders on examinations ordered for other indications can improve patient outcomes and should be explored.

Author Contributions: Conceptualization, Z.A., C.O., A.F.C. and M.T.W.; formal analysis, C.O., A.F.C. and M.T.W.; writing—original draft preparation, Z.A.; writing—review and editing, Z.A., M.W., C.O., A.F.C. and M.W.; supervision, M.T.W. All authors have read and agreed to the published version of the manuscript.

Funding: This research received no external funding.

Data Availability Statement: No new data were created or analyzed in this study. Data sharing is not applicable to this article.

Acknowledgments: The authors would like to acknowledge Sue Kaste for her contributions leading to a greater understanding of the effects of cancer and cancer treatment on dental development and for her mentorship of the first author of this manuscript.

Conflicts of Interest: The authors declare no conflict of interest.

References

1. Bailleul-Forestier, I.; Berdal, A.; Vinckier, F.; de Ravel, T.; Fryns, J.P.; Verloes, A. The Genetic Basis of Inherited Anomalies of the Teeth. Part 2: Syndromes with Significant Dental Involvement. *Eur. J. Med. Genet.* **2008**, *51*, 383–408. [CrossRef] [PubMed]
2. Schuurs, A. *Pathology of the Hard Dental Tissues*; John Wiley & Sons: Hoboken, NJ, USA, 2012; ISBN 9781118381342.
3. Vandenberghe, B.; Jacobs, R.; Bosmans, H. Modern Dental Imaging: A Review of the Current Technology and Clinical Applications in Dental Practice. *Eur. Radiol.* **2010**, *20*, 2637–2655. [CrossRef] [PubMed]
4. Scheinfeld, M.H.; Shifteh, K.; Avery, L.L.; Dym, H.; Dym, R.J. Teeth: What Radiologists Should Know. *Radiographics* **2012**, *32*, 1927–1944. [CrossRef] [PubMed]
5. Alves, I.D.S.; Vendramini, D.F.V.; Leite, C.D.C.; Gebrim, E.M.M.S.; Passos, U.L. Dental Findings on Face and Neck Imaging. *Radiol. Bras.* **2021**, *54*, 107–114. [CrossRef] [PubMed]
6. Steinklein, J.; Nguyen, V. Dental Anatomy and Pathology Encountered on Routine CT of the Head and Neck. *AJR Am. J. Roentgenol.* **2013**, *201*, W843–W853. [CrossRef]
7. Ash, M.J. *Wheeler's Dental Anatomy, Physiology and Occlusion*; WB Saunders Co.: Philadelphia, PA, USA, 1993.
8. Bs, M. Chapter-03 Tooth Numbering Systems. In *Textbook of Dental Anatomy and Oral Physiology*; Bs, M., Ed.; Jaypee Brothers Medical Publishers (P) Ltd.: New Delhi, India, 2013; pp. 24–29. ISBN 9789350259955.
9. Bäckman, B.; Wahlin, Y.B. Variations in Number and Morphology of Permanent Teeth in 7-Year-Old Swedish Children. *Int. J. Paediatr. Dent.* **2001**, *11*, 11–17. [CrossRef] [PubMed]
10. Altug-Atac, A.T.; Erdem, D. Prevalence and Distribution of Dental Anomalies in Orthodontic Patients. *Am. J. Orthod. Dentofacial Orthop.* **2007**, *131*, 510–514. [CrossRef]
11. Daugaard-Jensen, J.; Nodal, M.; Skovgaard, L.T.; Kjaer, I. Comparison of the Pattern of Agenesis in the Primary and Permanent Dentitions in a Population Characterized by Agenesis in the Primary Dentition. *Int. J. Paediatr. Dent.* **1997**, *7*, 143–148. [CrossRef]
12. Daugaard-Jensen, J.; Nodal, M.; Kjaer, I. Pattern of Agenesis in the Primary Dentition: A Radiographic Study of 193 Cases. *Int. J. Paediatr. Dent.* **1997**, *7*, 3–7. [CrossRef]
13. Ben Salem, M.; Chouchene, F.; Masmoudi, F.; Baaziz, A.; Maatouk, F.; Ghedira, H. Fusion or Gemination? Diagnosis and Management in Primary Teeth: A Report of Two Cases. *Case Rep. Dent.* **2021**, *2021*, 6661776. [CrossRef]
14. Piesco, N.; Avery, J. Development of Teeth: Crown Formation. In *Oral Development and Histology*; Thieme: New York, NY, USA, 2002.
15. Ghannam, M.G.; Alameddine, H.; Bordoni, B. Anatomy, Head and Neck, Pulp (Tooth). In *StatPearls*; StatPearls Publishing: Treasure Island, FL, USA, 2023.
16. Martos, J.; Lubian, C.; Silveira, L.F.M.; Suita de Castro, L.A.; Ferrer Luque, C.M. Morphologic Analysis of the Root Apex in Human Teeth. *J. Endod.* **2010**, *36*, 664–667. [CrossRef] [PubMed]
17. Gupta, M.; Madhok, K.; Kulshrestha, R.; Chain, S.; Kaur, H.; Yadav, A. Determination of Stress Distribution on Periodontal Ligament and Alveolar Bone by Various Tooth Movements—A 3D FEM Study. *J. Oral Biol. Craniofac. Res.* **2020**, *10*, 758–763. [CrossRef] [PubMed]
18. Tucker, A.S.; Sharpe, P.T. Molecular Genetics of Tooth Morphogenesis and Patterning: The Right Shape in the Right Place. *J. Dent. Res.* **1999**, *78*, 826–834. [CrossRef] [PubMed]
19. Thesleff, I. The Genetic Basis of Tooth Development and Dental Defects. *Am. J. Med. Genet. A* **2006**, *140*, 2530–2535. [CrossRef] [PubMed]
20. Rathee, M.; Jain, P. Embryology, Teeth. In *StatPearls*; StatPearls Publishing: Treasure Island, FL, USA, 2023.
21. Nanci, A. *Ten Cate's Oral Histology Development, Structure, and Function, 8/e*; Elsevier: New Delhi, India, 2012; ISBN 9788131233436.
22. Wang, X.-P. Tooth Eruption without Roots. *J. Dent. Res.* **2013**, *92*, 212–214. [CrossRef]
23. Billings, R.J.; Berkowitz, R.J.; Watson, G. Teeth. *Pediatrics* **2004**, *113*, 1120–1127. [CrossRef]
24. Proffit, W.R.; Frazier-Bowers, S.A. Mechanism and Control of Tooth Eruption: Overview and Clinical Implications. *Orthod. Craniofac. Res.* **2009**, *12*, 59–66. [CrossRef]
25. Kutesa, A.; Nkamba, E.M.; Muwazi, L.; Buwembo, W.; Rwenyonyi, C.M. Weight, Height and Eruption Times of Permanent Teeth of Children Aged 4–15 Years in Kampala, Uganda. *BMC Oral Health* **2013**, *13*, 1–8. [CrossRef]
26. Lakshmappa, A.; Guledgud, M.V.; Patil, K. Eruption Times and Patterns of Permanent Teeth in School Children of India. *Indian J. Dent. Res.* **2011**, *22*, 755–763.
27. Kunzendorf, B.; Diogo, M.C.; Covini, D.I.; Weber, M.; Gruber, G.M.; Zeilhofer, H.-F.; Berg, B.-I.; Prayer, D. Comparison of the Visibility of Fetal Tooth Buds on 1.5 and 3 Tesla MRI. *J. Clin. Med. Res.* **2020**, *9*, 3424. [CrossRef]
28. Bodenhoff, J.; Gorlin, R.J. Natal and neonatal teeth: Folklore and fact. *Pediatrics* **1963**, *32*, 1087–1093. [CrossRef] [PubMed]
29. Cunha, R.F.; Boer, F.A.; Torriani, D.D.; Frossard, W.T. Natal and Neonatal Teeth: Review of the Literature. *Pediatr. Dent.* **2001**, *23*, 158–162. [PubMed]
30. Haith, M.M.; Benson, J.B. *Encyclopedia of Infant and Early Childhood Development*; Elsevier Science: Amsterdam, The Netherlands, 2008; ISBN 9780123704603.
31. Pawelzik, J.; Cohnen, M.; Willers, R.; Becker, J. A Comparison of Conventional Panoramic Radiographs with Volumetric Computed Tomography Images in the Preoperative Assessment of Impacted Mandibular Third Molars. *J. Oral Maxillofac. Surg.* **2002**, *60*, 979–984. [CrossRef] [PubMed]

32. Puricelli, E.; Martins, G.L.; Ponzoni, D.; Corsetti, A.; Langie, R.; Morganti, M.A. Comparative Study of Puricelli's Panorametry in Conventional Panoramic Radiography and Cone Beam Computed Tomography Panoramic Reconstruction. *Rev. Fac. Odontol.-UPF* **2013**, *18*, 18–23. [CrossRef]
33. Pauwels, R.; Araki, K.; Siewerdsen, J.H.; Thongvigitmanee, S.S. Technical Aspects of Dental CBCT: State of the Art. *Dentomaxillofac. Radiol.* **2015**, *44*, 20140224. [CrossRef] [PubMed]
34. Abramson, Z.; Scoggins, M.A.; Burton, C.; Choudhri, A.F.; Holladay, C.; Pont Briant, N.R.; Sheyn, A.; Susarla, S. CT-Based Modeling of the Dentition for Craniomaxillofacial Surgical Planning. *J. Craniofac. Surg.* **2021**, *33*, 1574–1577. [CrossRef] [PubMed]
35. Maret, D.; Molinier, F.; Braga, J.; Peters, O.A.; Telmon, N.; Treil, J.; Inglèse, J.M.; Cossié, A.; Kahn, J.L.; Sixou, M. Accuracy of 3D Reconstructions Based on Cone Beam Computed Tomography. *J. Dent. Res.* **2010**, *89*, 1465–1469. [CrossRef]
36. Kapila, S.D. *Cone Beam Computed Tomography in Orthodontics: Indications, Insights, and Innovations*; John Wiley & Sons: Hoboken, NJ, USA, 2014; ISBN 9781118646595.
37. Lin, E.; Alessio, A. What Are the Basic Concepts of Temporal, Contrast, and Spatial Resolution in Cardiac CT? *J. Cardiovasc. Comput. Tomogr.* **2009**, *3*, 403–408. [CrossRef]
38. Hajizadeh, S.; Zadeh, R.Y.; Vatanparast, N. Pulp Revascularization in Three Immature Permanent Mandibular Molars with Necrotic Pulps: A Case Series. *Iran. Endod. J.* **2019**, *14*, 301.
39. Cohen, M.M., Jr. Syndromology: An Updated Conceptual Overview. VIII. Deformations and Disruptions. *Int. J. Oral Maxillofac. Surg.* **1990**, *19*, 33–37. [CrossRef] [PubMed]
40. Rathee, M.; Sapra, A. Dental Caries. In *StatPearls*; StatPearls Publishing: Treasure Island, FL, USA, 2023.
41. Sáenz Aguirre, M.; Gómez Muga, J.J.; Antón Méndez, L.; Fornell Pérez, R. CT Findings for Dental Disease. *Radiología* **2022**, *64*, 573–584. [CrossRef]
42. Kumar, K.; Merwade, S.; Prabakaran, P.; Ch, L.P.; Annapoorna, B.S.; Guruprasad, C.N. Magnetic Resonance Imaging versus Cone Beam Computed Tomography in Diagnosis of Periapical Pathosis—A Systematic Review. *Saudi Dent. J.* **2021**, *33*, 784–794.
43. Gliga, A.; Imre, M.; Grandini, S.; Marruganti, C.; Gaeta, C.; Bodnar, D.; Dimitriu, B.A.; Foschi, F. The Limitations of Periapical X-ray Assessment in Endodontic Diagnosis-A Systematic Review. *J. Clin. Med. Res.* **2023**, *12*, 4647. [CrossRef] [PubMed]
44. Ogura, I.; Minami, Y.; Sugawara, Y.; Mizuhashi, R.; Mizuhashi, F.; Oohashi, M.; Saegusa, H. Odontogenic Infection Pathway to the Parapharyngeal Space: CT Imaging Assessment. *J. Maxillofac. Oral Surg.* **2022**, *21*, 235–239. [CrossRef] [PubMed]
45. Gasner, N.S.; Schure, R.S. Periodontal Disease. In *StatPearls*; StatPearls Publishing: Treasure Island, FL, USA, 2023.
46. Zhao, H.J.; Pan, Y.P. Characteristics of alveolar bone loss in severe periodontitis and consideration of rehabilitation with implant. *Zhonghua Kou Qiang Yi Xue Za Zhi* **2023**, *58*, 298–304.

Disclaimer/Publisher's Note: The statements, opinions and data contained in all publications are solely those of the individual author(s) and contributor(s) and not of MDPI and/or the editor(s). MDPI and/or the editor(s) disclaim responsibility for any injury to people or property resulting from any ideas, methods, instructions or products referred to in the content.

MDPI AG
Grosspeteranlage 5
4052 Basel
Switzerland
Tel.: +41 61 683 77 34

Journal of Clinical Medicine Editorial Office
E-mail: jcm@mdpi.com
www.mdpi.com/journal/jcm

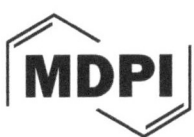

Disclaimer/Publisher's Note: The statements, opinions and data contained in all publications are solely those of the individual author(s) and contributor(s) and not of MDPI and/or the editor(s). MDPI and/or the editor(s) disclaim responsibility for any injury to people or property resulting from any ideas, methods, instructions or products referred to in the content.

www.ingramcontent.com/pod-product-compliance
Lightning Source LLC
LaVergne TN
LVHW072350090526
838202LV00019B/2512